SP Pvt. Ltd.

Dedicated to

Parents, Teachers and Students

Textbook of
Industrial Pharmacy

Third Year B. Pharmacy (Semester-V)

Baburao N. Chandakavathe
Department of Pharmaceutics
D. S. T. S. Mandal's College of Pharmacy, Solapur
Maharashtra – 413 004

&

Shivsharan B. Dhadde
Department of Pharmacology
D. S. T. S. Mandal's College of Pharmacy, Solapur
Maharashtra – 413 004

2019

Studium Press (India) Pvt. Ltd.

Textbook of
Industrial Pharmacy

ISBN: 978-93-85046-63-6

Published by:

Studium Press (India) Pvt. Ltd.
4735/22, 2nd Floor, Prakash Deep Building
(Near Delhi Medical Association)
Ansari Road, Darya Ganj, New Delhi-110 002
Tel.: + 91-11-43240200-15 (15 lines); Fax: 91-11-43240215
E-mail: pubdir@studiumpress.in

Printed at India

PHARMACY COUNCIL OF INDIA
(Constituted under the Pharmacy Act. 1948)

Prof. B. Suresh M.Pharm. Ph D, D Sc
President

Combined Councils' Building
Kotla Road, Aiwan-E- Ghalib Marg
P.B. No. 7020, New Delhi-110 002
Phone: 011 23239184, 23231348
Fax: 011 23239184

Pro-Chancellor, JSS University
Sri Shivarathreeshwara Nagar, Mysuru-570 015
Phone: 0821 2548391 Fax: 0821 2548394
sureshbhojraj@gmail.com
sureshjssuni@hotmail.com
www.jssuni.edu.in

FOREWORD

The present state-of-art book has been written as per B. Pharmacy (Semester-V) syllabus introduced by Pharmacy Council of India (PCI). This book has an inclusive content that covers the wider aspects of Basics of Industrial Pharmacy required by undergraduates, postgraduates, researchers and students preparing for various competitive exams.

The book is written in lucid, simple and easy to understand language. Each chapter of the book is accompanied with glossary of words and multiple choice, short answers and long answer type of questions for the self-evaluation and learning. In addition, the appendix of commonly used pharmaceutical additives, shortlisted questions from previous GATE/GPAT question papers and model question papers are also incorporated. All efforts have been taken to cover the answers of multiple choice and GATE/GPAT questions with relevant explanation collected from robust scientific materials.

Academicians may use the book as primary or additional teaching material for undergraduate and postgraduate pharmacy courses.

Dr. B. Suresh
President

About the Authors

Mr. Baburao N. Chandakavathe

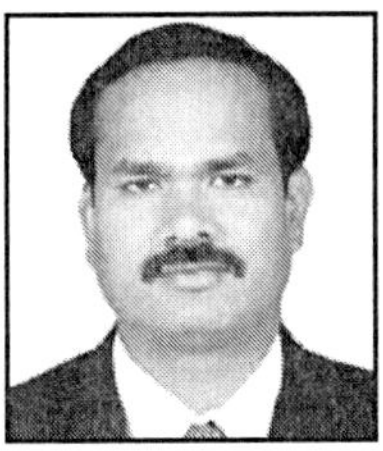

Baburao N. Chandakavathe working as Assistant Professor at D.S.T.S. Mandal's College of Pharmacy, Solapur, Maharashtra (India). He completed his graduation in Pharmacy from B.L.D.E.A's S.S.M. College of Pharmacy and Research Center, Vijaypur, Karnataka, and post graduation in Pharmaceutics from HKES Society's Matoshree Taradevi Rampure Institute of Pharmaceutical Sciences, Gulbarga, under Rajiv Gandhi University of Health Sciences, Karnataka, Bangalore. Mr. Baburao, qualified GPAT and received several scholarships and awards during his studies. His research interests are Polymeric science, Extraction and formulation of herbal preparations and novel drug delivery systems. He is serving as Editorial Board Member and Reviewer for many reputed national and international journals. Mr. Baburao, has more than 8 years of teaching and research experience. Mr. Baburao, taught Physical pharmacy and Pharmaceutics for under graduate students. He has presented scientific posters in national and international workshops/conferences. There are 12 publications in national and international journals with good impact factor. He also contributed two book chapters in reputed reference books in the area of nanotechnology and diabetes mellitus. Mr Baburao gained a good amount of knowledge in pharmaceutical additives and various pharmaceutical dosage forms. He has good command in formulation and evaluation of solid, liquid and semisolid dosage forms. Mr Baburao is life time member of professional bodies like Association of Pharmacy Teachers of India (APTI) and Indian Pharmaceutical Associations (IPA). Currently, he is pursuing his PhD in pharmacy from Punyashlok Ahilyadevi Holkar Solapur University, Solapur.

1 May 2019

Shivsharan B. Dhadde

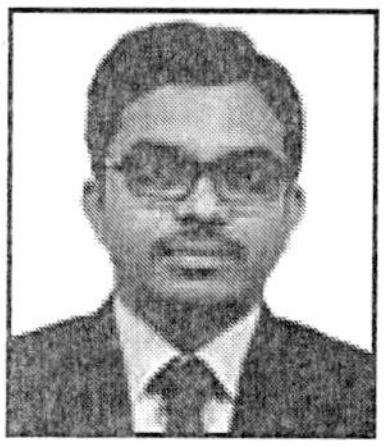

Shivsharan B. Dhadde is serving as Assistant Professor at D.S.T.S. Mandal's College of Pharmacy, Solapur, Maharashtra (India). He completed his graduation in Pharmacy from B.L.D.E.A's S.S.M. College of Pharmacy and Research Center, Vijaypur, Karnataka and post graduation in Pharmacology from Sree Siddaganga College of Pharmacy, Tumkur, Karnataka under Rajiv Gandhi University of Health Sciences, Karnataka, Bangalore. Mr Dhadde, qualified GATE (PY) 2009 and received several scholarships and awards during his studies. His research interests are Meta-Analysis of natural and synthetic pharmacological agents and evaluation of drugs for neurological and metabolic disorders. He is serving as Editorial Board Member and Reviewer for many reputed national and international journals. Mr Dhadde has more than 7 years of teaching and research experience. He worked as a resource person in more than six national and international workshops/conferences. Mr Dhadde has presented scientific posters in four national and six international workshops/ conferences. There are more than 20 publications in national and international journals in his credit with a cumulative impact factor of ~34 (Thomason Reuter). He also contributed four book chapters in reputed reference books in the area of diabetes mellitus, nanotechnology and polymer science. Recently Mr Dhadde published a book on experimental pharmacology entitled "Handbook of Experimental Pharmacology" Studium Press (India) Pvt. Ltd. Mr Dhadde has gained good citation index with H-Index of 10 and i10-index of 11.

10 May 2019

Preface

Purpose of the present book is to provide fundamental knowledge of Industrial Pharmacy aspects right from pre-formulation studies to pharmaceutical packaging sciences.

Today, the Industrial Pharmacy has tremendously drifted from the conventional approach to a highly digital and automated system. Fundamental principles of pharmaceutics deal with essential aspects of physicochemical properties of drugs and excipients, pharmacokinetic and pharmacodynamic properties of drugs, formulation and evaluation of dosage forms and its stability aspects.

Topics covered in this book are based on the syllabus designed by Pharmacy Council of India, New Delhi as per Bachelor of Pharmacy Course Regulations 2014. In this book, we made a sincere attempt to include as much relevant information as possible with illustrated points and suitable examples to make this book comprehensive.

This book is prepared by referring robust scientific materials available in the research and review articles and standard reference books. This book is reader-friendly, complex pharmaceutical concepts are elaborated in simple and easy language.

At the end of each chapter, we tried to incorporate a glossary of words and question bank including multiple choice questions, very short answer questions, short answer questions and long answer questions. Question bank is framed as per the examination pattern prescribed by Bachelor of Pharmacy Course Regulations 2014. Moreover, previous GATE/GPAT question papers have been taken into consideration and every effort has been made to cover the answers to those questions with relevant explanation. So that this book may help the students in various competitive examinations conducted national and international level in the field of pharmaceutical sciences.

We hope that the present book will be helpful for the graduate and postgraduate students and teachers of pharmacy.

Every care has been taken to ensure that the book is free from errors but absolute perfection is usually unattainable. Hence, errors if any may please be communicated to us.

Baburao N. Chandakavathe
(babu41126@gmail.com)
Shivsharan B. Dhadde
(sbdhadde@hotmail.com)

Table of Contents

Symbols and Abbreviations Used

α	Alpha
β	Beta
π	Pi
μ	Micro
°	Degree
θ	Theta
λ	Lambda
γ	Gamma
η	Eta
≥	Greater-than or equal to
≤	Less than or equal to
×	Multiplication
±	Plus-minus
<	Less-than
>	Greater-than
=	Equals
:	Colon
;	Semicolon
%	Percent
™	Trade mark
Σ	Summation
®	Registered
*	Asterisk
!	Exclamation mark
"	Quotation mark
#	Number
÷	Division
C	Celsius
F	Fahrenheit

MCC	Micro crystalline cellulose
DCP	Dicalcium phosphate
PVP	Polyvinylpyrrolidone
PEG	Polyethylene glycol
PVA	Polyvinyl alcohol
CMC	Carboxymethylcellulose
HPMC	Hydroxy propyl methyl cellulose
FD&C	Food drugs and cosmetics
D&C	Drugs and cosmetics
CAP	Cellulose acetate phthalate
GMP	Good manufacturing practices
IP	Indian pharmacopoeia
USP	United states pharmacopoeia
PhEr	European pharmacopoeia
QC	Quality control
QS	Quantity sufficient
SEM	Scanning electron microscopy
BCS	Biopharmaceutical classification system
SVP	Small volume parenterals
LVP	Large volume parenterals
WFI	Water for injection
EDTA	Ethylenediamine tetra acetic acid
HAS	Human serum albumin
IV	Intravenous
RBC	Red blood cells
CFU	Colony forming units
UV	Ultraviolet
PN	Parenteral nutrition
TPN	Total parenteral nutrition

ml	Millilitre
L	Litre
g	Gram
mg	Milligram
Kg	Kilogram
e.g.	Examples
i.e.,	That is
w/v	Weight/volume
v/w	Volume/weight
w/w	Weight/weight
v/v	Volume/volume
rpm	Rotation per minute
psi	Pounds per square inch
psig	Pounds per square inch gauge
ft	Feet
TPN	Total parenteral nutrition
mEq	Milli equivalent
GIT	Gastro-intestinal tract
GRAS	Generally recognized as safe
Vp	Vapour pressure
PVC	Polyvinyl chloride
EU	Endotoxin units
LAL	Limulus amoebocyte lysate
HEPA	High efficiency particulate air filter
LDPE	Low density polyethylene
HDPE	High density polyethylene
BHA	Butylated hydroxyl anisole
BHT	Butylated hydroxyl toluene
SPF	Sun protection factor
IPM	Isopropyl maleate
COPD	Chronic obstructive pulmonary disease
MDI	Metered dose inhalers
CFC	Chlorofluorocarbons
FDA	Food drug administration
HLB	Hydrophillic lipophillic balance
NDA	New drug application
GC	Gas chromatography
MS	Mass spectroscopy
GATE	Graduate aptitude test in engineering
GPAT	Graduate pharmacy aptitude test

UNIT-I

CHAPTER 1

PRE-FORMULATION STUDIES

INTRODUCTION

Formulation is the process of developing a drug candidate into drug product. Initially, there may be a number of potential drug candidate molecules, each with unique set of physicochemical properties and each showing activity towards a particular biological target. Ultimately, only one which is suitable will be developed into a drug product. The decision to select a successful drug candidate to be developed does not depend on pharmacological efficacy alone. In practice, the physicochemical properties of the molecule affect how a material will process pharmaceutically, its stability, its interaction with excipients, how it will transfer to the solution and ultimately, will determine its bioavailability. It follows that characterizing the physicochemical properties of drug candidates early in the development process will provide the fundamental knowledge. Based on which drug candidate selection and ultimately dosage form design, can be made by reducing development time and costs.

Pre-formulation is the stage in drug and dosage form development before formulation proper where pre-formulation scientist characterise physical, chemical and biological properties of new drug substances excipients in order to develop stable, safe and effective dosage form/s.

Pre-formulation studies are an important foundation tool in the early development of both active pharmaceutical ingredients (API) and dosage forms.

Pre-formulation study helps in:

- Selection of drug candidate
- Selection of excipients
- API and dosage form manufacturing process
- Selection of container and packaging materials which are inert towards formulation components
- Development of analytical method
- To test optimum storage conditions

Goals and Objectives of Pre-Formulation

The main goals of pre-formulation scientist during pre-formulation studies are:

i) To establish physicochemical properties of a new drug molecule.
ii) To establish the data on drug-excipient compatibility.
iii) To determine drug kinetic rate profile.
iv) To develop a stability indicating assay.

Pre-formulation aims to optimize the process of turning a drug candidate into a drug product. During preformulation, the physicochemical properties of drug candidates are studied. The data generated at this stage, allow decisions to be made on the likely ease of formulation of each drug candidate, indicate the most appropriate dosage form.

Solubility is the first parameter to be measured. An aqueous solubility greater than 10 mg/ml is optimal. The effects of low solubility may be mitigated by preparing a salt form or through using a novel formulation. The melting point and enthalpy of fusion are characteristic of polymorphic form and allow calculation of ideal solubility. Possession of pKa value indicates an ionizable group in the molecule. This means that its aqueous solubility will change with surrounding pH and that salt formation is possible. Salts enhance solubility by changing pH on dissolution. Salt formation ideally requires a difference of 3 pKa units between the free drug and the acid or base. Salts can also be used to enable isolation of the active or to enhance stability or processability of the drug.

Partition coefficients are determined between water and an organic phase (often n-octanol). Partition coefficients are usually quoted as a log P value. Lipophilic compounds have a positive log P value, hydrophilic compounds a negative log P value.

Particle shape affects flow. Flow is assessed using measure of compressibility (Carr's index or Hausner ratio) and angle of repose.

Compaction requires good compression and cohesion properties. As stated above, along with the evaluation of biologic activity of the compound, it is also evaluated with regard to chemical and physical properties that have a bearing on its ultimate and successful formulation.

Hence, preformulation study is essential in order to develop stable, safe and effective dosage forms, the following physical and chemical properties of the chemical compounds are considered:

Physicochemical Characteristics of Drug Substances

a. Physical Properties
   1. *Physical form:* (crystal and amorphous)
   2. Polymorphism
   3. Particle size
   4. Shape
   5. Flow properties
   6. *Solubility profile:* (pKa, pH, partition coefficient)

b. Chemical Properties
   1. Hydrolysis
   2. Oxidation
   3. Reduction
   4. Racemisation
   5. Polymerization

When sufficient information is collected on the compound's physical and chemical properties, initial formulations of the dosage form are developed for use in human clinical trials. During the course of the clinical trials, the proposed product is developed further, from initial formulation to final formulation and from small-scale production to scale-up, in preparation for large-scale manufacturing.

a) Physical Properties

Since solid dosage forms (tablets and capsules) account for approximately 70% of pharmaceutical preparations, an investigation into the solid-state properties of candidate drugs is an important task to be undertaken during preformulation. The determination of solid-state properties such as physical form, polymorphism, particle size, particle shape, powder flow and solubility profile of drug candidate is considered as important parameters for preformulation studies.

1. Physical form

The crystal or amorphous forms of a powdered drug can affect the dissolution rate, thus the rate and extent of absorption, for a number of drugs.

Crystal: Crystals are characterized by the repetitious arrangement of atoms, molecules or ions in a regular three-dimensional structure.

Characterization of crystal morphology can be done by 1) optical microscopy and 2) scanning electron microscopy (SEM).

Crystals may have different external structures (outer appearance) with a single internal structure. These external structures are known as crystal habits. Crystal habits are influenced by the environment of the growing crystals. Five types of crystal habits are generally recognized during crystallization.

i) *Platy:* Plates, crystal growth in length and width and moderate height.
ii) *Acicular:* Needle-like, crystal growth in one direction.
iii) *Tabular:* Moderate expansion of two parallel faces.
iv) *Bladed:* Flat acicular
v) *Prismatic:* Columns

Factors affecting crystal habit

1. Excessive super saturation tends to transform a prism into a needle shape.

2. Cooling rate and agitation changes habit as it changes the degree of supersaturation, *e.g.,* naphthalene gives thin plates (platy) if rapidly recrystallized in cold ethanol or methanol, whereas slow evaporation yields prisms.
3. The crystallising solvent affects habit by preferential absorption on to certain faces, inhibiting their growth. Resorcinol produces needles from benzene and squat prisms from butyl acetate.
4. The addition of co-solvents or other solutes and ions which change habit by poisoning crystal growth in one or more directions. Sodium chloride is usually cubic but urea produces an octahedral habit.

Different crystal habits change the dissolution rate and cause changes in powder flow (which is important as the die of a tabletting machine is filled by volume and requires good powder flow in order to guarantee content uniformity of the product) and sedimentation and caking of suspensions.

The molecular complex has incorporated the crystallizing solvent molecules into specific sites within the crystal lattice and has a stoichiometric number of solvent molecules complexed. When the incorporated solvent is water, the complex is called hydrates and when the solvent is other than water, the complex is called solvates. Depending on the ratio of water molecules within a complex the following nomenclature is followed.

(i) *Anhydrous:* 1 mole compound + 0 mole water
(ii) *Hemihydrate:* 1 mole compound + ½ mole water
(iii) *Monohydrate:* 1 mole compound + 1 mole water
(iv) *Dihydrate:* 1 mole compound + 2 moles water

Properties of solvates / hydrates

(i) Generally, the anhydrous form of a drug has greater aqueous solubility than its hydrates. This is because the hydrates are already in equilibrium with water and therefore have less demand for water. *e.g.,* anhydrous form of the ampicillin has higher aqueous solubility than the hydrates.
(ii) Non-aqueous solvates have greater aqueous solubility than the non-solvates. *e.g.,* chloroform solvates of griseofulvin are more water soluble than their non-solvate forms.

Evaluation of crystal structure, polymorphism and solvate form is an important pre-formulation activity. The solubility of these pseudopolymorphs may be arranged in ascending order: The changes in crystal characteristics can infiuence bioavailability and chemical and physical stability and can have important implications in dosage form process functions.

There is a correlation between the melting point of the different polymorphs and the rate of dissolution because the one with the lowest melting point will most easily give up molecules to dissolve, whereas the most stable form (highest melting point) will not give up molecules to the solvent so readily.

High melting point = strong lattice = hard to remove a molecule = low dissolution rate

Low melting point = weak lattice = easy to remove a molecule = high dissolution rate

Various techniques are used to determine crystal properties. The most widely used methods are hot stage microscopy, thermal analysis, infrared spectroscopy and X-ray diffraction.

Amorphous form: If a solid does not have any fixed internal structure, that form is called *amorphous form*. They have molecules randomly placed as in a liquid. Amorphous forms are prepared by rapid precipitation, lyophilization or rapid cooling of molten liquids.

Characteristics of amorphous forms:

- *Melting point:* Stable > metastable form > unstable form > amorphous form of the same drug
- *Dissolution rate:* Stable < metastable form < unstable form < amorphous form of the same drug.

The amorphous or crystalline character of a drug substance may be of considerable importance to its ease of formulation and handling, its chemical stability, even its biologic activity. Certain medicinal agents may be produced to exist in either a crystalline or an amorphous state. The energy required for a molecule of the drug to escape from a crystal is much greater than is required to escape from an amorphous powder. Therefore, the amorphous form of a compound is always more soluble than a corresponding crystal form. Hence, different extents of drug absorption may result in consequent differences in the degree of pharmacologic activity obtained from each. Two antibiotic substances, Novobiocin and chloramphenicol palmitate, are essentially inactive when administered in crystalline form, but, when they are administered in the amorphous form, absorption from the gastrointestinal tract proceeds rapidly, with a good therapeutic response. In other instances, crystalline forms of drugs may be used because of greater stability than the corresponding amorphous forms. For example, the crystalline forms of penicillin-G as the potassium salt or sodium salt are considerably more stable than the analogous amorphous forms. Thus, in formulation work on penicillin-G, the crystalline forms are preferred and result in an excellent therapeutic response.

2. Polymorphism

Polymorphism is existence of drug molecule in more than one crystalline forms. Polymorphic forms usually exhibit different physicochemical properties, including melting point and solubility. Polymorphic forms in drugs are relatively common, it has been estimated that at least one-third of all organic compounds exhibit polymorphism.

Many organic molecules, including drugs and excipients, exhibit polymorphism. Often this is of a form called *monotropic polymorphism*, which means that only one polymorphic form is stable and any other polymorph that is formed will eventually convert to the stable form. However, some materials exhibit *enantiotropic polymorphism*, which means that under different conditions (temperature and pressure) the material can reversibly transform between alternative stable forms; this type of behaviour will not be considered further here. Considering monotropic polymorphism, the true stable form has the highest melting point and all other forms are described as metastable. This means that the other forms exist or a period of time and thus appear stable, but given a chance they will convert to the true stable form. Different metastable forms can exist or very short times or many months before they convert to the stable form, depending upon the conditions under which they are stored. In general, there will be a correlation between the melting point of the different polymorphs and the rate of dissolution, because the one with the lowest melting point will most easily give up molecules to dissolve, whereas the most stable form (highest melting point) will not give up molecules to the solvent so readily.

Examples for polymorphism:

1) Theobroma oil exist in four polymorphic forms. The unstable gamma form which melts at 18° C. the alpha form melts at 22° C, the beta prime form melts at 28° C and the stable beta form melts at 34.5° C.
2) Chloramphenicol palmitate has three polymorphs A, B and C out of which B polymorph which is more soluble form and has more absorption in humans.

Methods to identify polymorphism:

1. *Optical crystallography:* It is used in the identification of polymorphs. Crystal exist in isotropic and anisotropic forms. When isotropic crystals are examined the velocity of light is same in all directions while anisotropic crystals have 2 or 3 different light velocities or refractive indices. Video recording systems have made it possible to record the events visualized during the heating and cooling stages.
2. *Polarizing microscope:* The polarizing microscope fitted with a hot and cold stage is very useful for investigating polymorph. It is useful to know: i) The degree of stability of metastable form. ii) Transition temperature. iii) Melting point iv) Rates of transition under various thermal and physical conditions. v) Whether to persue polymorphism as a route to an improved dosage form.
3. *Hot stage microscopy:* Using this technique fluid phase transformation as a function of temperature is observed. Generally, silicone oil hot stage microscopy is used for detection of pseudo polymorphs.
4. *X-ray diffraction method:* Using Bragg's equation: $n\lambda = 2d \sin \theta$ where d = distance for different planes of crystal, λ = wavelength of X-ray used, θ = angle of incoming beam, n = order of spectrum.

X-ray diffraction

a) Powder x-ray diffraction → basically focusing on packing pattern of the atom.
b) Exact relative location of atom in crystal is determined.

5. *NMR technique:* In this technique, powder sample must be rotated at a special angle with respect to magnetic field.

6. *FTIR technique:* It has been used to quantify binary mixtures of polymorphs. In identification of polymorphs, only solid samples (as mineral oil mulls and KBr pellets) can be used.
7. *Dilatometry:* Measure change in volume caused by thermal or chemical effect. Using dilatometry the melting behaviour of *Theobroma oil* was studied. Extremely accurate but tedious, time consuming and not widely used.
8. *Microcalorimetry:* Used to characterize thermodynamic properties of different molecules.
9. Thermal methods:
   a) DSC [Differential Scanning Calorimetry]
   b) DTA [Differential Thermal Analysis]
   c) TGA [Thermal Gravimetric Analysis]

This method measures heat loss or gain from physical or chemical changes occurring in sample which is recorded as a function of temperature as substance is heated at uniform scale. Advantage: i) Thermodynamic parameter can be evaluated. ii) Heat of Transition from one polymorph to the other. Polymorphs can also be determined by its melting point.

3. Particle size

Certain physical and chemical properties of drug substances, including dissolution rate, bioavailability, content uniformity, taste, texture and stability, are affected by the particle size and particle size distribution. In addition, flow characteristics and sedimentation rates, among other properties, are important factors related to particle size. It is essential to establish as early as possible how the particle size of the drug substance may affect formulation and efficacy. Particle size significantly influences the oral absorption profiles of certain drugs *e.g.,* griseofulvin, nitrofurantoin, spironolactone and procaine penicillin. Also, satisfactory content uniformity in solid dosage forms depends on particle size and the equal distribution of the active ingredient throughout the formulation.

A number of techniques can be used to determine particle size and size distributions include the microscopic method, sedimentation method using the Andreasen pipette, sieving method. Other methods of particle size determinations include elutriation, centrifugation, permeation, adsorption, electronic sensing zone (the Coulter counter) and light obstruction, etc.

4. Particle shape

Particle size determinations techniques discussed above are based on the assumption that particles can be adequately represented by an equivalent circle or sphere. Whereas this is often the case, in some pharmaceutically relevant cases, particles deviate markedly from circularity and sphericity and the use of a single equivalent diameter measurement may be inappropriate. For example, a powder consisting of monosized fibrous particles would appear to have wide size distribution according to statistical diameter measurements. However, the use of an equivalent diameter based on the projected area would also be misleading.

However, particle shape influences the surface area, flow of particles, packing and compaction properties of particles. A sphere has a minimum surface area per unit volume. Therefore these properties can be compared for spheres and asymmetrical particles in order to decide the same. Some typical powder shapes are shown in Fig. 1.1.

5. Flow properties

Flow property is important physical property considered in tablet manufacturing and filling of the solid dosage form (*e.g.,* dry powder) in the containers. Formulation should have sufficient flow ability to ensure that the appropriate quantity of powder flows into the dies of tablet machine on a consistent basis. While the tests described for powder flow are useful development tools, the ultimate test of a formulation is the uniformity of weight of tablets manufactured on a production tablet machine.

To improve the flow property of powder usually, glidants are added to the formulation. Examples of glidants are talc, CAB-O-SIL, starch, calcium silicate etc.

Flow property of powder can be expressed by Carr's index, Hausner's ratio and angle of repose.

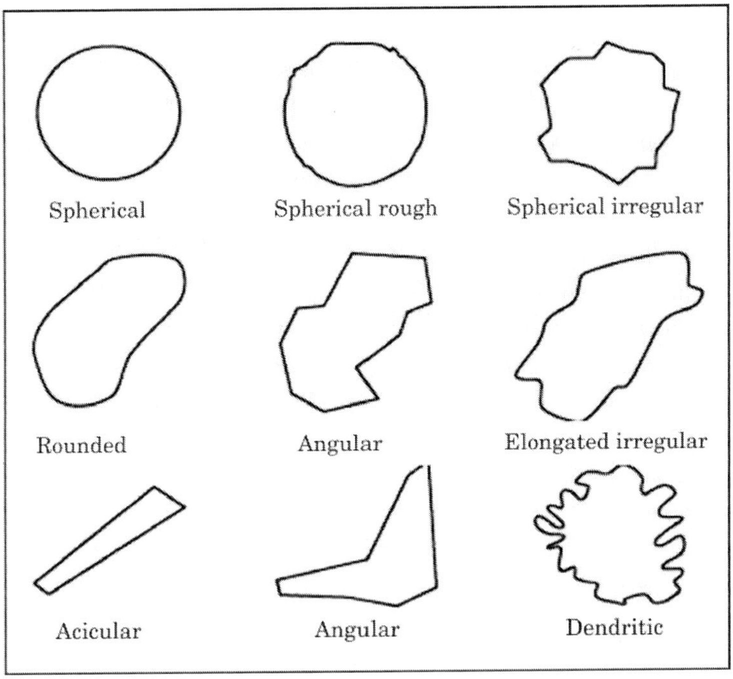

Fig.1.1: Some typical powder shapes

Carr's index: Carr and Neumann developed a simple test to evaluate the flowability of powder by comparing poured (fluff) density and tapped density of powder and rate at which it packed down. Carr's index (X) can be determined by the formula:

$$\text{Carr's index (X)} = \frac{\text{Tapped density} - \text{bulk density}}{\text{Tapped density}} \times 100$$

Carr's index values of powder and its flow property are given in Table 1.1.

Hausner's ratio: Similar to the Carr's index, Hausner also correlated the density ratio of powder and its flow property. Hausner's ratio values and flow property is given in Table 1.2. Hausner's ratio is calculated by the formula:

$$\text{Hausner ratio} = \frac{\text{Tapped density}}{\text{Bulk density}}$$

Table 1.1: Carr's index values and flow property

Carr's index	*Type of flow*
5 – 15	Excellent
12 – 16	Good
18 – 21	Fair to passable*
23 – 35	Poor
33 – 38	Very poor
> 40	Extremely poor

**Maybe improved by the addition of glidants*

Table 1.2: Hausner's ratio values and flow property

Hausner's ratio	*Type of flow*
< 1.25	Good glow
> 1.5	Poor flow
1.25 to 1.5	Added glidant improves the flow

Angle of repose: Angle of repose is a relatively simple technique for estimating the flow properties of a powder. It can easily be determined by allowing a powder to flow through a funnel and fall freely onto a surface. The height and diameter of the resulting cone are measured and the angle of repose is calculated from this equation:

$$\theta = \tan^{-1} \frac{h}{r}$$

Where; h is the height of the powder cone and r is the radius of the powder cone.

Hence, the angle of repose is the maximum angle possible between the surface of pile of powder and horizontal plane. Powders with a low angle of repose flow freely, and powders with a high angle of repose flow poorly. The angle of repose and type of flow is given Table 1.3.

6. Solubility profile

pKa (dissociation constants or ionization constant)

pKa is important in preformulation study because the extent of dissociation or ionization has a significant effect on the formulation and pharmacokinetic parameters of the drug. For a compound containing basic or acidic functional groups, solubility at a given pH is influenced by the compound's ionization characteristics. Solubility of a compound in aqueous media is greater in the ionized state than in the neutral state. Thus, the solubility of ionizable compounds is dependent on the pH of the solution. Many drugs are weak acids or bases and thus are ionizable within the pH range of the gut.

Table 1.3: Angle of repose and type of flow

Angle of repose (°)	*Type of flow*
< 20	Excellent
20 – 30	Good
30 – 34	Passable
> 40	Very poor

Solubility and dissolution and therefore absorption of a weak base can be altered by changes to gastric pH (*e.g.,* when coadministered with antacids). While a weakly basic compound might fully dissolve in the acidic environment of the stomach and result in high exposure levels under such conditions, coadministration of drugs that raise the stomach pH can lead to greatly decreased solubility, leading to significantly lower exposure. Other considerations for an ionizable compound include the impact of ionization on stability and permeability and for compounds containing both acidic and basic functional groups the formation of zwitterions, for which the solubility at the isoelectric point is typically the lowest over the entire pH range.

The Henderson-Hasselbalch equation provides an estimate of the ionized and un-ionized drug concentration at a particular pH.

For acidic compounds:

pH = pKa + log ([ionized drug]/[un-ionized drug])

For basic compounds:

pH = pKa + log ([un-ionized drug]/[ionized drug])

pKa of a compound is thus a measure of drug un-ionized at a certain pH. If a compound is ionizable, a salt can be formed, which may have better dissolution or an improvement in other physical properties such as hygroscopicity, solid-state stability, or the potential for polymorphism. Methods for determination of pKa include: a) potentiometric method; b) spectrophotometric method; c) solubility method; d) conductometric method.

pH

Two areas of critical importance are the effects of pH on solubility and stability. The effect of pH on solubility is critical in the formulation of liquid dosage forms (oral, topical solutions, intravenous solutions and admixtures). The solubility of a weak acid or base is often pH dependent.

The total quantity of a monoprotic weak acid (HA) in solution at a specific pH is the sum of concentrations of free acid and salt (A) forms. If excess drug is present, the quantity of free acid in solution is maximized and constant because of its saturation solubility. As the pH of the solution increases, the quantity of drug in solution increases because water-soluble ionizable salt is formed. The expression is

$$HA \overset{Ka}{\leftrightarrow} H^+ + A^-$$

Where Ka is the dissociation constant.

Partition coefficient

The partition coefficient is a measure of a molecule's affinity for the hydrophilic or lipophilic phase. If a solute is added to a mixture of two immiscible liquids, it will distribute between the two phases and reach equilibrium at a constant temperature. Hence, partition coefficient is defined as the ratio of the un-ionized drug distributed between the organic and aqueous phases at equilibrium.

$$P_{o/w} = \frac{C_{organic}}{C_{water}} \text{ at Equilibrium}$$

Where P is the distribution constant or partition constant, $C_{organic}$ is the concentration of the drug in the organic phase and C_{water} is the concentration of the drug in the aqueous phase.

Drugs having values of partition coefficient much greater than 1 are classified as lipophilic, whereas those with partition coefficient much less than 1 are indicative of a hydrophilic drug.

For a series of compounds, the partition coefficient can provide an information in screening for some biologic properties. For drug delivery, the lipophilic/hydrophilic balance has been shown to be a contributing factor for the rate and extent of drug absorption. Although partition coefficient data alone does not provide an understanding of *in vivo* absorption, it does provide a means of characterizing the lipophilic/hydrophilic nature of the drug. Since biological membranes are lipoidal in nature, the rate of drug transfer for passively absorbed drugs is directly related to the lipophilicity of the molecule. The partition coefficient is commonly determined using an oil phase of octanol or chloroform and water.

Partition law can effectively used for:

1. Extraction of crude drugs
2. Recovery of antibiotics from the fermentation broth
3. Recovery of biotechnology-derived drugs from bacterial cultures
4. Extraction of drugs from biologic fluids for therapeutic drug monitoring
5. Absorption of drugs from dosage forms (ointments, suppositories, transdermal patches)

The solubility range of a solute as per USP and IP is given in Table 1.4.

Table 1.4: Solubility criteria as per USP and IP

Description	*Parts of solvents required for one part of the solute*
Very soluble	< 1
Freely soluble	1 – 10
Soluble	10 – 30
Sparingly soluble	30 – 100
Slightly soluble	100 – 1000
Very slightly soluble	1000 – 10,000
Insoluble	> 10,000

b) Chemical Properties

Chemically, drug substances are alcohols, phenols, aldehydes, ketones, esters, ethers, acids, salts, alkaloids, glycosides and others, each with reactive chemical groups having different susceptibilities to chemical instability. Chemically, the most frequently encountered destructive processes are hydrolysis and oxidation. The other chemical process such as reduction, racemisation and polymerization also plays important role in the instability of drug candidates.

1. Hydrolysis

Hydrolysis is a solvolysis process in which (drug) molecules interact with water molecules to yield breakdown products. For example, aspirin, or acetylsalicylic acid, combines with a water molecule and hydrolyzes into one molecule of salicylic acid and one molecule of acetic acid. Hydrolysis is probably the most important single cause of drug decomposition, mainly because a great number of medicinal agents are esters or contain such other groups as substituted amides, lactones and lactams, which are susceptible to the hydrolytic process.

There are several approaches to the stabilization of pharmaceutical preparations containing drugs subject to hydrolysis. Perhaps the most obvious is the reduction or elimination of water from the pharmaceutical system. Even solid dosage forms containing water-labile drugs must be protected from humidity in the atmosphere. Decomposition by hydrolysis may be prevented in other liquid drugs by suspending them in a non-aqueous vehicle rather than dissolving them in an aqueous solvent. Use of complexing agent, it forms complex with drug and prevents hydrolysis and self-life of drug is prolonged.

2. Oxidation

Another destructive process is oxidation, which destroys many drugs, including aldehydes, alcohols, phenols, sugars, alkaloids and unsaturated fats and oils. Chemically, oxidation is a loss of electrons from an atom or a molecule. Each electron lost is accepted by some other atom or molecule, reducing the recipient. Many of the oxidative changes in pharmaceutical preparations have the character of autoxidations. Autoxidations occur spontaneously under the initial influence of atmospheric oxygen and proceed slowly at first and then more rapidly. The process has been described as a type of chain reaction commencing with the union of oxygen with the drug molecule and continuing with a free radical of this oxidized molecule participating in the destruction of other drug molecules and so forth.

Pharmaceutically, oxidation of a susceptible drug substance is most likely to occur when it is not kept dry in the presence of oxygen or when it is exposed to light or combined with other chemical agents without proper regard to their influence on oxidation. Oxidation of a chemical in a pharmaceutical and the stability of the drug is preserved by agents called antioxidants, which react with one or more compounds in the drug to prevent the progress of the chain reaction. In general, antioxidants act by providing electrons and easily available hydrogen atoms that are accepted more readily by the free radicals that are those of the drug being protected. Various antioxidants are employed in pharmacy. Among those most frequently used in aqueous preparations are sodium sulfite (Na_2SO_3, at high pH values), sodium bisulfite ($NaHSO_3$, at intermediate pH values), sodium metabisulfite ($Na_2S_2O_5$ at low pH values), hypophosphorous acid (H_3PO_2) and ascorbic acid. In oleaginous (oily or unctuous) preparations, alpha-tocopherol, butyl hydroxyanisole and ascorbyl palmitate find application.

3. Reduction

Reduction is elimination of water from the pharmaceutical system. Even solid dosage forms containing water-labile drugs must be protected from humidity in the atmosphere. This may be accomplished by applying a waterproof protective coating over tablets or by keeping the drug in a tightly closed container. It is fairly common to detect hydrolyzed aspirin by noticing an odour of acetic acid upon opening a bottle of aspirin tablets. In liquid preparations, water can frequently be replaced or reduced in the formulation through the use of substitute liquids such as glycerin, propylene glycol and alcohol. In certain injectable products, anhydrous vegetable oils may be used as the drug's solvent to reduce the chance of hydrolytic decomposition.

4. Racemization

Different isomers of a drug often have differing pharmacological activity or toxicity. Optically active molecules with one chiral centre are known as enantiomers. The conversion of one enantiomer into its mirror-image is known as racemization. In racemization, the optically active compound loses its optical activity without changing its chemical composition and converted into its inactive form that is a racemic mixture. This reaction is important in the stability of pharmaceutical formulation since the biological effect of dextro form can be considerably less than that of the levo form. For example, levo adrenaline is 15 to 20 times more active than dextro-adrenaline.

In drug molecules with more than one chiral centre (diastereomers), racemization at one of the chiral centres is known as epimerization.

The antibiotic tetracycline, or instance, forms the 4-epi-tetracycline epimer, which is not active against microorganisms and is more toxic than tetracycline.

Retinol and all other related molecules, which together are known as vitamin A, contain an unsaturated hydrocarbon chain. The double bonds in the chain are all in the trans configuration. On storage of all-trans-retinol or on subjecting it to heat, the molecule changes configuration at the double bond at the 13-position of the molecule, to form 13-cis-retinol, which has no activity as a vitamin.

The kinetics of racemisation may be studied in a manner similar to hydrolytic reactions. By determining the rate constant, the temperature dependency of the reaction and dependence of the reaction on the pH, it is possible to establish the optimal conditions for storage of preparation. Racemisation reactions, in general, undergo degradation in accordance with first order kinetic principles. The racemization of compound appears to depend on the functional group bound to the asymmetric carbon atom; aromatic groups tend to accelerate the racemisation process.

5. Polymerization

The reaction of a drug molecule with another molecule of the same drug may result in the formation of a dimer or polymer. In other words, Polymerization is a reaction between two or more identical molecules that form a new and generally larger molecule.

The penicillin antibiotic amoxicillin, besides undergoing hydrolysis of the β-lactam ring, also undergoes dimerization by nucleophilic attack on the β-lactam ring by the amino group, especially in more concentrated solutions. The reaction can continue to produce a trimer and tetramer.

Polymerization is a major mechanism of degradation of the disinfectant glutaraldehyde at alkaline pH. Because glutaraldehyde undergoes keto-enol tautomerism, an aldol condensation reaction between the keto and enol forms of the molecule results in the production of a dimer. Further reaction to produce a polymer then occurs. In order to avoid polymerization on storage, glutaraldehyde solution needs to be formulated at an acidic pH, where polymerization does not occur. Its disinfectant activity is optimal at a slightly alkaline pH, so an alkaline buffer is added immediately before used.

Formaldehyde is another example of a drug capable of polymerization. In solution, it may polymerize to paraformaldehyde $(CH_2O)n$, a slowly soluble white crystalline substance that may cloud the solution. The formation of paraformaldehyde is enhanced by cool storage, especially in solutions with high concentrations of formaldehyde.

Biopharmaceutics Classification System (BCS) of Drugs

By considering the physicochemical properties of drugs, a scientific basis or Biopharmaceutics Classification System (BCS) classifies drugs into four classes according to their dose, their aqueous solubility over the gastrointestinal pH range and their permeability across the gastrointestinal mucosa.

The classification system is based on Fick's first law applied to a membrane:

$$J_W = P_W C_W$$

Where J_W is the drug flux (mass/area/time) through the intestinal wall at any position and time, P_W is the permeability of the membrane and C_W is the drug concentration at the intestinal membrane surface.

This approach assumes that no other components in the formulation affect the membrane permeability and/or intestinal transport. Using this approach studied the solubility and permeability characteristics of various representative drugs and obtained a biopharmaceutic drug classification for predicting the *in-vitro* drug dissolution of immediate-release solid oral drug products with *in-vivo* absorption.

Biopharmaceutics Classification System of drugs is mentioned in Table 1.5.

A drug is considered to be highly soluble where the highest dose strength is soluble in 250 ml or less of aqueous media over the pH range 1-8. The volume is derived from the minimum volume anticipated in the stomach when a dosage form is taken in the fasted state with a glass of water. If the volume of aqueous media needed to dissolve the drug in pH conditions ranging from 1 to 8 is greater

Table 1.5: Biopharmaceutics classification of drugs

Class	*Solubility*	*Permeability*	*Comments*
Class 1	High	High	Drug dissolves rapidly and is well absorbed. Bioavailability problem is not expected for immediate release drug products
Class 2	Low	High	Drug is dissolution limited and well absorbed. Bioavailability is controlled by the dosage form and rate of release of the drug substance
Class 3	High	Low	Drug is permeability limited. Bioavailability may be incomplete if drug is not released and dissolved within absorption window
Class 4	Low	Low	Difficulty in formulating a drug product that will deliver consistent drug bioavailability. An alternate route of administration may be needed

than 250 ml then the drug is considered to have low solubility. The classification, therefore, takes into account dose of the drug as well as its solubility.

A drug is considered to be highly permeable when the extent of absorption in humans is expected to be greater than 90% of the administered dose. Permeability can be assessed by comparing with known standard compounds or by pharmacokinetic studies.

Class I Drugs: Class I drugs will dissolve rapidly when presented in immediate-release dosage forms and are also rapidly transported across the gut wall. Therefore (unless they form insoluble complexes, are unstable in gastric fluids or undergo pre-systemic clearance) it is expected that such drugs will be rapidly absorbed and thus show good bioavailability. Examples of class I drugs are the β-blockers propranolol and metoprolol.

Class II Drugs: The dissolution rate is liable to be the rate-limiting step in oral absorption in class II drugs. Hence, it should be possible to generate a strong correlation between *in vitro* dissolution and *in vivo* absorption in class II drugs. This class of drug should be amenable to formulation approaches to improve the dissolution rate and hence oral bioavailability. Examples of class II drugs are the non-steroidal anti-inflammatory drug ketoprofen and the antiepileptic carbamazepine.

Class III Drugs: Class III drugs are those that dissolve rapidly but which are poorly permeable. It is important that dosage forms containing class III drugs release them rapidly in order to maximize the amount of time these drugs, which are slow to permeate the gastrointestinal epithelium, are in contact with it. Examples are the H_2-antagonist ranitidine and the β-blocker atenolol.

Class IV Drugs: Class IV drugs are those that are classed as poorly soluble and poorly permeable. These drugs are liable to have poor oral bioavailability, or the oral absorption may be so low that they cannot be given by the oral route. Forming prodrugs of class IV compounds, the use of novel drug delivery technologies or finding an alternative route of delivery approaches that have to be adopted to significantly improve their absorption into the systemic circulation. Examples are diuretics hydrochlorothiazide and furosemide.

Significance of BCS Classification

- BCS provides information about pharmacokinetic property of drug, so one can manipulate in the chemical structure of the drug so as to optimize the physicochemical properties of the lead drug molecules for desired drug delivery and targeting.
- If the formulator is aware of the solubility and permeability characteristics of the drug, then he can easily decide the drug delivery technology for that drug to get optimum pharmacokinetic characteristics.
- It is applicable to both pre-clinical and clinical drug development process.
- BCS provides basic information for determining the conditions under which *in-vitro* and *in-vivo* correlations are expected.
- Because of high solubility and high permeability of class I drugs, targeted drug delivery becomes difficult. Formulation approaches include both the control of release rate and physicochemical characteristics of drugs like pH- solubility profile of the drug.
- The dosage forms containing class II drugs require micronization, lyophilisation, addition of surfactants, use of complexing agents etc. approaches to improve the solubility or dissolution.

- Class III drugs are required for technologies that address the fundamental limitations of absolute or regional permeability. Peptides and proteins constitute solely class III drugs and these are now centre of focus for research in drug delivery.
- Class IV present a major challenge for the development of drug delivery system and route of choice due to their poor solubility and permeability characteristics. These are often administered by parenteral route with formulation containing solubility enhancers.

Application of Pre-Formulation Considerations

Pre-formulation testing is considered as the first step before the rational development of a dosage form with a drug molecule. It involves the exploitation of biopharmaceutical principles in selecting the right excipients, right composition, right processing steps and right packaging materials. Obviously, the ultimate aim is to design an optimum drug product which is cost-effective, safe, stable, patient-friendly and therapeutically effective.

The pre-formulation testing is considered the fundamental aspect of developing robust formulations and can be considered as an alarming process before actually developing the dosage forms. The overall objective of pre-formulation testing is to gather enough data in order to develop a chemically stable and therapeutically effective drug product that can be commercially produced at a large scale. It also shortens the time of drug development process.

- Pre-formulation is a stage of product development during which the physicochemical properties of drug substance being analysed. Before the formulation of a drug substance into a dosage form, it is essential that to be chemically and physically characterized.
- Pre-formulation begins with calculation/prediction *'in silico'* (computer simulated) of many of the important physicochemical characteristics of the active pharmaceutical ingredients.
- Pre-formulation influences on the selection of the drug candidate itself, selection of formulation components, active pharmaceutical ingredients and drug product manufacturing processes, determination of the most appropriate container closure system, development of analytical methods, assignment of active pharmaceutical ingredients retest periods, the synthetic

route of the active pharmaceutical ingredients and toxicological strategy.

Solid Dosage Forms

Virtually all solid dosage forms are manufactured from powders and an understanding of the unique properties of powder systems is necessary for their rational formulation and manufacture.

Powders consist of solid particles surrounded by spaces filled with fluid (typically air) and uniquely possess some properties of solids, liquids and gases.

- Powders are not solids, even though they can resist some deformation
- Powders are not liquids, although they can be made to flow.
- Powders are not gases, even though they can be compressed.

Powder technology is concerned with solid/fluid interactions, interparticle contact and cohesion between particles. These are strongly influenced by physicochemical properties of powder drug and excipients.

When formulating any pharmaceutical dosage form, it is important to remember that there is an equilibrium between the bioavailability of the product, its chemical and physical stability and the technical feasibility of producing it.

The most important function of pre-formulation stage solid dosage forms formulation is solid state characterization which determines the next step in the formulation work of the studied active pharmaceutical ingredients.

- Physical properties of the studied active pharmaceutical ingredients influence on its physical and chemical stability.
- It influences on the route of administration, delivery system and the drug activity. Moreover, chemical stability of the drug is affected by the physical properties.
- Crystal morphology, polymorphism, amorphous forms and hygroscopicity are usually studied.
- In addition, solubility, salt form, melting point, dissolution of the active pharmaceutical ingredients are also studied.

- Certain properties such as particle size, its distribution, its surface area and porosity are studied in the pre-formulation stage of the solid dosage forms. These properties relate mainly to the ability of the powder to flow in the compressing machine and subsequently its compressibility.
- They influence the dissolution rate of the active pharmaceutical ingredients, stability, bioavailability, degradation rate and purity.
- Pre-formulation studies also include true density, flowability, the colour of the active pharmaceutical ingredient/s, electrostaticity, caking and polymorphism. These properties influence on the dosage form appearance, stability and solubility.

Liquid Dosage Forms

Liquid dosage forms are essential pharmaceutical products which involve a mixture of active drug components and nondrug components (excipients). Liquid dosage forms are prepared by:

a) Dissolving the active drug substance in an aqueous or non-aqueous (*e.g.,* glycerin, ether, alcohol) solvent *e.g.,* syrups, elixirs, solution etc.

b) Suspending the drug in appropriate medium *e.g.,* suspension.

c) Incorporating the drug substance into an oil or water phase *e.g.,* emulsion.

Liquid dosage forms are meant for the administration of drugs through the oral route, parenteral route and instillation in the body cavity.

Liquid orals

- Pre-formulation studies have a significant part to play in anticipating formulation problems and identifying a logical path in dosage form technology. The need for adequate drug solubility cannot be overemphasized. The most appropriate salt for development. Stability studies in solution will indicate the feasibility of parenteral or other liquid dosage form and can identify methods of stabilization.
- As compared with the dry form, the degradation is much rapid in solution form hence, stability of drug in the solution form is important when drug is intended to formulate in liquid dosage

form. Pre-formulation study data of solubility and liquid state stability plays an important role in development of liquid dosage form.

- Moreover, it is important to ascertain that the drug doesn't degrade when exposed to GI fluid when administered orally. Based on the pH based stability study, using different stimulator GI condition can be designed.
- In addition, a poor solution stability of drug may urge the formulator to choose a less soluble salt form, provided the bioavailability is not compromised.

Parenteral Dosage Form

Parenteral preparations are defined as sterile preparations containing one or more active ingredients intended for administration by injection, infusion or implantation into the body. They are packaged in either single-dose or multi-dose containers.

Pre-formulation Consideration for Parenterals

Formulation of parenteral products involves prior consideration of physicochemical properties of the drug and excipients. The preformulation study involves the evaluation of:

- *Active drug substance:* These properties include physical state (crystal characteristics), polymorphism, solubility, pharmacokinetics, pH, stability and compatibility of the drug.
- *Route of administration:* Pre-formulation studies help to decide the route of administration of injections.
- *Selection of injection volume:* One of the first steps in the formulation of a solution product is to select the administration volume and concentration.
- *pH and tonicity requirements*
- *Choice of excipients*
- *Sterility considerations*
- *Desired type of packaging*

The detailed preformulation consideration for parenteral preparations is discussed in Chapter 6.

Glossary

Crystal forms	The repetitious spacing of constituent atoms or molecules in three-dimensional array
Amorphous form	The atoms or molecules are arranged in a random manner
Glidant	One which improves the flow property of powder or granules
Partition-coefficient	The distribution of the solute (undissociated) between the two immiscible layers
Polymorphism	Existence drug molecule more than one crystalline forms
Hydrolysis	Drug molecules interact with water molecules to yield break-down products
Oxidation	Chemically, oxidation is a loss of electrons from an atom or a molecule
Reduction	Elimination of water molecule from the pharmaceutical system
Polymerization	Polymerization is a reaction between two or more identical molecules that form a new and generally larger molecule
Pre-formulation	It is a stage of product development during which the physicochemical properties of drug substance are analysed
Hygroscopicity	It is the ability of a compound to absorb the atmospheric moisture
Solubility	The concentration of solute in solution when it is in equilibrium with a solid substance at a particular temperature
Permeability	Passage of drug molecule across a biological membrane
Dissolution	The particle of the solute leaving the solid and passing into solution

QUESTION BANK

Q. I: Multiple Choice Questions

1 If Carr's index of powder is 10% then the type of powder flow is

a) Poor
b) Excellent
c) Very poor
d) Good

2 pH of the buffer system can be calculated by using

a) pH-partition theory
b) Noyes-Whitney law
c) Henderson-Hasselbalch equation
d) None of the above

3 The amorphous form of the drug is prepared by

a) Rapid precipitation
b) Lyophilisation
c) Rapid cooling of liquid melts
d) All of the above

4 Among the following which has higher solubility

a) Amorphous form of drug
b) Crystalline form of drug
c) Both (a) and (b)
d) None of the above

5 The solvent present in crystal lattice of drug molecule is water then it is known as

a) Solvates
b) Hydrates
c) Clathrates
d) Molecular adduct

6 If the solvent present within a crystal lattice of the drug is other than water then it is known as

a) Solvates
b) Hydrates
c) Clathrates
d) Adduct

7 The ability of compound to exist in more than one crystalline form is known as

a) Crystallization
b) Amorphous formation
c) Polymorphism
d) None of the above

8 Flow property of powder can be determined by

a) Angle of repose
b) Carr's index
c) Hausner's ratio
d) All of the above

9 _______ provides an estimate of the ionised and unionised drug concentration at a particular pH

a) Henry's law
b) Raoult's law
c) Henderson Hasselbalch equation
d) Nearest' equation

10 The distribution of an unionised drug between the organic phase and aqueous phase at equilibrium is known as

a) Partition law
b) Henderson Hasselbalch equation
c) Raoult's law
d) None of the above

11 It is the stage of product development where scientist characterise physicochemical property of the drug substance is known as

a) Formulation
b) Pre-formulation
c) Production
d) None of the above

12 Potentiometric titration is used for determination of

a) Dissociation constant
b) Partition coefficient
c) Solubility
d) Permeability

13 The rate and extent of absorbed drug available at the site of action is referred as

a) Bioequivalence
b) Bioavailability
c) Absorption
d) None of the above

14 Biopharmaceutics Classification system (BCS) is done based on

a) Solubility
c) Dissolution characteristics of the drug

b) Permeability
d) All of the above

15 Biopharmaceutics Classification system (BCS) is used for determination of

a) Equilibrium solubility
b) Ionisation constant
c) Bioequivalence
d) All of the above

16 Determination of particle size is done by

a) Microscopic method
c) Coulter- Counter method
b) Seiving method
d) All of the above

Q. II: Very Short Answer Questions **2 Marks**

1. Define pre-formulation. Enlist different pre-formulation parameters.
2. Write the goals and objectives of pre-formulation.
3. Give BCS classification of drugs
4. Give physical and chemical parameters of pre-formulation.

Q. III: Short Answer Questions **5 Marks**

1. Add a note on BCS classification of drugs.
2. Write the significance of BCS classification of drugs.
3. Give the difference between crystal and amorphous substances.
4. What is polymorphism? Add a note on polymorphism of drugs.
5. Discuss hydrolysis and oxidation of drugs as pre-formulation parameters.
6. Discuss the impact of pre-formulation study on the stability of dosage forms.
7. Give the importance of powder flow in solid dosage form.
8. Give an account on applications of preformulation in development of solid dosage forms.

Q. IV: Long Answer Questions **10 Marks**

1. Discuss the importance of pKa and partition coefficient in the pre-formulation studies.
2. Explain the role of pre-formulation studies at various levels of formulation.
3. Explain in detail pre-formulation parameters.
4. Explain the applications pre-formulation in the development of solid dosage forms.

UNIT-II

CHAPTER 2

TABLETS

INTRODUCTION

Tablets are solid unit dosage forms of a medicament comprising of one or more active ingredients along with suitable pharmaceutical excipients.

Tablets may vary in size, shape, weight, hardness, thickness, disintegration and dissolution characteristics and in other aspects, depending on their intended use and method of manufacture. Most tablets are used in the oral administration of drugs. Many of these are prepared with colourants and coatings of various types. Other tablets, such as those administered sublingually, buccally, or vaginally are prepared to have features most applicable to their particular route of administration. Tablets are prepared by compaction of powdered or granular medicament alone or in combination with other excipients by exerting high pressures with the aid of tablet compression machines.

Advantages

1. Tablets are more widely used solid unit dosage form of medicaments.
2. Tablets are more stable than liquid dosage forms.
3. They provide an accurate and stable dose precision.
4. Tablets are less expensive among all the solid oral dosage forms.
5. Tablets can be suitably coated to modify drug release.

6. Tablets are suitable for large scale economic production.
7. The drug release from a tablet can be varied from rapid to sustained release.
8. Embossed or monogrammed punches used for tablet compression enables easy product identification.

Disadvantages

1. Some amorphous, hygroscopic and low-density drugs are difficult to compress into tablets.
2. Drugs having unpleasant colour, odour and taste requires coating of tablets.
3. Tablets have slow onset of action when compared to parenteral dosage forms.
4. Some drugs may affect the gastric mucosa or cause local irritation when administered as tablets.
5. Tablets cannot be administered to unconscious or comatose patients.
6. Tablets are difficult to be swallowed by children and seriously ill patients.
7. The novel drug delivery system is preferred over tablets when drugs undergo hepatic first-pass metabolism.

Ideal Characteristics of Tablets

An ideal tablet should possess the following properties.

1. Tablets should have uniform weight, size and elegant appearance.
2. It should have sufficient strength and must be resistant to shocks, fracture and erosion encountered during its manufacture, transportation and usage.
3. Tablets should retain its physical and chemical stability throughout its shelf life.
4. Tablets should be formulated into reasonable size and shape to enable easy administration.
5. The active medicament(s) should be uniformly distributed in the tablet.
6. The release rate of the drug from tablet should be in a controlled and reproducible manner.

7. Tablets should be devoid of any manufacturing defects like lamination and capping etc.
8. The tablet should be devoid of any harmful micro-organisms, contaminants, excipients etc.
9. The tablet should enable easy and economical manufacturing.

Classification of Tablets

(A) ***Tablets ingested orally***

1. Compressed tablets *e.g.,* Paracetamol tablets, Metformin hydrochloride tablets etc.
2. Multiple compressed tablets
3. Delayed release tablets, *e.g.,* Enteric coated Bisacodyl tablets
4. Sugar-coated tablets, *e.g.,* Multivitamin tablets
5. Film-coated tablets, *e.g.,* Metronidazole tablets
6. Chewable tablets, *e.g.,* Antacid tablets

(B) ***Tablets used in the oral cavity***

1. Buccal tablets, *e.g.,* Vitamin - C tablets
2. Sublingual tablets, *e.g.,* Nitroglycerin tablets
3. Troches or lozenges *e.g.,* Amylmetacresol and dichlorobenzyl alcohol tablets (Strepsils)
4. Dental cones

(C) ***Tablets administered by other route***

1. Implantation tablets
2. Vaginal tablets, *e.g.,* Clotrimazole tablets

(D) ***Tablets used to prepare solution***

1. Effervescent tablets, *e.g.,* Disprin tablets (Aspirin)
2. Dispersible tablets, *e.g.,* Enzyme tablets (Digiplex)
3. Hypodermic tablets
4. Tablet triturates *e.g.,* Enzyme tablets (Digiplex)

(E) ***Prolonged release tablets***

1. Sustained release tablets *e.g.,* Diclofenac sustained release tablets
2. Controlled release tablets *e.g.,* Glipizide controlled release tablets

Compressed tablets: Compressed tablets are prepared by wet granulation or dry granulation and direct compression method. Compressed tablets are administered orally for rapid disintegration and drug release for systemic and local effects.

Multiple compressed tablets: Multiple compressed tablets are prepared by subjecting the fill material to more than a single compression. The result may be a multiple-layer tablet or a tablet within a tablet, the inner tablet being the core and the outer portion being the shell.

A) *Layered tablet*- Either two layered (for two components) or three layered (for three components) tablets.

B) *Compressed coated type*- Either tablet within a tablet or tablet coated with two layers of compressed material.

Tablets in this category are usually prepared for two reasons;

1. To separate physically or chemically incompatible ingredients.
2. To produce repeat action or prolonged action of the drug.

Delayed action tablets: This dosage form is intended to release the drug after some time delay or after the tablet has passed one part of the GIT into another. All enteric coated tablets are type of delayed action tablet but all delayed action tablets are not enteric or not intended to produce enteric action.

Sugar coated tablets: Compressed tablets may be coated with a coloured or an uncoloured sugar layer. The coating is water soluble and quickly dissolves after swallowing. The sugarcoat protects the enclosed drug from the environment and provides a barrier to objectionable taste or odour. Primary role sugar coating is to produce an elegant, glossy, easy to swallow, widely utilized in preparing multivitamin and multivitamin-mineral combination.

Enteric-coated tablets: Enteric-coated tablets have delayed-release features. They are designed to pass unchanged through the stomach to the intestines, where the tablets disintegrate and allow drug dissolution and absorption. Enteric coatings are employed when the drug substance is destroyed by gastric acid or is particularly irritating to the gastric mucosa or when bypass of the stomach substantially enhances drug absorption.

Chewable tablets: These are intended to be chewed in the mouth before swallowing, example antacid tablets but bitter or foul testing drugs are not suitable for this type of tablets.

Buccal and sublingual tablets: These tablets are small, flat and are intended to be held between the cheek and teeth or in cheek pouch (buccal tablets) or below the tongue (sublingual tablets). Drugs used by this route are for quick systemic action. The tablets are designed not to be disintegrated rapidly but to dissolve slowly.

Troches or lozenges: Troches or lozenges are disc-shaped solid dosage forms containing a medicinal agent and generally a flavouring substance in a hard candy or sugar base. They are intended to be slowly dissolved in the oral cavity, usually for local effects, although some are formulated for systemic absorption. They are commonly used to treat a sore throat or to control coughing in common cold. They may contain local anaesthetics, antiseptic, antibacterial agents, demulcents, astringent and antitussive.

Dental cone: These tablets are designed to be placed in the empty socket remaining after tooth extraction. The main purpose is to prevent microbial growth in the socket or to reduce bleeding.

Implantation tablets: These tablets are designed for implantation in the body to provide prolonged drug effect from one month to a year, tablets are usually small, cylindrical not more than 8 mm in length. This method requires a special surgical technique for implantation and discontinuation of therapy.

Vaginal tablets: These are designed to undergo slow dissolution and drug release in the vaginal cavity. Tablets are wide or pear-shaped, these include antibacterials, antiseptics and astringents to treat vaginal infection.

Effervescent tablets: Effervescent tablets are prepared by compressing granular effervescent salts that release gas when in contact with water. The tablets are prepared by compressing the active ingredient with a mixture of organic acids such as citric acid or tartaric acid and sodium bicarbonate.

Dispersible tablets: Tablets are intended to be added to a given volume of water to produce a solution of a given drug concentration.

Hypodermic tablets: These tablets are composed of one or more drugs with water-soluble ingredients. The drug is added to sterile water to prepare a sterile solution, which is injectable.

Tablet triturates: Tablet triturates are small, usually cylindrical, moulded or compressed tablets containing small amounts of usually potent drugs. Today, only a few tablet triturate products are available commercially, with most of these produced by tablet compression. Since tablet triturates must be readily and completely soluble in water, only a minimal amount of pressure is applied during their manufacture. A combination of sucrose and lactose is usually the diluent. The few tablet triturates are used sublingually, such as nitroglycerin tablets.

***Sustained release tablets*:** Sustained-release tablets are designed to release the drug at a predetermined rate in order to maintain a constant drug concentration for a specific period of time with minimum side effects.

Controlled release tablets: Controlled release tablets are designed to release (zero order) the drug at a predetermined rate and predetermined time with minimum side effects.

FORMULATION OF TABLET

A tablet consists of an active ingredient/s (therapeutically active components) and the excipients (therapeutically inactive or non-drug components). The formulation of tablet determines its tensile strength, disintegration and dissolution characteristics and drug content uniformity. In formulation of tablet, followings must be taken into consideration a) Physical and chemical properties of the active ingredient/s and the excipients b) Incompatibilities between the drug and excipients and bioavailability of the drug. General formulation for tablets is given in Table 2.1

Active Pharmaceutical Ingredient

This is the pharmacologically active ingredient in the dosage form. Active pharmaceutical ingredients are classified into two types based upon their solubility *i.e. insoluble drugs* and *soluble drugs*.

Excipients or Additives

Following are the ideal characteristics of the excipients

Table 2.1: General Formulation of tablets

1. Active pharmaceutical ingredient (Drug)
2. Excipients or additives
(a) Diluents (or) fillers
(b) Binders
(c) Disintegrants
(d) Dissolution modifiers
(e) Anti-frictional agents
i) Lubricants
ii) Glidants
(f) Anti-adherents
(g) Wetting agents
(h) Adsorbents
(i) Organoleptic agents

- They must be physically and chemically stable.
- They must be biologically inactive.
- They must not affect drug bioavailability.
- They must be free from microbial contamination.
- Excipients must meet the pharmaceutical standards.
- The excipients used in the tablet formulation must be accepted by regulatory agencies.
- Excipients used in food drug products must be approved to be used as food excipients.
- The excipient used in a formulation must be considered for its incompatibility problems.
- They must be economical.

(a) *Diluents or fillers*

Diluents are inert substances which add the necessary bulk to a formulation to prepare tablets of the desired size. Certain drugs like aspirin, antibiotics etc, exert their therapeutic action in sufficiently high doses, hence do not require diluents. Highly potent drugs such as digoxin, clonidine hydrochloride etc., exerts their therapeutic effect in very low doses, hence their bulk is increased by adding diluents.

Apart from increasing the bulk of the tablet, the diluents may also be used for:

(i) Enhance tablet properties like improved cohesion between tablet components.

(ii) The easy flow of tablet formulation ingredients during manufacturing.

(iii) Ease in direct compression of tablets during manufacturing.

(iv) Adjustment of weight of the tablet according to the capacity of the die of tablet press.

Types of Diluents

I. *Organic diluents:*

These are carbohydrates or derivatives of carbohydrates. These diluents exhibit the following properties like compactibility (the ability of the particles to be held closely and tightly), flowability (ability of the particles to flow), hygroscopicity (tendency to absorb moisture), lubricity, solubility and stability.

(1) Dextrose: It is an odourless, white and sweet crystalline powder which imparts a cool mouth feeling. It is free-flowing and water soluble. Dextrose is available as hydrous dextrose (dextrose monohydrate) and anhydrous dextrose. Anhydrous form of dextrose is used when low moisture is desired but granules prepared from this dextrose are of hard in nature. Dextrose turns brown in the presence of alkaline compounds and undergoes reaction with amines resulting in its discolouration (also seen with lactose and sucrose). Commercially dextrose is available in both hydrous and anhydrous forms under the brand name Cerelose.

(2) *Lactose*: It is a white, odourless powder, slightly sweet in taste. It is soluble in water (1 g of lactose in 4.63 ml of water) and insoluble in alcohol. Lactose is commercially available in different particle size ranges. Lactose is a reducing sugar and undergoes *Maillard reaction.* This is a type of chemical reaction which occurs between reactive carbonyl group of reducing sugar and amine group of amino acid or drugs (such as aminophylline and amphetamine). This reaction is faster in an alkaline environment as the amine group do not undergo neutralization. *Maillard reaction* gives a poor characteristic odour. This odour depends upon the type of amino acid involved in the reaction. Chemically lactose is an isomeric compound containing α-lactose and β-lactose which are in equilibrium with each other. Depending upon

the temperature of crystallization, α-lactose (at low temperature) or β-lactose (above 93°C) is produced. Lactose is available in different forms such as hydrous lactose, anhydrous lactose and spray – dried lactose.

Hydrous lactose: It is α -lactose monohydrate and is generally used in wet granulation process. In this process, wetting of lactose leads to its dissolution. This dissolved lactose forms a coat over the drug and decreases the release of drug. This is advantageous when slow dissolution of drug is required, hydrous lactose has the particle size of 100 mesh sieve and contains about 5% w/w water. It has good flow properties but poor binding characteristics. The binding properties can be increased by thermal or chemical dehydration. The mechanical strength of the tablet is inversely proportional to the particle size of hydrous lactose. Hydrous lactose is often used in combination with microcrystalline cellulose.

Anhydrous lactose: Compressibility and flow properties of anhydrous lactose are low when compared to other lactose forms, hence gets affected upon long time storage. This form of lactose absorbs moisture from the atmosphere under elevated humidity conditions. Hence, tablets containing anhydrous lactose as diluents must be carefully packed to protect from moisture absorption.

Advantages of anhydrous lactose over hydrous lactose:

1. Anhydrous lactose has less tendencies to undergo a *Maillard reaction.*
2. Anhydrous lactose form is of particular importance during the process of direct compression (In direct compression, moisture content should be low), due to its better stability.

   Anhydrous lactose is available as anhydrous *α* -lactose and anhydrous β-lactose forms.

Anhydrous α-lactose: Is obtained by dehydration of hydrous *α*-lactose. Anhydrous *α* -lactose is available as aggregates of *α* -lactose units. This form of lactose is less elastic, softer and weaker. Hence, upon application of even small stress leads to its brittle fracture readily (in comparison with hydrous lactose). The disintegration time of tablet containing anhydrous *α* -lactose is high.

Anhydrous β-lactose: Consists of very fine crystals of anhydrous β-lactose in the form of agglomerates. This form of lactose has very good compaction properties and it is less sensitive to lubricants. It is an ideal diluent for active ingredients which are moisture sensitive, as anhydrous β-lactose has low moisture content.

Anhydrous β-lactose, when compared with α -lactose monohydrate, has ten times greater solubility, higher dissolution rate and less brittle fracture.

Spray dried lactose: It is α-lactose monohydrate in crystal form. These crystals are present as agglomerates (crystals stick to each other). Spray-dried lactose also contains up to 10% of the amorphous material.

Spray dried lactose has good compression and flow characteristics. These properties are seen even when the concentration of active ingredient is as high as 20-25%. But the compression characteristics of this diluents is lost when its moisture level falls below 3% of normal moisture. The fall in moisture content is seen when drying occurs for long periods of time.

Fast-Flo lactose (NF Hydrous): It is hydrous lactose in the form of spherical crystals or amorphous agglomerates. Spherical crystals of this form of lactose are easily compressible when compared with agglomerates of spray dried lactose.

(3) *Mannitol*: It is an odourless, white, crystalline powder with a slight sweet pleasant taste. It dissolves slowly and imparts a cooling sensation in the mouth due to its negative heat of solution, hence preferably used as a diluent for chewable tablets. Mannitol is an inert and non-hygroscopic, hence used as a diluent in vitamin formulation which is moisture sensitive. Formulations containing mannitol requires more amount of lubricants as they have less flowability. Mannitol softens granules when compared with sucrose or dextrose. Commercially mannitol is available under the brand name Mannogem 2080.

(4) *Microcrystalline cellulose (MCC):* It is a white, odourless, a tasteless crystalline powder containing porous microfibers of cellulose. As the length of cellulose polymer increases, the tensile strength of the tablet also increases. It is an inert insoluble powder with good flowability.

It is used as diluent, disintegrating agent, glidant, lubricating agent and pore/channel former. The static and dynamic coefficient of friction of MCC is very less; hence it is used as the lubricating agent. The lubricating property of MCC is lost, when the concentration of active ingredient is more than 20% or when the concentration of powder tablet blend excluding MCC is more than 20% hence, additional lubrication is required. In low dose drugs, microcrystalline cellulose can also act as a secondary binder. This secondary binding nature controls the drug content uniformity, avoids migration of dyes that are water soluble and enhances uniform evaporation of the liquid from wet granules. MCC is used in both direct compression and wet granulation methods of tabletting. Commercially MCC is available under the brand names Avicel, Emcocel and Vivacel.

(5) *Sorbitol*: Sorbitol is a white granular powder which is soluble in water. Sorbitol and mannitol are optical isomers. Sorbitol and mannitol have low caloric value. They are non-carcinogenic (does not cause tooth decay). Sorbitol is used as a hygroscopic substance to maintain a proper moisture level during compression of moisture-critical granules. Commercially sorbitol is available under the brand names Neosorb 60, Sorbogen and Sorbidex P.

(6) *Starch*: Starch is a white water-insoluble and odourless substance. It is obtained from different sources like corn, potato, tapioca, wheat etc. Among these, potato starch mucilage possess maximum viscosity. Starch is available in different form like dry powder, granules, swollen granules and as a solution. Starch (USP grade) possesses poor compression and flowability characteristics. Starch contains 11-14% moisture. It is also available in a specially dried form which contains about 2-4% of moisture. Upon exposure to moisture, dried starch shows an increase in moisture content up to 6-8%.

Starch is used for many purposes such as diluents, binding agent, disintegrating agent and film-former. A possible mechanism by which starch exhibits disintegrant action includes:

1. Improved capillary force for rapid uptake of water or GI fluids in the entire tablet matrix, resulting in disintegration of the tablet.
2. Swelling of starch when in contact with water or GI fluids resulting in tablet disintegration.
3. Particles of starch deform upon compression. This deformed starch particles in the presence of water try to regain its shapes. This creates stress on the tablet, resulting in tablet disintegration.

Various modified forms of starch available are Sta-Rx 1500, Emdex, Celutab, National 78-1551 or starch 1551 (partially hydrolysed or pregelatinised starch). These modified forms of starch provide mechanical strength to the tablet and also aids in rapid release of the drug from the tablet.

(7) *Sucrose or sugar*: It is a white, odourless and sweet tasting substance available in different particle sizes like granular (table sugar), fine granular, fine, superfine and confectioners sugar (very fine sugar of which 80% should pass through 325 number mesh). Confectioners sugar with 3% cornstarch is used for wet granulation process to avoid caking of tablets.

Sucrose is hygroscopic and soluble in water and alcohol. It has good compactibility and stability. Tablets containing sucrose has long disintegration time. Sucrose granules when used in the form of dry powder, then either water or hydroalcoholic binder is added.

Sucrose is water-soluble diluents, hence used in combination with water-insoluble diluents else hard sucrose granules are formed. These hard sucrose granules when used in tablet formulation, causes dissolution of the tablet but not disintegration. Some brand names of sucrose-based diluents are Dipac which contains 97% sucrose +3% modified dextrins, Nutab which is having 95% sucrose + 4% invert sugar + small quantities of corn starch and magnesium stearate and Sugar tab having 90-93% sucrose + 7-10% invert sugar.

Disadvantages

- It is hygroscopic.
- Though sucrose is not a reducing sugar, upon ageing it turns brown in presence of alkaline compounds.
- If sucrose is present in large amounts in tablet, the tablet hardens upon ageing.
- Sucrose forms cake upon standing.
- Sucrose based tablets cannot be advised for hyperglycemic patients.

Comparative properties of some organic diluents on a scale of 1 (low grade) to 5 is shown in Table 2.2.

Table 2.2: Comparative properties of some organic diluents.

Types of organic diluents	*Properties*						
	Compac-tibility	*Disinteg-ration*	*Flow ability*	*Hygrosc-opicity*	*Lubri-city*	*Solubi-lity*	*Stabi-lity*
Dextrose	3	2	2	1	2	4	3
MCC	5	2	1	2	4	0	5
Sucrose	4	4	3	4	1	5	4

II. *Inorganic type diluents:*

Inorganic diluents are salts of metals of calcium and magnesium. These diluents exhibit the following properties like abrasiveness, absorbency, lubricity, mechanical strength, pH and solubility.

(1) *Calcium phosphate (dibasic):* It consists of small microcrystals of calcium phosphate (dibasic) or dicalcium phosphate (DCP) in the form of free-flowing aggregates. It is a fine white powder, insoluble in water, neutral and alkaline medium and slightly soluble in dilute acids. It is stable both physically and chemically and it is relatively inexpensive. Some of the commercially available brand names of DCP are Emcompress, Fujicalin, DiTab etc.

Disadvantages:

- Tablet formulations containing inorganic acetates and DCP as diluents develop an acetic odour upon long time storage.
- Absorption profile of many drugs (*e.g.,*: tetracycline) can be adversely affected by calcium salts.

Emcompress – It contains unmilled dicalcium phosphate and 5-20% of other excipients. The other excipients used improves the compaction and disintegration of tablets. Emcompress cannot be used with drugs such as ascorbic acid and thiamine hydrochloride, as it affects the hardness and disintegration times of these tablets. Emcompress also causes chemical decomposition of ascorbic acid.

Fujicalin – It is anhydrous dibasic calcium phosphate in the form of spherical granules. It has small size granular particles, hence have a large surface area. The porosity of Fujicalin is also high. It enhances faster dissolution perhaps due to its anhydrous nature.

(2) *Calcium phosphate (Tribasic):* It has properties similar to dibasic calcium phosphate. It is a fine white powder, insoluble in water, slightly alkaline in nature and abrasive. It is also non-hygroscopic. It finds limited use in wet granulation process. These diluents should not be used with salts of strong acids with weak organic bases, acetate salts and vitamin E or vitamin A esters of palmitate or acetates. Commercially calcium phosphate (tribasic) is available under the brand name Tritab.

(3) *Calcium sulphate dihydrate:* It is available as white or greyish or yellowish white, insoluble, non-hygroscopic powder with mild abrasiveness. It is used with acidic, neutral and basic drugs. It is a low-cost diluent. It is used with polymeric binders like polyvinylpyrrolidone, methylcellulose starch paste etc. The absorptive capacity of calcium sulphate dihydrates for oils are high.

(4) *Calcium carbonate*: It is available as dense, fine white powder which is usually insoluble. Its solubility depends upon pH. It is comparatively more soluble than its calcium salt form, It is obtained from ground oyster and mined limestone. It is available in various ranges of particle size and impurities. It is non-hygroscopic. Physically and chemically inert and it is inexpensive.

It is a directly compressible diluent. This diluent exerts pharmacological action which is significant as an antacid and also as a nutritional supplement.

Disadvantage

It encounters the same problem as that of MCC when over wetted or mixed, leading to formation of hard granules which disintegrate slowly. Hence, this problem can be overcome by using calcium carbonate with other diluents like starch, microcrystalline cellulose etc.

(b) *Binders*

Binders are also called as pharmaceutical glue, as they cause adhesion of powder particles to form granules. They are incorporated to produce cohesive bonding between granules during the process of compaction to form a tablet. Formation of granules depends largely upon the type of binder used. This is because the binder determines the granule size uniformity, appropriate hardness of granules and quality of the tablet.

The selection of binder is done by considering the following criteria:

- The binder should provide appropriate hardness to the tablet.
- The binder should maintain its integrity even after compression.
- The binder should allow proper release of drug from the tablet after disintegration.

Types of binders

Dry binders: These are added in the form of powder to the powder blend of tablet. This tablet blend is wetted with a suitable liquid like water or hydroalcoholic solution.

Wet binders: These are added in the form of a solution which is prepared by dissolving in an appropriate solvent like water or hydroalcoholic solution. This binder solution is then added to the powder tablet blend by four ways *i.e.,* low shear, high shear, atomization and extrusion.

Addition of a plasticizer to binder solution has shown to improve the wet massing properties of granules and tablet. The tablet properties which were improved are a tensile strength, capping pressure and decreased friability. Plasticizers which were used to study the effect on binders were glycerin, propylene glycol and polyethylene glycol 400.

Sugar as binder

Sucrose (or sugar): Apart from diluent, sucrose is also used as a binder in both forms: dry and wet. Sucrose solution (wet binder) produces hard granules depending upon the concentration of sucrose. Sucrose as a binder can be used in the range of 20-85%. The more the amount of binder, harder the granules and hence, harder the tablet. If sucrose solution is made using hydroalcoholic solution, comparatively softer granules can be obtained. The sugar solution must be of high concentration to avoid bacterial multiplication.

Sucrose is used in granulation of tablets containing tribasic calcium phosphate as diluents and for drugs such as acetophenetidin, aminophylline, meprobamate and paracetamol. In iron-tablets containing ferrous sulphate, sucrose plays the dual role: As binder and also prevents oxidation of ferrous sulphate.

Natural polymers as binder

1. *Gelatin*: 2 to 10% of gelatin solution is a strong binder, earlier gelatin was widely used as a binder, but now it has been replaced by synthetic polymeric binders like methylcellulose, polyvinyl pyrrolidone etc. Tablets containing gelatin as a binder are hard and need addition of disintegrants are required to ease disintegration of tablet.

Preparation of gelatin solution: Gelatin is hydrated by soaking in cold water for hours or by keeping it overnight. This soaked gelatin is heated to boil, so as to form gelatin solution. This hot gelatin solution must be used as early as possible, else it gels upon cooling. One of the disadvantages of gelatin is it acts as a media for growth of microorganisms, hence preservatives are to be added.

2. *Gums*: Certain natural gums such as acacia and tragacanth are used as binders in tablet formulation.

3. *Acacia*: It is used as a binder at the concentrations of 5 to 10% acacia is being replaced by synthetic polymers like polyvinylpyrrolidone (PVP) and certain cellulose derivatives. Acacia is a suitable binder in case where the drug concentration to be used is high and granulation is difficult *e.g.,* Mephenesin. The granules produced from acacia are hard.

4. *Tragacanth*: It is used as a binder at the concentrations of 5 to 10%, granules produced by tragacanth are not hard as that of acacia.

5. *Starch:* Various forms of starch which can be used as binders are starch 1500, starch paste and pregelatinised starch.

Starch 1500: It is used for multiple purposes like dry binder, wet binder and as disintegrating agent, starch 1500 contains 20% of cold water soluble portion. This cold water soluble portion serves as an efficient binder whereas remaining 80% (cold water insoluble portion) helps in tablet disintegration. Starch 1500 in dry form is mixed with powder tablet blend and is then granulated using water of appropriate temperature. In order to achieve tablet hardness similar to that obtained from starch paste, 3-4 times amount of starch 1500 is required.

Starch paste: It is one of the most widely used binder, it has some advantages like the tablet containing starch paste as binder disintegrates rapidly, starch when used as an internal binder and water as a granulating liquid, then also the tablet disintegrates rapidly.

Preparation of starch paste:

Method I: In this method, starch is taken with 1 or 1 ½ parts of cold water and suspended in it. To this suspension of starch, add 2 to 4 times of boiling water with constant stirring. This causes swelling of starch and a translucent paste is formed. This paste can be further diluted with cold water to get the desired concentration of starch paste.

Method II: In this method, a suspension of starch in cold water is prepared. This suspension is then transferred to a steam jacketed kettle. In the kettle, the suspension is heated to boiling with constant stirring forming starch paste. A properly made starch paste is translucent rather than transparent.

Pregelatinised starch: This starch is obtained by cooking the starch and drying it subsequently. Pregelatinised starch can be added in dry form to the powder blend of the tablet followed by wetting with water. This starch can cause over wetting and thickening of granules. It can be used instead paste. In contrast to starch, it is soluble in water without the need of boiling.

Synthetic polymers as binder:

1. *Ethyl cellulose*: It is insoluble in water but soluble in alcohol. It is available in various viscosity grades. 2-10% of low viscosity grade ethylcellulose in ethanol is used as a binder.

It is a non-aqueous binder, hence suitable for drugs which are sensitive in the presence of water, powders with poor compression characteristics (*e.g.* drugs likes paracetamol, caffeine, meprobamate and ferrous fumarate) can be granulated using ethylcellulose.

2. *Methylcellulose*: The binding strength of methyl cellulose depends on the viscosity grades. It is available in low (10 to 50 cps) and high viscosity (1000 to 10000 cps) grades. Granules produced using methylcellulose compress easily and the tablets produced from these granules do not become hard upon storage. A 5% solution of methylcellulose and 10% starch paste produces granules of same hardness. It acts as a comparatively better binder for soluble excipients like mannitol, lactose etc.

3. *Polyethylene glycol (PEG) 6000:* It is white to yellow solid having melting range of 70 to 75°C. It solidifies at 56 to 63°C. It may be used in a situation where the tablet formulation is sensitive to water or alcohol, hence acting as an anhydrous granulating agent.

4. *Polyvinyl alcohol (PVA):* They are water-soluble film forming agents which are used as binders. They are available in different viscosity grades. PVA with a viscosity of 10 to 100 cps is used as a granulating agent. It produces soft granules (when compared to acacia) that undergo easy disintegration and usually do not harden upon long time storage. Granulation properties of polyvinyl alcohols are similar to that of acacia, but offer an advantage that they are not highly contaminated with bacteria.

5. *Polyvinylpyrrolidone (PVP):* It is a versatile inert binder, soluble in both water and alcohol, slightly hygroscopic and expensive. It is used in the concentration of 5 to 10%. It is used as both dry binder and wet binder. Granules of insoluble powders are prepared by dissolving PVP in aqueous or hydroalcoholic solutions.

It is used as a binder to prepare granules of effervescent tablets (Effervescent tablets which contain sodium bicarbonate and citric acid can be prepared by wet granulation using 5% of PVP in anhydrous ethanol) and chewable tablets. The granules made of fine powder of sodium bicarbonate and citric acid show good compression characteristics, hence these tablets produce vigorous effervescence and rapidly undergoes dissolution.

PVP can be dissolved in both anhydrous ethanol and anhydrous isopropanol, to use as a binder in effervescent tablets. Anhydrous ethanol is more appropriate in effervescent tablet granulation because it does not undergo acid-base reactions in the absence of water, whereas anhydrous isopropanol levels behind its odour in the tablet irrespective of the duration and the drying method of tablets.

PVP is also used as a very good binder in chewable tablets. It is of more importance as a binder in chewable tablets containing aluminium hydroxide-magnesium hydroxide. Addition of 2 to 3% of glycerin to these tablets decreases tablet hardening upon long time storage.

6. *Sodium CMC:* It is used in the concentrations of 5 to 15% to produce soft granules, which generally show good compression. It can be used

to granulate both soluble and insoluble powders. The granules produced are softer when compared with the granules produced using PVP.

(c) Disintegrants

Disintegrating agents are added to promote tablet breakup after administration. This is seen when the tablet comes in contact with an aqueous environment or GI fluid.

Disintegrating agents act in opposition to binding agents. Stronger the binder used stronger the disintegrating agent is required to disintegrate the tablet so as to release the medicament.

Disintegrating agents can be added by two methods:

(i) Intra-granular (internal addition): Disintegrating agent is added to the tablet powder blend along with other ingredients. This mixture is granulated and the granules so produced are compressed to form tablets.

(ii) *Extra-granular (external addition):* In this method, to the powder tablet mixture, granulating liquid is added to form granules. To the above formed granules, disintegrating agent is added. These granules are then subjected to compression to form tablets. This method is widely used for addition of disintegrants.

Mechanism of disintegrating agents

(i) Improved capillary forces for rapid uptake of water or GI Fluids in this mechanism, the pore structure of the tablet is an important criteria. Disintegrating agents in the concentration of 5 to 20% are used for the continuous breakdown of tablet matrix by this mechanism.

(ii) Swelling of disintegrating agents when in contact with water or GI fluids. In this mechanism the tablet matrix should be rigid which is an important criteria, as there should be no accommodation of the swollen disintegration agent within it.

(iii) Release of gas to disintegrate the tablet: In this mechanism, the disintegrants are used in such tablets which have poor disintegration characteristics. This is done to allow rapid disintegration or to make the formulation easily soluble. These

Table 2.3: Examples for disintegrating agents and their concentrations.

Disintegrants	***Concentration***	***Comments***
Alginic acid	5–10% w/w	Obtained from the seaweed, consisting of D-mannuronic and L-glucuronic units. It is insoluble in water and slightly acidic in nature. Due to its good affinity for water and high absorptivity, it acts as a good disintegrant.
Microcrystalline cellulose (MCC)	5–15% w/w	It is one of the most effective disintegrants
Guar gum	2–8% w/w	It is natural gum consisting of sugar units. Its colour ranges from off-white to tan and is not always pure white. Upon ageing, it discolours in alkaline tablets. It is unaffected by pH, moisture content and tablet matrix solubility. It is an excellent disintegrant in the concentration range of 2-8% w/w.
Sodium starch glycolate	2–8% w/w	It is a semisynthetic disintegrant obtained by cross-linking and carboxy methylating potato starch. The granules containing sodium starch glycolate rapidly absorbs water and swells, resulting in rapid and uniform disintegration of tablets.
Starch	Cornstarch USP (5–20% w/w), starch 1500 (5–15% w/w)	It is one of the most widely used disintegrating agent
Hydroxy propyl methyl cellulose (HPMC)	5–10% w/w	They exert their disintegrating action by swelling on exposure to water, but they are not more advantageous compared to starch or MCC.
Methylcellulose and sodium CMC	5–10% w/w	They exert their disintegrating action by swelling on exposure to water, but they are not more advantageous compared to starch or MCC.

disintegrants are required in low concentration compared to other disintegrants.

(iv) *Enzymatic destruction of Binders*: In this mechanism, the non-cohesives tablets are disintegrated by adding little quantity of suitable enzyme. This is done by incorporating binders by wet granulation process, hence making the tablets of cohesive nature and then adding enzymes.

Examples for disintegrating agents and their concentration are given in Table 2.3.

Super disintegrating agents: These are the newer class of disintegrating agents which are required in less quantity compared to starch. Since they are used in small quantities, they do not have much influence on flowability and compressibility of powder tablet blend. Based on the chemical nature there are three types of super disintegrating agents

a. Sodium starch glycolate (modified starch or Primogel)
b. Croscarmellose (modified cellulose)
c. Cross-linked polyvinylpyrrolidone (modified cellulose)

d) Dissolution modifiers:

These are added to the tablet formulation in order to change the drug release pattern from the tablet. They are of particular importance in controlled release drug delivery systems.

e) Anti-frictional agents:

Anti-frictional agents can be classified as follows:

1. *Lubricants*: These are added to a tablet formulation to decreases the friction between the granules and the die wall of tablet press. Lubricants are required during tablet compression and ejection. The selection of lubricant is done by considering the following points:

- Type of the tablet (immediate release or sustained release).
- Desired disintegrating and dissolution characteristics.
- Problems associated with lubrication and flow of powder blend.
- Formulation requirements.
- Physical properties of granules or powder blend, which is to be compressed into tablets.
- Compatibility between drug and lubricants.

Generally, with increased concentration of lubricants increases the disintegration and dissolution time. This is because of decreased penetration of water in the tablet (as lubricants are generally hydrophobic in nature).

Methods of addition of lubricants: Lubricants can be added to a tablet formulation in the form of dry powders, alcohol solutions, suspensions or emulsions. After additions of lubricant, the tablet powder blend is mixed for two to five min. The two methods by which lubricants are added to tablet formulation are:

(i) Incorporation method: The lubricant is added to the powder blend of the tablet. This type of addition promotes uniforms distribution of lubricant throughout the powder blend of the tablet and also forms a coat on the particles of the powder. This powder blend is then subjected to granulation. The granules so produced are more or less intact upon compression into tablets. The coating of lubricants may also be seen on tablet surface. The best lubricants are hydrophobic in nature and may tend to increase disintegration and dissolution rate of the tablet.

(ii) Mixing method: In this method, lubricants are added to the final granules before compression into tablet. This method provides ease of tablet ejection from die cavity. The effectiveness of a lubricant depends upon its particles size, as in turn it influences the dissolution and disintegration properties of the final tablet. Inappropriate lubrication results in tablet processing defects such as binding and sticking (filming), whereas over lubrication results in capping and lamination. This is usually seen in stearate lubricants.

Mechanism of Lubricants: Lubricants exert their action by two mechanisms:

(i) *Fluid lubrication or hydrodynamic lubrication*: In this type, the lubricating agents form a finite and continuous layer between the moving surfaces of tablet and die press during compression and ejection. Example: liquid paraffin (mineral oil)

(ii) *Boundary lubrication*: In this type, the polar portion of a lubricating agent which contains long carbon chains adheres to the metal surface of the die wall. These lubricants are better than fluid lubricants as they show good adherence to the die wall of the tablet press. Example: magnesium stearate.

Lubricants are two types (i) soluble lubricants and (ii) insoluble lubricants.

Soluble lubricants: *e.g.,* sodium and magnesium lauryl sulfates, sodium benzoate, PEG 4000 (carbowax 4000) and PEG 6000 (carbowax 6000) and sodium chloride.

They are used in the concentration range of 1-5%. Sodium benzoate and sodium chloride have limited application in the field of pharmaceuticals.

Insoluble lubricants: *e.g.,* calcium or magnesium stearate (0.25-2%), mineral oil, talc (1-5%), stearic acid (0.25-2%).

2. *Glidants*: These are the agents which are added to tablet formulation to improve the flow property of granules. These agents have the capacity to improve the flow property of granules from hopper to the die cavity. The uniformity in tablet weight depends upon the uniform filling of granules into the die cavity. The efficiency of glidant in the powder blend can be determined by compressing the powder blend into the tablet and then determining the tablets weight variation.

Mechanism of glidants: Glidants exhibit their action by any of the following mechanism.

- Electrostatic charge which is present on the granules is dispersed by glidants. This decreases the aggregation of granules and enhances the flow properties of granules.
- Glidants distributes itself in the granules and enhances the flow property of granules.
- Adsorption of gases onto the glidants is more when compared to granules; hence flow of granules is promoted.
- Glidants adhere to the surface of the granules forming a film, reducing the friction between granular particles and reducing surface roughness of the granules.
- Glidants decrease Vander Waal's forces of attraction by separating the granules.

Types of glidants

CAB-O-SIL: It consists of very fine particles of fumed silica. It is a pure white and free-flowing powder, which is insoluble in water, because of its very fine particle nature, it forms agglomerates hence, it is mixed with other excipients. CAB-O-SIL coats the tablet blend (powder or granules) thereby decreasing the frictional force and enhancing flowability.

CAB-O-SIL is used as an anti-adherent in concentration of 1 to 2% and as a glidant in the concentration of 0.1 to 0.5%. If higher concentration of CAB-O-SIL is used, then the flowability of tablet material is affected leading to weight variation of the final tablet.

Corn-starch: It is used as both glidant (5-10%) and anti-adherent (3-10%). It is used as a secondary lubrication in wet granulation process. For example metallic stearates like calcium, magnesium and sodium etc.

f) Anti-adherents

These agents prevent the sticking of tablet material (powder or granules) to the punch and to some extent to the tablet die wall. Hence, it avoids the tablet processing problems of sticking and picking which occurs due to the presence of excess moisture.

Lubricants used in the tablet formulation can act as anti-adherents but sometimes to overcome friction it may require addition of some more lubricants, for example, CAB-O-SIL (0.1–0.5%), Syloid (0.1–0.5%), SLS (<1%), metallic stearates like calcium, magnesium and sodium (<1%), talc (1–5%), corn starch (3–10%) etc.

g) Wetting agents

These agents are added to a tablet formulation containing the poorly soluble components (such as active ingredient, preservative or antioxidant). These are used to enhance the dissolution rate of the components of tablet. They act by reducing the interfacial tension existing between solid and liquid components and promote colloidal dispersion. Some of the wetting agents like alginates, bentonite, cellulose derivatives, tragacanth, sodium lauryl sulphate (SLS), polysorbates, sorbitan esters etc.

h) Adsorbents

In tablet formulation, a little quantity of adsorbent is added. The added adsorbent adsorbs the semisolid or liquid excipients and avoids cohesiveness of tablet powder to allow proper tablet compression. Some of the commonly used adsorbents are fuller's earth and kaolin (hydrated aluminium silicate).

i) ***Organoleptic agents***

1. *Colouring agents:* These are the agents which impart colour to the tablet. They are used for the following reasons. (a) They help in easy identification of the tablet. (b) They give elegance to the tablet appearance.

Insoluble colouring agents such as lakes are added to the dry powder blend of the tablet. This mixture is then directly compressed to form tablet.

Water-soluble colouring agents such as dyes are dissolved in the granulating solvent (water, alcohol or hydroalcoholic solution). This solvent is then added to the powder tablet blend to form granules. This method assures uniform mixing. But these dyes may undergo mottling upon drying. These dyes can also be mixed with an excipient in dry state before mixing with final tablet blend. Care must be taken to avoid migration of colouring agent during drying of granules.

Types of colouring agents:

Artificial colouring agents: The artificial colouring agents which are commonly used are FD &C dyes. These approved dyes are used in the form of solutions or in the form of powders (lakes of these dyes).

Natural colouring agents: Natural colouring agents do not require FD& C and D & C approval for incorporation into drug products.

Dyes: They are soluble colouring agents which becomes insoluble after application.

Lakes: They are dyes in the form of dry powders adsorbed on hydrous oxide such as aluminium hydroxide.

Pigments: They are insoluble colouring agents available as powders. They are to be mixed with water, oil or other solvents. Some examples of FD & C approved colouring agents used in tablets are blue 1(brilliant blue), red (erythrosine), green 3 (fast green) and yellow 6 (sunset yellow) etc.

2. *Flavouring agents*: Flavouring agents are added just before compression in order to prevent volatilization as they are volatile oils. If there is a possibility of oxidation, then the flavouring oil is emulsified.

Emulsifying agent used may be starch or acacia gum giving rise to dry flavouring agent in aqueous solution or specially encapsulated (using spray drying) to avoid oxidation. The flavouring agent used should not show any incompatibility with drug. Flavouring agents are added to the tablet:

(i) To make chewable tablet palatable which are intended to dissolve in the mouth. Dissolution in mouth enhances drug bioavailability of these tablets.

(ii) When the tablet is difficult to swallow for children chewable tablet may be used containing a flavouring agent.

The water-soluble flavouring agents have poor stability. Flavour oil in the concentration of 0.5 to 0.75% added during granulation which does not affect tablet characteristics.

3. *Sweetening agents:* These agents are added to tablet formulation to impart sweet taste and to mask bitter taste. Examples saccharin, aspartame, sucrose, mannitol, dextrose, maltose etc. Saccharin is 450 times sweeter compared to sucrose. But disadvantages associated with saccharin are bitter aftertaste and it is carcinogenic. This bitter aftertaste can be reduced to some extent by adding a small quantity of sodium chloride. Aspartame is nearly 200 times sweeter than table sugar.

MANUFACTURING OF TABLETS

Tablets are prepared by moulding method or compression method. Tablets are prepared primarily by compression, a limited number prepared by moulding. Moulded tablets are prepared on a large scale by tablet machinery or on a small scale by manually forcing dampened powder material into a mould from which the formed tablet is then ejected and allowed to dry.

Compressed tablets are manufactured with tablet machines capable of exerting great pressure in compacting the powdered or granulated material. Their shape and dimensions are determined by the use of various shaped punches and dies. Compressed tablets may be made by three basic methods: direct compression, wet granulation and dry granulation.

Direct compression

Direct compression is a simple method since it involves less processing steps compared to other tablet manufacturing methods. Direct compression is a dry process wherein the powdered material is compressed directly into the tablets.

For direct compression method, some granular chemicals like potassium chloride, possess free-flowing and cohesive properties that enable them to be compressed directly in a tablet machine without any need of granulation. For chemicals lacking this quality, special pharmaceutical excipients may be used to impart the necessary qualities for the production of tablets by direct compression. These excipients include fillers, such as spray-dried lactose, microcrystals of alpha-monohydrate lactose, sucrose–invert sugar–starch mixtures, microcrystalline cellulose, crystalline maltose and dicalcium phosphate; disintegrating agents, such as direct compression starch, sodium carboxymethyl starch, cross-linked carboxymethylcellulose fibers, and cross-linked polyvinylpyrrolidone; lubricants, such as magnesium stearate and talc; and glidants, such as fumed silicon dioxide.

Ideal characteristics of vehicles used in direct compression

- It should possess good compressibility and flow properties.
- It should be physiologically inert.
- Must be compatible with other ingredients of tablet
- It must retain its compression characteristics even in the presence of other drugs and additives.
- The particle size of the excipients should be equivalent to that of the active ingredient.
- It should possess appreciable disintegration characteristics.
- It should not hinder the release of drug from the tablet.
- The vehicle must remain stable in the presence of air, moisture and elevated temperatures.
- It should be cost-effective and tasteless

Procedure for direct compression

The various steps involved in direct compression of tablets (Fig. 2.1) is illustrated as below:

1. Drug is added to the size reduction equipment and ground.
2. The suitable directly compressible excipients are added in a blender and mixed thoroughly.
3. The blended powder material is compressed by tablet compression machine.

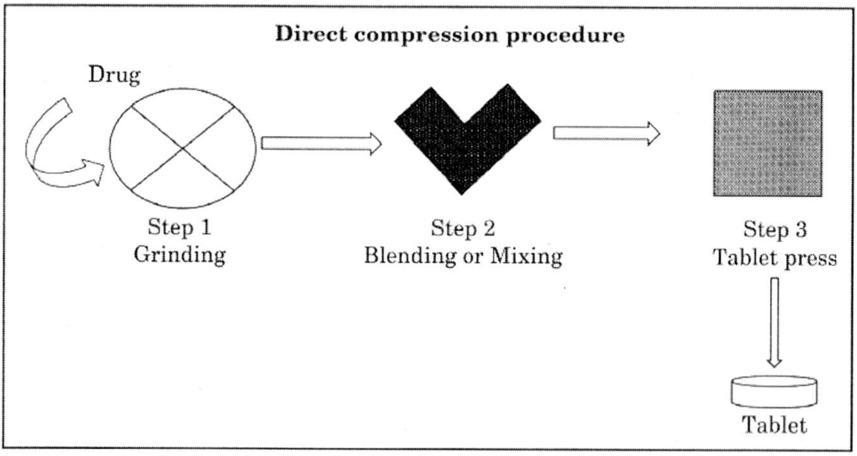

Fig. 2.1: Various steps involved in direct compression of tablets.

Example: Formulation table for direct compression method is given in Table 2.4.

Table 2.4: Formulation table for direct compression method.

Ingredients	*For 1 tablet*	*For 100 tablets*
Ascorbic acid	255 mg	25.5 g
Microcrystalline cellulose	159 mg	15.9 g
Stearic acid	9 mg	0.9 g
Colloidal silica	2 mg	0.2 g

All the ingredients mentioned in the above table are weighed and properly mixed in a suitable blender. This mixture is compressed to form tablets by using a standard concave punch.

Advantages

1. Direct compression technique is less time consuming.
2. It requires less labour, equipment and space area.

3. It requires the fewest processing steps for tablet manufacturing.
4. Being a dry process, it is suitable for heat and moisture sensitive substances.
5. The microbial contamination of tablets is prevented due to absence of water.
6. The wear and tear of tablet press tooling (*i.e.,* dies and punches) is reduced.

Disadvantages

1. This method is not suitable for large dose drugs
2. Direct compression is not preferred when drugs have poor flow properties.
3. Occasionally, an interaction between the drug and directly compressible filler (diluents) can occur, *e.g.,* yellow colouration of tablets occur due to the reaction between spray-dried lactose (diluents) and amine compounds.
4. The dry nature of this technique results in the development of static charges within the drug during processing steps. This, in turn, results in poor drug content uniformity.
5. The pre-processing of directly compressible adjuvant makes them expensive.

GRANULATION

Granulation may be defined as a process in which small particles adhere together by forming bonds, resulting in the formation of large aggregates called granules.

Reasons for Granulation

The powder is converted into granules for the following reasons.

1. The granulation process improves the flow properties of the resultant granules.
2. Granulation process prevents the problem of dust during compression
3. Granulation prevents segregation of drug particles.
4. The ability of the drug to undergo compression is improved.

5. The drug release rates from the tablet can be controlled.
6. It helps in densifying the materials.
7. The process helps to get elegant tablets.
8. The granulation process can be utilized to produce particles of uniform size.
9. It helps to achieve and control the bulk density of the powder within desired limits.

Techniques of Granulation

The tablet formulation ingredients prior to granulation are milled to achieve uniform sized particles. This prevents their segregation into a layer which is usually seen during the various processing steps of tablet manufacture. The granules can be prepared by following methods:

1. Dry granulation
2. Wet granulation or moist granulation.

1. *Dry granulation method*

This method is also known as double compression or compression granulation or pre-compression granulation. By the dry granulation method, the powder mixture is compacted into large masses and subsequently broken down or sized into granules. For this method, either the active ingredient or the diluent must have cohesive properties.

The process of dry granulation involves the formation of tablet by first converting the tablet formulation into slugs or compact masses. These formed masses are screened to form uniform-sized fine granules. This technique is suitable for those drugs which are moisture sensitive, undergoes degradation at high temperature encountered during the drying process and the drugs administered in high doses.

The various steps involved in the dry granulation (Fig. 2.2) of the tablets is illustrated below:

1. Drug is added to the granulator and ground
2. The suitable diluents and other excipients are added and mixed in a blender
3. After mixing the powder mixture is slugged or compressed into large flat tablets or pellets.

4. These large tablets or slugs are broken down by hand or crushed to form granules.
5. The granules undergo dry screening through the desired mesh for sizing (mesh no. 16).
6. Finally, the lubricating agent is added and mixed thoroughly in a blender.
7. The resultant granules are compressed by a tablet press.

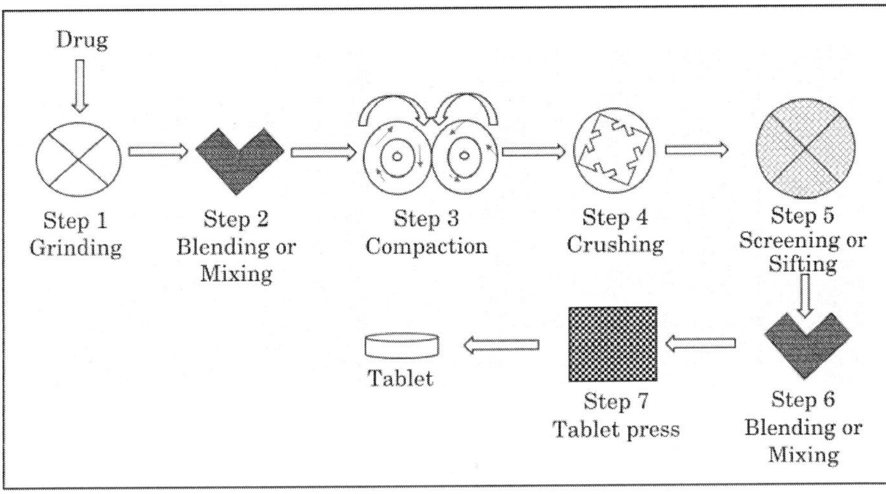

Fig. 2.2: Various steps involved in dry granulation.

Example of tablet formulation prepared by dry granulation method (Table 2.5).

Table 2.5: Formulation of acetylsalicylic acid tablet

Ingredients	***For 1 tablet***	***For 100 tablets***
Acetyl salicylic acid	0.325 g	32.5 g
Starch	0.0325 g	3.25 g

Starch is dried until the moisture content is about 10%. This dried starch is thoroughly mixed with acetylsalicylic acid. The mixture is compressed in the form of slugs. The formed slugs are ground to a size of 14-16 mesh. The ground starch is again recompressed in the form of tablets. Recompression is carried out by using a tablet compression machine.

The dry granulation is achieved by:

- Slugging (slug formation)
- Roller compaction method

Slugging (slug formation): After weighing and mixing the ingredients, the powder mixture is slugged or compressed, into large flat tablets or pellets about 1 inch in diameter using specially designed tablet press. The slugs are broken up by hand or by mill and passed through a screen for sizing of granules. The granules are then mixed with the remaining portion of the lubricant and undergo final compression to form tablets.

Slugging serves to expel the air entrapped in the powdered material, thus making the mass dense and simultaneously enhancing the flow properties of the formed granules.

Application: The slugging process is suitable for drugs like aspirin and its combinations, acetaminophen, antacids, ascorbic acid, magnesium hydroxide, thiamine hydrochloride etc.

Roller compaction method: In roller compaction method, ribbon-shaped compact masses are formed. The roller compaction method requires a specially designed equipment *i.e.,* Roller compactor. Roller compaction method is suitable for large-scale production of tablets by compression granulation.

Roller compactor

Construction: The roller compactor comprises the following components. Powder feed, feed hopper, screw conveying system (vertical feed screw and horizontal feed screw), compaction rolls, a hydraulic actuator, a device for prebreak mechanism, attritor, screens and product receiver (Fig. 2.3).

The two compaction rolls are closely arranged which revolve towards each other by hydraulic actuator. The surface of these compaction rolls can be smooth or toothed. The feed reservoir is connected to the feed hopper *via* suitable tubes. This hopper is connected to the horizontal feed screw which is various shapes and sizes. A device for pre-break mechanism is provided which helps in pre-break of the compact masses of powdered material. An attritor is also present along with three

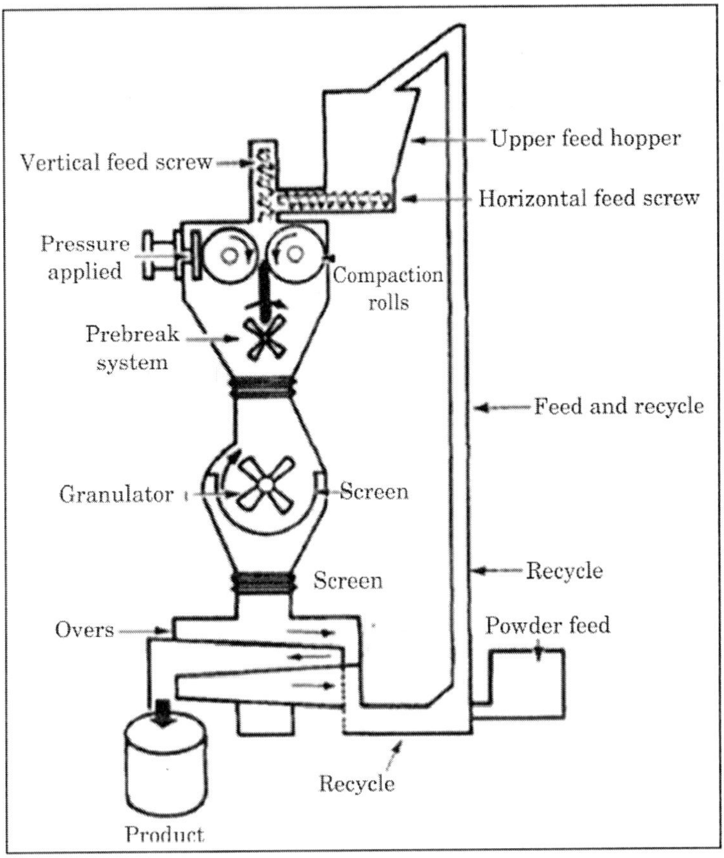

Fig. 2.3: Roller compactor

screens, which segregate the compact particles present along with three screens. Which segregate the compacted particles according to their particle size. A separate provision is provided for the collection of product (ribbon-shaped compact masses.) fines and overs. The latter two *i.e.,* fines and overs are recycled *via* the recycling system.

Working: The powder blend is fed into the hopper from the feed reservoir this hopper directs the powdered feed into the horizontal feed screw which in turn transfers it into the vertical feed screw in a continuous manner. The vertical feed screw serves two functions i) Initially it expels the air from the powdered material. ii) Also helps to maintain a constant powder flow rate to the compaction rolls. This is achieved by setting the vertical screw at a speed higher than the compaction rolls resulting in their overload.

The rotational speed of both the screws can be varied. The powdered feed is then passed onto the compaction rolls which exert a prefixed constant pressure on the material. This result in the formation of ribbon-like compact masses which are comparable to the slugs formed during slugging. That compact mass passes into the pre-break device which provides an initial breakup of the compact mass (like chips and flakes). These are then lead into the attritor. The attritor along with the screens functions in further breaking of the masses to the desired particle size. Thes milled mass consists of overs (materials whose particle size exceeds the upper limit of the desired particle size), product and fines (material whose particle size is lower than the lower limit of the desired particle size). Theses collected fines and overs are recycled into the upper feed hopper *via* the tubing which also serves to transfer the feed. The product consisting of desired particle size is collected in the product receiver. This product is then suitably lubricated and compressed into tablets.

2. *Wet granulation (or) moist granulation*

Wet granulation is a most widely used method for the preparation of compressed tablets. The steps required are (a) weighing and blending the ingredients, (b) preparing a damp mass, (c) screening damp mass into granules, (d) drying the granulation, (e) sizing the granulation by dry screening, (f) adding lubricant and blending, and (g) forming tablets by compression.

Wet granulation is the most conventional, versatile and it imparts all the physical properties to the granules. This technique differs from direct compression and dry granulation as it involves the use of liquids to form compact masses.

The various steps involved in the wet granulation (Fig. 2.4) of the tablets is illustrated as below:

1. Drug is added to the grinder and ground.
2. The suitable adjuvants (*e.g.,* diluents and other excipients) are added and mixed in a blender.
3. Granulating liquids (*e.g.,* alcohols) are added to form a damp mass.

4. The mass is screened to form granules.
5. These granules are dried to remove excess of the liquid.
6. Dry screening of granules results in size reduction and granules become spherical.
7. The lubricating agent is added and the mixture is mixed thoroughly in a blender.
8. The resultant granules are compressed by machine tooling (*i.e.*, dies and punches) of a tablet press.

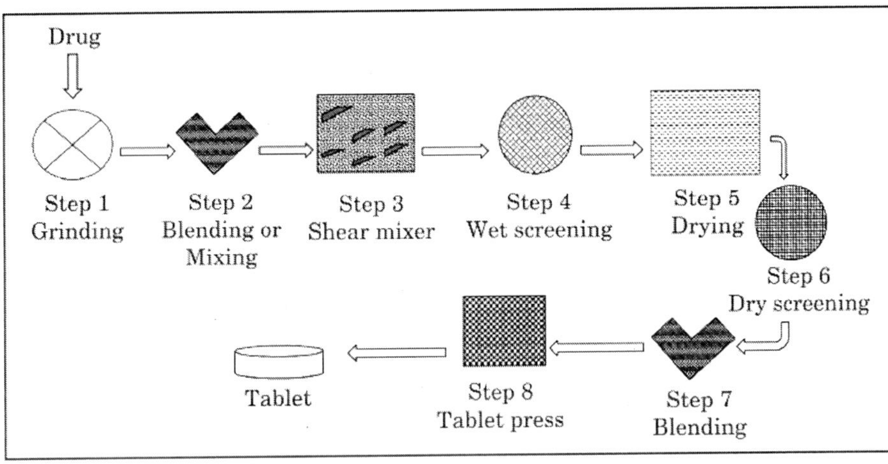

Fig. 2.4: Various steps involved in wet granulation.

MECHANISMS OF GRANULE FORMATION

Mechanism of granule formation can be discussed in two mechanisms i) Particle bonding mechanisms ii) Granulation proper. In particle bonding mechanisms the interparticular bonding takes place and leads to nucleation and in granulation proper the deposition of powder particle over the nuclei or combining of two or more nuclei to form granules.

Particle Bonding Mechanisms

To form granules, bonds must be formed between powder particles so that they adhere and these bonds must be sufficiently strong to prevent breakdown of the granule to powder in subsequent handling operations. The five primary bonding mechanisms between particles are:

1. Adhesion and cohesion forces in the immobile liquid films between individual primary powder particles
2. Interfacial forces in mobile liquid films within the granules
3. The formation of solid bridges after solvent evaporation
4. Attractive forces between solid particles
5. Mechanical interlocking.

Adhesion and cohesion: If sufficient liquid is present in a powder it forms a very thin film immobile layer, there will be an effective decrease in interparticle distance and increase in contact area between the particles.

Interfacial forces in mobile liquid films: During wet granulation liquid is added to the powder mix and will be distributed as films around and between the particles. Sufficient liquid is usually added to exceed that necessary for an immobile layer and produce mobile film. At low moisture level termed as pendular state, the particles are held together by lens shaped rings of liquid. When all air is displaced between the particles the capillary state is reached and particles are held by capillary suction at the liquid air interface.

Funicular state represents an intermediate stage between pendular and capillary state.

In massing process during wet granulation, continued kneading/ mixing of material originally in the *pendular state* will densify the wet mass, decreasing the pore volume occupied by air and eventually producing funicular or capillary state without further addition of liquids.

Droplet is important in the process of granulation because moist granules will be dried. They are however a prerequisite for the formation of solid bridges formed by binders present in the liquid or materials which dissolve in the granulating liquids.

Solid bridges are formed by partial melting, hardening binder and crystallisation of dissolved substances. In the absence of liquids and solid bridges formed by binders, there are two types of attractive forces which operate between the particles such as electrostatic forces, Vander Waal's forces etc.

Water distribution between particles of granule during formation and drying is shown in Fig. 2.5.

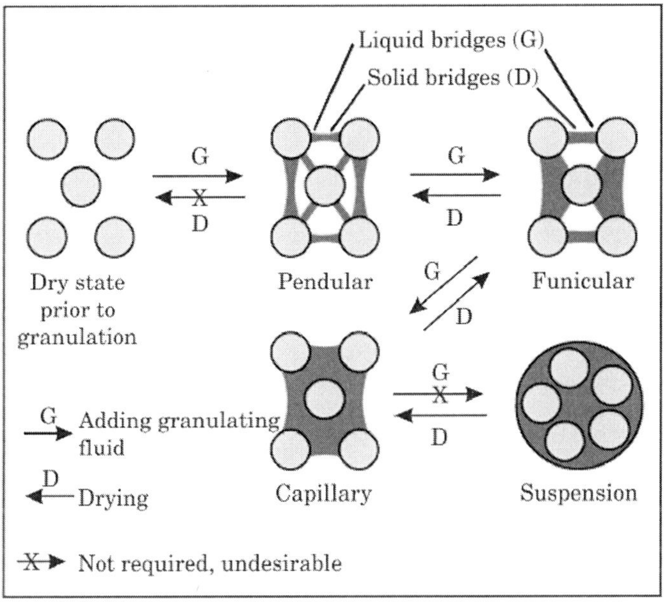

Fig. 2.5: Water distribution between particles of a granule during formation and drying.

Granulation Proper

In dry granulation method, adhesion of particles takes place because of applied pressure. A compact or sheet is produced which is larger than the granule size required and therefore the required size can be attained by milling and sieving. In wet granulation methods, liquid added to dry powders has to be distributed through the powder by the mechanical agitation produced in the granulator. The particles adhere to each other because of liquid films and further agitation and/or liquid addition causes more particles to adhere. The precise mechanism by which a dry powder is transformed into a bed of granules varies for each type of granulation equipment but the mechanism discussed below serves as a useful broad generalization of the process. The proposed granulation mechanism can be divided into three stages: nucleation, transition and ball growth.

Nucleation: Granulation starts with particle–particle contact and adhesion due to liquid bridges. Number of particles will join to form the pendular state. Further agitation densities the pendular bodies to form the capillary state and these bodies act as nuclei for further granule growth.

Transition: Nuclei can grow by two possible mechanisms: either single particles can be added to the nuclei by pendular bridges or two or more nuclei may combine. The combined nuclei will be reshaped by the agitation of the bed. This stage is characterized by the presence of a large number of small granules with a fairly wide size distribution. Providing that the size distribution is not excessively large, this point represents a suitable endpoint for granules used in capsule and tablet manufacture as relatively small granules will produce a uniform tablet die or capsule fill. Larger granules may give rise to problems in small-diameter dies due to bridging across the die and uneven fill.

Ball growth: Further granule growth produces large, spherical granules and the mean particle size of the granulating system will increase with time. If agitation is continued, granule coalescence will continue and produce an unusable, over-massed system, although this is dependent upon the amount of liquid added and the properties of the material being granulated. Although ball growth produces granules which may be too large for pharmaceutical purposes, some degree of ball growth will occur in planetary mixers and it is an essential feature of some spheronizing equipment. The four possible mechanisms of ball growth are illustrated in Fig. 2.6.

i) Coalescence: Two or more granules join to form a larger granule.

ii) Breakage: Granules break into fragments which adhere to other granules, forming a layer of material over the surviving granule.

iii) Abrasion transfer: Agitation of the granule bed leads to attrition of material from granules. This abraded material adheres to other granules, increasing their size.

iv) Layering: When a second batch of powder mix is added to a bed of granules, the powder will adhere to the granules, forming a layer over the surface and thus increasing the granule size. This mechanism is only of relevance to the production of layered granules using spheronizing equipment.

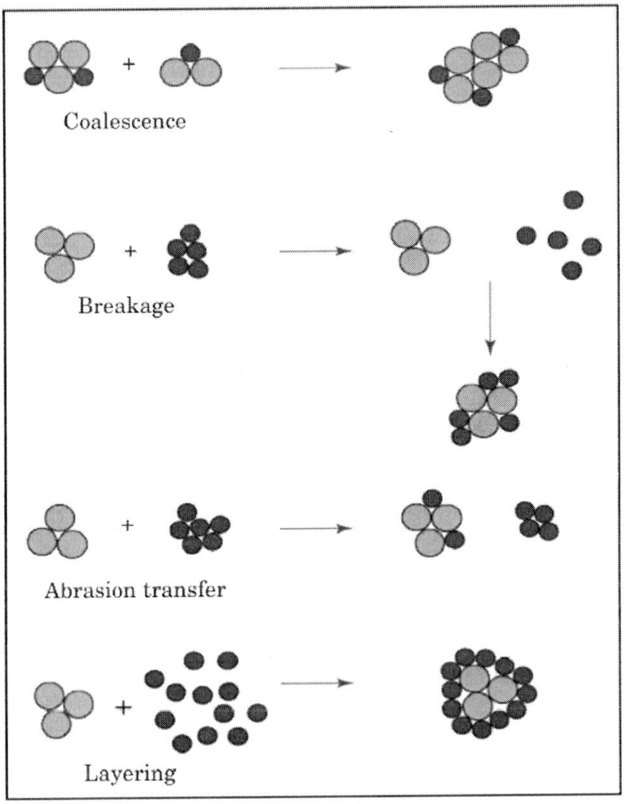

Fig. 2.6: Mechanisms of ball growth during granulation.

EVALUATION OF GRANULES OR POWDERS

1. Particle size and size distribution
2. Surface area
3. Density
   - Bulk density
   - Tapped density
   - Granular density

4. Granule strength and friability
5. Flow properties
   - Angle of repose
   - Percentage compressibility index
   - Hausner's ratio
6. Moisture content
7. Percentage fines

1. Particle Size and Size Distribution

i) Size affect the average weight of tablet, disintegration time, weight variation, friability, flowability and drying rate. ii) The size and shape depends upon processing requirements during granulation.

The methods for determination of particle size and size distribution are: a) sieving b) sedimentation rate c) microscopy (SEM) d) by light scattering.

2. Surface Area

It is not commonly used for granules but generally used for drug substances. If required particle size is measured and from this surface area is measured. Mostly used methods are gas adsorption method and air permeability method. In gas adsorption, gas is adsorbed as monolayer on particles. This is in turn calculated and converted to surface area. In air permeability, the rate of air permeates a bed of powder is used to calculate surface area of powder sample.

3. Density

Density may influence compressibility, tablet porosity and dissolution. Dense hard granules may require higher load to produce cohesive compact to reduce free granules seen on the surface of tablets. Dense granules have less friability but cause a problem in releasing the drug.

a. *Bulk density*:

$$\text{Bulk density} = \frac{\text{Mass}}{\text{Bulk volume}}$$

Where, bulk density of granules is mass of granules in gm and volume of granules in measuring cylinder in ml. If more compressible bed of particulate – less flowable powder or granules. If less dense or compressible – more flowable powder or granules

b. *Tapped density:*

$$\text{Tapped density} = \frac{\text{Mass}}{\text{Tapped volume}}$$

c. *Granular density*: Granular density is determined by using pycnometer, two methods are used to determine the granular density i) In one, intrusion fluid used mercury, and ii) Any solvent of low surface tension *e.g.,:* benzene

The accuracy of these methods depends upon ability of intrusion fluid to penetrate the pores of granules. Liquids should not masks granules solubilities in it, and having property to penetrate the pores. Density is then determined from volume of intrusion fluid displaced in pycnometer by given mass of granulation. It is calculated by using equation:

$$\text{Granular density (D)} = \frac{\text{Mass}}{\text{Total volume of pycnometer (Vp)} - \text{volume of intrusion fluid in ml (Vi)}}$$

Where, Vp – total volume of pycnometer, Vi – volume of intrusion fluid (ml) containing mass (in gm) of granules required to fill pycnometer.

4. Granule Strength and Friability

Granule strength and friability changes in the particle size distribution of granulations and compressibility into cohesive tablets. Granule strength and friability are measured by i) Compressive strength/ hardness, ii) Using friability measurements/apparatus.

5. Flow Properties

It is an ability of the granule to flow from hopper to die cavity for tablet uniformity. If flow property of granules is not uniform we are not getting tablet of uniform size. Flow property of material results from many forces: 1. Frictional force 2. Surface tension force 3. Mechanical force caused by interlocking of irregular shape particles 4. Electrostatic forces 5. Cohesive/Vander Waal's forces.

- Forces also affect granule property such as particle size and shape, particle size distribution, surface texture, roughness and surface area.
- If particle size of powder is </= 150 μ the magnitude of frictional and Vander Waal's force predominate.
- When particle size increases mechanical and physical properties become more important with packing properties.

Flow properties of granules are determined by measuring:

a. Angle of repose
b. Percentage compressibility index
c. Hausner's ratio

Determination of angle of repose, Hausner's ratio and percentage compressibility index are discussed in detail in Chapter 1.

6. Moisture Content

The amount of moisture present in the granule is called moisture content. Generally granules contain 2% moisture. It is required for the binding of the powder or granules during compression in die cavity. Percentage of moisture is calculated by using moisture balance or IR balance. IR balance consist of simple balance which is placed in the casing in which the IR bulb is attached which produce heat inside the chamber.

The small amount of sample taken to measure moisture content and placed it in the moisture balance. Initial reading is noted and IR bulb is switched on. The heat generated due to IR bulb the moisture is removed from the granules. The final reading is recorded and calculated the % moisture content using the formula:

$$\%\ \text{moisture content} = \frac{\text{Initial weight} - \text{final weight}}{\text{Initial weight}} \times 100$$

7. Percentage Fines

% fines means amount of powder remained in the granule. Generally 10-15% of fines accepted in granules. It is necessary for the tablet compression because if 100% granules are used then it is difficult to maintain hardness of tablet. Since they have free space in the die cavity and after compression tablet will crack due to air entrapment. % fines can be calculated by using sieve method. % of fines should not be more than 15%.

TABLET COMPRESSION MACHINE

Tablets are made by compressing a formulation containing a drug or drugs with excipients on a stamping machine called presses. Tablet presses (tablets compression machine) are classified as either single punch or multi-station rotary presses.

Single Punch Press

In case of single punch machine, all of the compression force is applied by the upper punch, making the single punch machine a "stamping press". A single punch press possesses one die and one pair of punches that is a set of tabletting tools (Fig. 2.7). The powder is held in a hopper which is connected to hopper shoe located at the die table. The hopper shoe moves to and fro over the die, by either a rotational or translational movement. When the hopper shoe is located over the die, the powder is fed into the die by gravitational powder flow. The amount of powder filled into the die is controlled by the position of the lower punch. When the hopper shoe is located beside the die, the upper punch descends and the powder is compressed. The lower punch is stationary during compression and pressure is thus applied by the upper punch and controlled by the upper punch displacement. After ejection, the tablet is pushed away by the hopper shoe as it moves back to the die for the next tablet. The output of tablet from a single punch press is around 200 tablets per minute.

Application

Single punch press thus has its primary use in the production of small batches of tablets such as formulation development and during the production of tablets for clinical trials.

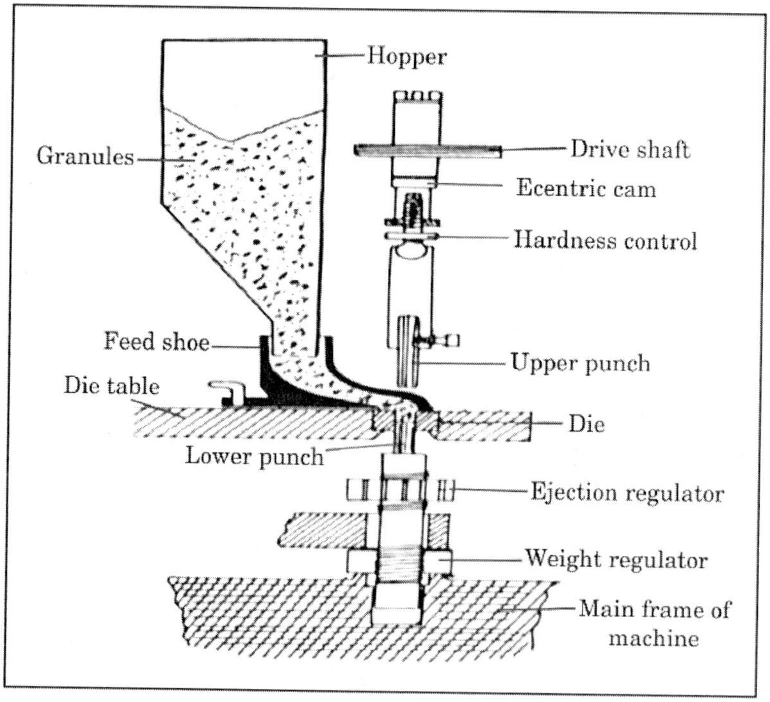

Fig. 2.7: Single punch compression machine

Rotary Tablet Compression Machine

Tablet presses are designed with following basic components:

1) Hopper for holding and feeding granulation
2) Dies that define the size and shape of the tablet.
3) Punches for compressing the granulation within the dies.
4) Cam tracks for guiding the movement of the punches.
5) A feeding mechanism for moving granulation from hopper into the dies.

Multi-station presses are termed rotary because the head of the tablet machine that holds the upper punches, dies and lower punches in place rotate. As their head rotates, the punches are guided up and down by fixed cam tracks, which control the sequence of filling, compression and ejection. The portion of the head that hold the upper and lower punches are called upper and lower turrets ‘respectively, the one which controls the movement of upper and lower punches is called an upper and lower cams respectively and the portion holding the dies is called the die table. At the start of compression cycle granulation stored in a hopper emptied into the feed-frame, which has several interconnected compartments.

The pull-down cam (fill cam) guided the lower punches to the bottom of their vertical travel, allowing the dies to overfill. The punches are then passed over a weight control cam (weight adjustment ramp), which reduces the fill in the dies to the desired amount. A blade (scrapper) at the end of the feed frame removes the excess granulation and directs it around the turret and back into the front of the feed-frame. Next, the lower punches travel over the lower compression roll (pre-compression and main compression roll) while simultaneously the upper punches ride beneath the upper compression roll (pre-compression and main compression roll). The upper punches enter a fixed distance into the dies, while the lower punches are raised to squeeze and compact the granulation within the dies. To regulate the upward movements of the lower punches, the height of the lower pressure is changed. After the moments of compression, the upper punches are withdrawn as they follow the upper punch raising cam (upper lifting cam); the lower punches ride up the cam (ejection cam), which brings the tablets to flush with or slightly above the surface of the dies. The tablets strike a sweep off blade affixed to the front of the feed- frame and slide down a chute into the receptacle. At the same time, the lower punches re-enters the pull-down cam and the cycle is repeated (Fig. 2.8).

In general, all rotary presses are engineered for fast and economical production of all kind of tablets. Larger machines can readily produce several million tablets in a working day.

Mechanism of Tablet Compression

The events that occur during the compression of tablet as follows

1. Particle rearrangement or transitional repacking
2. Deformation at the point of contact
3. Fragmentation and deformation
4. Bonding

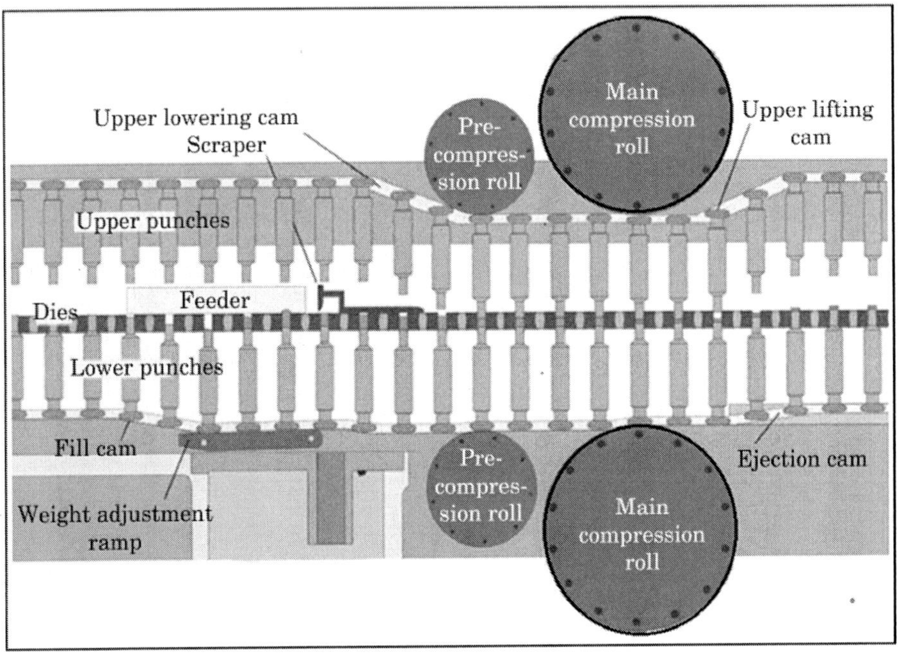

Fig. 2.8: The compression cycle of rotary tablet press

5. Deformation of the solid body
6. Decompression

1. *Particle rearrangement or transitional repacking*

The granulation to be compressed is placed in the hopper of the tablet press, the formulation and processing are designed to ensure that the desired volume of granulation is fed into each die cavity. Particle size distribution of granulation and shape of granule determine the initial packing as granulation is delivered into the die cavity.

2. *Deformation at the point of contact*

When stress is applied to a material deformation occurs (change in form). If deformation disappears completely upon release of the stress it is known as elastic deformation. Deformation that does not completely recover after release of stress is known as plastic deformation. The force required to initiate a plastic deformation is known as yield stress. When the particles of granules closely packed that no further filling of void occurs. Further increase of compressional force causes deformation at point of contact.

3. *Fragmentation and deformation*

At higher pressure, fracture occurs when the stresses within the particle become great enough to propagate cracks. Fragmentation increases the number of particles and forms new clean surface areas that are potential bonding areas.

4. *Bonding*

Several mechanisms of bonding in the compression process has been observed these are a) mechanical theory b) intermolecular theory c) liquid surface film theory

a) Mechanical theory: Mechanical theory proposes that under pressure the individual particle undergo plastic, elastic or brittle deformation so edges of the particles intermesh forming a mechanical bond.

b) Intermolecular theory: Intermolecular theory proposes molecules or ions at the surface of solid have unsatisfied intermolecular forces (surface free energy) which interact with other particles.

c) Liquid surface film theory: Liquid surface film theory proposes that bonding is the presence of thin liquid film which may be a consequence of fusion or solution.

5. *Deformation of the solid body*

Applied pressure is further increased, the bonded solid is consolidated towards limiting density.

6. *Decompression*

As upper punch is withdrawn from the die cavity, the tablet is confined in the die by radial pressure. Consequently, any dimensional change during decompression must occur in axial direction that may further leads to capping of tablets.

Tablet Tooling (Punches and Dies)

Tablet compression machines are made in keeping in view the type of dies and punches will be used on them. The punches and dies and their setup on compression machine is called tooling. Punches and dies are a key element of the tablet pressing process. They are responsible for the final appearance and shapes of manufactured tablets, therefore they must be designed and produced with high precision and accuracy. During work they are exposed to strong compression, they often press powders of abrasive and corrosive properties, which requires using high-quality steel, an appropriately selected heat treating, and sometimes covering with special coatings which prevent tablets from wear and tear or becoming gluey or using other materials such as sintered carbides.

The tablet tooling, it is classified as B and D mainly. The B tooling dies and punch can further have specifications as BB and D tooling dies and punches can be utilised on B tooling machine which is called as DB. Different types of tablet tooling are given in Table 2.6.

Different types of Toolings are as follows:

- 'B' -Tooling
- 'D' -Tooling
- 'BB' -Tooling
- 'DB' -Tooling

Punch: The job of the upper punch is to control compression position within the die. The job of the lower punch is more complex than that of the upper.

Table 2.6: Different types of tablet tooling

Type of tooling	*Punch length (mm)*	*Punch diameter (mm)*	*Die diameter (mm)*	*Height of dies (mm)*	*Max. Tab. size (mm)*
B	133.6	19	30.15	22.22	16/19
D	133.6	25.4	38.1	23.82	25/25
BB	133.6	19	24.0	22.22	13/14
DB	133.6	25.4	30.15	23.22	19/19

1. The lower punch first overfills the die with too much powder.
2. Then to achieve final and proper tablet weight the lower punch is moved up to allow the scrapper to sweep the excess powder off the surface of the die table.
3. Then the powder in the die is moved downward into the die which is called underfill to prevent the effects of centrifugal force from slinging powder back out of the die. This feature is not found on all rotary presses.
4. Pre-compression is a feature found on most modern tablets presses. It's designed to help tamp the powders together lightly compressing the powder and driving the air out of the die prior to final compression.
5. The main compression is where the final tablet is compressed.
6. Ejection is achieved by simply pushing the tablet up out of the die.

Terminology related to punch

Head	: The end of the punch that guides it through the cam track of tablet machine during rotation.
Head flat (Dwell flat)	: The flat area of the head that receives the compression force from Rollers (in upper punches) and determines the weight and ejection height (in lower punches).
Outside head angle	: The area gets in touch with the roller prior to head flat, while compression.
Inside head angle	: This is the area, which pulls down the lower punches after ejection and lifts the upper punches after compression.
Neck	: The relieved area between the head and barrel, which provides clearance for the cams.
Barrel	: This area guides the punch (while going up and down) with reference to turret guides.
Stem	: The area of the punch opposite the head, beginning at the tip and extending to the point where the full diameter of the barrel begins. If the chamfer is present the barrel usually reaches its full diameter just above the chamfer.
Tip	: This determines size, shape and profile
Tip face	: This area of punch is where the tablet is formed. Good surface finish is required here to get quality tablets.
Working length	: This distance between bottom of the cup and the head flat is called as working length which determines weight and thickness of the tablet.

Table 2.7: *(Contd...)*

Overall length	: Distance between top of the cup and the head flat.
Key angle	: The relationship of the punch key to the tablet shape. The keys position is influenced by the tablet shape, take-off angle, and turret rotation.
Domed heads	: Increases the dwell time and hence help to achieve the better tablet hardness.
Dwell time	: The time punches spends below the pressure roller while rotating in the machine.
Clearance	: Die bore dia – punch tip dia = Clearance.
Hardness	: Usually measured in HRC (Rockwell 'C' scales)

***Die*:** Hardened steel (HCHC) mould to make the shape of a tablet.

Terminology related to Die

Die O.D.	: The outside diameter of the die, which is compatible with the die pockets in the press
Die height	: The overall height of the die
Die bore	: The cavity where the tablet is made. The Cavity's shape and size determine the same form of tablet
Chamfer	: Entry angle of the die bore
Taper dies	: Dies with tapered bore on one or both sides. They are used for easy ejection of tablets (mainly for double-layered tablets)
Die groove	: The groove around the periphery of the die, which allows the die to be fixed in the press
Lined (insert) dies	: Dies fitted with a linear insert made from a much harder, more wear resistant material such as tungsten, carbide and ceramic

PROCESSING PROBLEMS (TABLET MANUFACTURING DEFECTS AND REMEDIES)

1. *Capping*: Capping is the term used, when the upper or lower segment of the tablet separates horizontally, either partially or completely from the main body of a tablet and comes off like a cap, during ejection from the tablet press, or during subsequent handling. Capping is usually due to the air–entrapment in a compact during compression and subsequent expansion of tablet on ejection of a tablet from a die.

2. *Lamination:* Lamination is the separation of a tablet into two or more distinct horizontal layers. Air-entrapment during compression and subsequent release on ejection. The condition is exaggerated by higher speed of turret.

3. ***Chipping:*** Chipping is defined as the breaking of tablet edges, while the tablet leaves the press or during subsequent handling and coating operations. Reason: Incorrect machine settings, specially mis-set ejection take-off.

4. ***Cracking:*** Small, fine cracks observed on the upper and lower central surface of tablets, or very rarely on the sidewall are referred to as cracks. Reason: It is observed as a result of rapid expansion of tablets, especially when deep concave punches are used.

5. ***Sticking:*** Sticking refers to the tablet material adhering to the die wall. Filming is a slow form of sticking and is largely due to excess moisture in the granulation. Reason: Improperly dried or improperly lubricated granules.

6. ***Picking*:** Picking is the term used when a small amount of material from a tablet is sticking to and being removed off from the tablet-surface by a punch face. The problem is more prevalent on the upper punch faces than on the lower ones. The problem worsens if tablets are repeatedly manufactured in this station of tooling because of the more and more material getting added to the already stuck material on the punch face. Reason: Picking is of particular concern when punch tips have engraving or embossing letters, as well as the granular material is improperly dried.

7. ***Binding*:** Binding in the die is the term used when the tablets adhere, seize or tear in the die. A film is formed in the die and ejection of tablet is hindered. With excessive binding, the tablet sides are cracked and it may crumble apart. Reason: Binding is usually due to excessive amount of moisture in granules, lack of lubrication and/or use of worn dies.

8. ***Mottling:*** Mottling is the term used to describe an unequal distribution of colour on a tablet, with light or dark spots standing out in an otherwise uniform surface. Reason: One cause of mottling may be a coloured drug, whose colour differs from the colour of excipients used for granulation of a tablet.

9. ***Double Impression:*** Double Impression involves only those punches, which have a monogram or other engraving on them. Reason: At the moment of compression, the tablet receives the imprint of the punch.

Now, on some machines, the lower punch freely drops and travels uncontrolled for a short distance before riding up the ejection cam to push the tablet out of the die, now during this free travel, the punch rotates and at this point, the punch may make a new impression on the bottom of the tablet, resulting in Double Impression.

10. *Tablet Weight Variation*: The tablet weights are mainly affected by following reasons:

This type of variation can be due to inconsistent powder density, flow properties and particle size distribution. Density can change on the press, often because of overfilling of the die and re-circulation of the powder on the tablet press, whereas particle size distribution may change when the product becomes unblended during transfer or because of static electricity. This may also change because the product cannot withstand the handling mechanical stress that undergoes before it reaches tablet press.

Various tablet defects, their causes and remedies related to formulation and punching machine are given in Table 2.7.

Table 2.7: Tablet defects, their causes and remedies related to formulation and punching machine.

Tablet defects	***Related to formulation***	***Related to puniching machine***
1. Capping		
Causes:	i) Large amount of fines in the granulation ii) Too dry or very low moisture content iii) Not thoroughly dried granules iv) Insufficient amount of binder or improper binder v) Insufficient or improper lubricant.	i) Poorly finished dies ii) Deep concave punches or iii) Lower punch remains below the face of die during ejection iv) Incorrect adjustment of the sweep-off blade v) High turret speed
Remedies	i) Remove some or all fines ii) Moisten the granules properly by adding hygroscopic substance *e.g.*, sorbitol, methyl-cellulose or PEG4000	i) Polish dies properly. Investigate other steels or other materials ii) Use flat punches

Table 2.7: *(Contd...)*

Table 2.7: *(Contd...)*

Tablet defects	*Related to formulation*	*Related to puniching machine*
	iii) Dry the granules properly iv) Increasing the amount of binder v) Increase the amount of lubricant or change the type of lubricant.	iii) Make proper setting of lower punch during ejection iv) Adjust sweep-off blade correctly to facilitate proper ejection v) Reduce speed of turret.
2. Lamination		
Causes:	i) Oily or waxy materials in granules ii) Too much hydrophobic lubricant (magnesium stearate).	i) Rapid relaxation of the peripheral regions of a tablet, on ejection from a die ii) Rapid decompression
Remedies:	i) Modify mixing process. Add adsorbent or absorbent ii) Use a less amount of lubricant or change the type of lubricant.	i) Use tapered dies, *i.e.*, upper part of the die bore has an outward taper of 3° to 5° ii) Use pre-compression step iii) Reduce turret speed and reduce the final compression pressure.
3. Chipping		
Causes:	i) Sticking on punch faces ii) Too dry granules iii) Too much binding causes chipping at bottom.	i) Groove of die worn at compression point. ii) Barreled die (center of the die wider than ends) iii) Edge of punch face turned inside/inward iv) Concavity too deep to compress properly.
Remedies:	i) Dry the granules properly or increase lubrication ii) Moisten the granules to plasticize. Add hygroscopic substances. Optimize binding, or use dry binders.	i) Polish to open end, reverse or replace the die ii) Polish the die to make it cylindrical iii) Polish the punch edges iv) Reduce concavity of punch faces and use flat punches.

Table 2.7: *(Contd...)*

Table 2.7: *(Contd...)*

Tablet defects		*Related to formulation*	*Related to puniching machine*
4. Cracking			
	Causes:	i) Large size of granules ii) Too dry granules iii) Tablets expand iv) Granulation too cold.	i) Tablet expands on ejection due to air entrapment ii) Deep concavities cause cracking while removing tablets
	Remedies:	i) Reduce granule size. Add fines ii) Moisten the granules properly and add proper amount of binder iii) Improve granulation. Add dry binders iv) Compress at room temperature	i) Use tapered die ii) Use special take-off.
5. Sticking			
	Causes:	i) Granules not dried properly ii) Too little or improper lubrication iii) Too much binder iv) Hygroscopic granular material v) Oily or waxy materials vi) Too soft or weak granules.	i) Concavity too deep for granulation. ii) Too little pressure. iii) Compressing too fast.
	Remedies:	i) Dry the granules properly ii) Make moisture analysis to determine limits. iii) Increase or change lubricant. iv) Reduce the amount of binder or use a different type of binder. v) Modify granulation and compress under controlled humidity. vi) Modify mixing process. Add an absorbent. vii) Optimize the amount of binder and granulation technique.	i) Reduce concavity to optimum. ii) Increase pressure. iii) Reduce speed.
6. Picking			
	Causes:	i) Excessive moisture in granules. ii) Too little or improper lubrication. iii) Low melting point substances, may soften from the heat of compression and lead to picking.	i) Rough or scratched punch faces. ii) Bevels or dividing lines too deep. iii) Pressure applied is not enough; too soft tablets.

Table 2.7: *(Contd...)*

Table 2.7: (*Contd...*)

Tablet defects	***Related to formulation***	***Related to puniching machine***
	iv) Low melting point medicament in high concentration. v) Too warm granules when compressing. vi) Too much amount of binder.	
Remedies:	i) Dry properly the granules, determine the optimum limit. ii) Increase lubrication; use colloidal silica as a polishing agent‘, so that material does not cling to punch faces. iii) Add high melting-point materials. Use high melting point lubricants. iv) Refrigerate granules and the entire tablet press. v) Compress at room temperature. Cool sufficiently before compression. vi) Reduce the amount of binder, change the type or use dry binders.	i) Polish faces to high lustre. ii) Design lettering as large as possible. iii) Plate the punch faces with chromium to produce a smooth and non-adherent face. iv) Reduce depths and sharpness. v) Increase pressure to optimum.
7. Binding		
Causes:	i) Too moist granules and extrudes around lower punch. ii) Insufficient or improper lubricant. iii) Too coarse granules. iv) Too hard granules for the lubricant to be effective. v) Granular material very abrasive and cutting into dies. vi) Granular material too warm. vii) Sticks to the die.	i) Poorly finished dies. ii) Rough dies due to abrasion and corrosion. iii) Undersized dies and too little clearance. iv) Too much pressure in the tablet press.
Remedies:	i) Dry the granules properly. ii) Increase the amount of lubricant or use a more effective lubricant. iii) Reduce granular size, add more fines and increase the quantity of lubricant.	i) Polish the dies properly. ii) Investigate other steels or other materials iii) Rework to proper size. iv) Increase clearance. v) Reduce pressure

Table 2.7: (*Contd...*)

Table 2.7: *(Contd...)*

Tablet defects		*Related to formulation*	*Related to punching machine*
	iv)	Modify granulation.	
	v)	Reduce granular size.	
	vi)	If coarse granules, reduce its size.	
	vii)	Use wear-resistant dies.	
	viii)	Reduce temperature.	
	ix)	Increase clearance if it is extruding.	
8. Mottling			
Causes:	i)	A coloured drug used along with colourless or white-coloured excipients.	
	ii)	A dye migrates to the surface of granulation while drying.	
	iii)	Improperly mixed dye, especially during direct compression.	
	iv)	Improper mixing of a coloured binder solution.	
Remedies:	i)	Use appropriate colourants.	
	ii)	Change the solvent system, change the binder, reduce drying temperature and use a smaller particle size.	
	iii)	Mix properly and reduce size if it is of a larger size to prevent segregation.	
	iv)	Incorporate dry colour additive during powder blending step, then add finely powdered adhesives such as acacia and tragacanth and mix well and finally add granulating liquid.	
	v)	Use lake dyes	
9. Double impression			
Causes:		Free rotation of either upper punch or lower punch during ejection of a tablet.	
Remedies:	i)	Use keying in tooling, *i.e.,* inset a key alongside the punch, so that it fits the punch and prevents punch rotation.	
	ii)	Newer presses have anti-turning devices, which prevent punch rotation.	
10. Weight variation			
Causes:	i)	Poor flow properties and particle size distribution.	
	ii)	Inconsistent powder density	
	iii)	Unblended powder mixture	
Remedies:	i)	Improving flow properties	
	ii)	Complete blending of powder mixture	
	iii)	Optimum powder density	

TABLET COATING

Tablets are coated for a number of reasons, including to protect the medicinal agent against destructive exposure to air and/or humidity; to mask the taste of the drug; to provide special characteristics of drug release (*e.g.,* enteric coatings); and to provide aesthetics or distinction to the product.

Types of Tablet Coating

I. Sugar coating

Sugar coating is the process which involves the application of sugar (sucrose) based coating solution to the tablets. The process is carried out in mechanically operated coating pans of stainless steel. These pans are about 1-4 feet in diameter having variable capacities and mounted at a certain angle during the coating process, the pans are rotated mechanically at desired speed so that the tablets inside the pan cascade over each other and get coated with the coating solution. For sugar coating, tablets should be a smooth convex surface and thin edges so that the coating is uniform and tablets should be resistant to abrasion, breakage and chipping.

Advantages

- Unpleasant taste, odour and colour of the tablet can be masked
- Protect the medicinal agent from destructive environmental conditions
- Sugar-coated tablets have good consumer appeal.
- It requires inexpensive and simple equipment.
- The raw materials used in the coating solution are readily available and cost-effective.
- The tablets produced are of high quality, smooth and have an elegant appearance.

Disadvantages

- Sugar coating is a time consuming and lengthy process.
- It requires several hours to days to complete the process.
- It requires highly skilled manpower.

- Sugar coating increases the tablet weight by 50-100% of the original weight.
- Sugarcoated tablets may vary slightly in size from batch to batch and within a batch.
- Increased size and weight of the tablets increases the cost of packaging and shipping.
- For sugar-coated tablets imprinting becomes difficult due to highly glossed surface.

Steps of sugar-coating: Process of sugar coating encompasses following steps:

1. *Sealing*

Sealing is the first step in sugar coating of tablets which is done to protect the tablet core from adverse effects of moisture. The major component used in the formulation of sugar coating solution is water. Tablet cores are porous and absorb water which leads to their softening and disintegration. This adversely affects their physical and chemical stability.

Sealing is achieved by applying a polymer-based water impermeable coating solution by either ladling or spray techniques. The polymers used for this purpose are natural gums such as zein, shellac, although the use of synthetic polymers, such as cellulose acetate phthalate or polyvinyl acetate phthalate and hydroxy propyl methyl cellulose (HPMC) is now favoured.

Among polymers, shellac is considered to be an effective sealant. But it lengthens the tablet disintegration and dissolution time because it gets polymerized on storage. This problem can be overcome by adding polyvinylpyrrolidone or any other suitable polymer along with shellac. Zein, which is an alcohol-soluble protein derivative obtained from corn is also an effective sealant. It does not reflect any polymerization on prolong storage hence, does not change the solubility characteristics of the coating.

This step of coating involves dissolving the polymer in a suitable solvent (usually ethanol) in a concentration of 15-30% w/w which is then ladled or sprayed on the tablets rotating in the coating pan. A stream of warm air is blown simultaneously to facilitate drying and to prevent the tablets from sticking to each other.

A dusting powder such as talc is applied during the seal coating process to prevent the tablet from sticking to each other or to the walls of the coating pan. Excessive use of dusting powder should be avoided; else it may impart slippery nature to the tablets and prevents their proper rolling in the pan. It also makes the tablet surface difficult to wet in the subsequent sub-coating step.

2. *Sub-coating*

Sub-coating is the next major step of sugar coating process. It is done to provide the sealed tablet cores with round edge and to build up the core weight. This step also serves as the basis for the remaining sugar coating process. Sub-coating involves alternate applications of a solution of binding agents followed by dusting with a dusting powder and then subjecting the tablets to drying this process is continued until the tablet core attains the desired shape and weight.

During the sub-coating process, care should be exercised in selecting the appropriate ratio of binder and dusting powder. Excessive amounts of dusting powder may result in brittle and rough coating while less amounts may cause sticking and lump formation of the tablets.

Example for binder formulation used during sub-coating process is given in Table 2.8.

Table 2.8: Example for binder formulation

Ingredients	*Quantity (% w/w)*
Gelatin	3.3
Sucrose	55.3
Gum Acacia	8.7
Distilled water	Q. S. to 100%

Example for dusting powder formulation used during sub-coating process is given in Table 2.9.

Table 2.9: Example dusting powder formulation

Ingredients	*Quantity (% w/w)*
Calcium carbonate	40
Gum Acacia	2
Talc	25
Titanium Dioxide	5
Sucrose	28

Thus, sub-coating is regarded as a sandwich of alternate layers of binders and dusting powder. This is a complex step and requires highly skilled operators. The excess dusting powder is removed by rolling the tablets on a screen or sieve.

Sub-coating can be achieved by two methods a) lamination method and b) suspension method

a. *Lamination method:* This method involves alternate application of a solution of binding agents and then, dusting with a suitable dusting powder such as talc, titanium dioxide, calcium carbonate, powdered sucrose, powdered gum acacia, kaolin, cocoa powder, dextrin, corn starch, calcium sulphate etc.

b. *Suspension method:* In this method, a sub-coating suspension of the binder and dusting powder is sprayed over the tablets. This method is less complex than the lamination method and can be carried out by less experienced personnel.

3. *Grossing / smoothing / syruping*

In order to prepare a good quality sugar-coated product, it is imperative that the surface of the coating be smooth and free from irregularities prior to application of the colour coat. While the requisite smoothness may be achieved during the application of the sub-coat, it is not unusual to find that further smoothing is necessary. Depending on the degree of smoothing required, the smoothing coating may simply consist of a 70% sucrose syrup, often containing titanium dioxide as an opacifier or whitening agent, and possibly tinted with other colourants to provide a good base for subsequent application of the colour coat. If a substantial amount of smoothing is required, as in the case in which the sub-coat tablets have a pitted surface, other additives like talc, calcium carbonate, corn starch may be used in low concentrations to speed-up the smoothing process.

4. *Colour coating*

Almost all the sugar-coated tablets are coloured as it adds to their aesthetic value and also increases patient acceptability. The colours used for this purpose should be approved by FD and C. Generally water-soluble dyes and water-insoluble inorganic pigments and lakes are used as colouring agents.

Colour coating of tablets is done by two processes:

a) *Dye coating process:* In this process, the tablets are coated with coating syrups containing water-soluble dye (natural or synthetic) in a suitable concentration. The final colour is obtained by applying nearly 50-60 individual coats of coloured syrup with a drying time of 15-30 min between each coat. Natural water-soluble dyes are riboflavin, turmeric, caramel, carotenoids, indigo, flavones, carminic acid, chlorophyll and anthocyanins. Synthetic water-soluble dyes are FD&C yellow # 5 and FD&C blue # 2.

Dye coating process has certain disadvantages such as:

(i) It requires highly skilled operators and it is time consuming process.
(ii) Tablet to tablet colour variability may arise due to non-uniform distribution of the colour.
(iii) Batch to batch colour variation may occur
(iv) Certain dyes are photosensitive and fade away on storage.
(v) Certain water-soluble dyes affect the bioavailability of drugs.
(vi) Overdrying, under drying or rapid drying may cause colour migration giving the tablet a mottled appearance.

(b) *Pigment coating process:* In this process, inorganic pigments like titanium dioxide, iron oxides and certain lakes (water-insoluble pigments) like aluminium lakes are used as colouring agents. These are dispersed in a suitable solvent along with an opacifier like titanium dioxide. The resultant opacified lake suspension is then used for colour coating. Titanium dioxide is used to impart opaqueness and to optimize the colour shade as lakes are not totally opaque. Various shades of the same colour can be produced by varying the ratio of opacifier and lake.

The advantages of using lakes and inorganic pigments over water-soluble dyes are:

(i) They impart batch to batch and tablet to tablet colour uniformity.
(ii) Their processing time is short.
(iii) Their water-insoluble nature prevents colour migration during drying.

(iv) They are photostable.

(v) They prevent moisture permeation hence, mottled appearance of tablets is not seen.

(vi) Unlike water-soluble dyes, they do not interfere with the bioavailability of the drug.

5. *Polishing*

After colour coating, the tablets show a dull or mottled appearance. Thus, they require polishing or finishing imparting the desired gloss and lustre. This is accomplished by drying the colour coated tablets overnight in trays so that the moisture is removed which may otherwise lead to blooming or sweating. The dried tablets are then transferred to clean polishing pans lined with canvas or cheesecloth and polished by applying mixtures of waxes like beeswax, carnauba wax, candelilla wax or hard paraffin wax. The canvas lining transfers the waxes to the tablet surface and provides buffing action as the tablets roll in the pan, they take up wax from the canvas and achieve their lustre. Waxes can also be applied by dusting their powdered form on the rolling tablets or by placing pieces of wax in the pan and allowing the tablets to roll until they achieve the desired lustre. Another method of polishing the tablets is dissolving the waxes in a non-aqueous solvent and pouring or spraying this solution on the tablets.

6. *Printing*

Sugar-coated tablets are imprinted with manufacturers name, code or logo for identification purpose either before or after their polishing. The printing process is known as Rotogravure.

II. Film coating

Film coating is application of a thin film of polymeric solution around the tablet core. The coating solution is an aqueous or organic solvent based medium containing a suitable polymer as the main ingredient together with other additives like opacifiers, plasticizers, colourants etc. Coating solution is sprayed over a rotating/fluidized bed of tablets. The coated tablets are dried by passing hot air which evaporates the solvent leaving a thin deposit of coating material around the tablet core.

Advantages

(i) Film coating has better mechanical elasticity, flexibility and strength compared to sugar coating.

(ii) Film-coated tablets are suitable for diabetic patients.

(iii) Sugar coating which increases the tablet weight by 50 to 100% but in film coating weight gain is only 2-6%.

(iv) Film coating helps to retain the debossed/embossed markings on the tablet surface.

(v) Film coating process requires just few hours for completion compared to the lengthy and cumbersome sugar coating.

Disadvantages

(i) Film-coated tablets have less consumer appeal.

(ii) They don't have the elegance as that of the sugar-coated tablets.

The process of film coating

Film coating process is similar to sugar coating process. They share the common equipment and process parameters. Like sugar coating, a film coating is also carried out by pan spray method and fluidized bed methods.

Pan spray film coating of tablets

Typically, pan-coating processes are preferred method of tablet film coating. Various parameters considered during pan spray film coating of tablets are related to the coating pan, drying air and spray pattern.

Coating pan related parameters

(a) *Size and shape of the pan*: The shape design, capacity, presence or absence of baffles in pan plays an important role in mixing of the tablet mass. Poor movement of the tablets within the pan results in poorly coated tablets which lacks uniformity in colour and coating.

(b) *Speed of pan rotation:* Speed of pan rotation is selected depending on the design of pan, the type of tablets being coated and the properties of the coating solution. Larger pans which are used for non-aqueous film coating are rotated at speeds of 10-15 rpm, while those which are used for aqueous film coating and rotated at slow speed of 3-10 rpm since aqueous solution require much time for drying. The speed of pan rotation should be optimum. Slow rotation speed causes over wetting of tablets resulting in sticking of the tablets to each other or to the surface to the pan. On the other hand, high-speed rotation does not allow sufficient drying time resulting in tablets with a coarse surface.

Drying air related parameters

(a) Quality of the incoming air: The drying air should be free from humidity, the presence of moisture in the air alters the rate of coating and drying which ultimately affects the quality of the coating.

(b) Temperature of the air: The temperature of the air should be optimum, so as to obtain a suitable drying environment. The temperature should neither be too high nor low. High temperature causes rapid drying of the sprayed coating solution before it reaches the tablet bed surface, whereas low temperature causes inadequate drying of tablets.

(c) Rate of air flow: The air flow rate should be controlled so that the volume of air supplied and exhausted should be balanced.

Spray related parameters

(i) Spray application rate: The rate at which the coating solution is sprayed depends, on the tablet core characteristics, composition of the solution, mixing of tablets and drying air efficiency. Spray rate is controlled by the fluid stream pressure, design of the spray nozzle, orifice size and viscosity of the coating solution.

(ii) Method of spraying: The spray should be such that the coating solution should spread evenly over the entire mass of tablets. Too wide spray pattern results in direct application of the coating solution to the pan surface. This causes wastage of the material and inefficient coating. Too narrow spray pattern leads to over wetting of the tablets causing variation in coating from tablet to tablet.

(iii) Distance between sprayer and bed: During the coating operation, care should be exercised to maintain a proper distance between the spray nozzle and the tablet bed. This parameter affects the spray pattern as well as the quantity of coating solution being applied to each tablet during each rotation of the pan.

(iv) Degree of atomization of the coating solution: Atomization is defined as the process by which a liquid jet is divided into a spray of fine droplets. The degree of atomization is directly proportional to the parameters such as the pressure and volume of the atomizing air as the shape and design of the spray nozzles with respect to the stream of coating solution.

Degree of atomization can be controlled by adjusting the above given parameters. Poor degree of atomization results in quality defects in film coating. Examples (a) too fine atomization causes early drying of the coating solution before it reaches tablet bed. This gives the tablet a rough appearance. (b) Improper atomization results in large droplets, which causes over wetting of the tablet leading to coating defects like sticking, picking or orange peel effects.

Formulation of film coating

Ideal properties of film coating materials

- Coating materials should be compatible with other excipients.
- They should have the efficiency to mask the bad taste and odour of the drug.
- They should be non-toxic
- They should be capable to produce a pharmaceutically elegant product.
- They should be pharmacologically inert.
- They should be resistant towards heat, light, air and moisture.
- They should be soluble in the chosen solvent.
- The film former or polymer should not change with ageing and should be resistant to cracking.
- The film former or polymer should not cause bridging or filling of the debossed tablet surface.
- They should be colourless, odourless and tasteless. Film-coating solutions may be nonaqueous or aqueous. The nonaqueous solutions contain the following types of materials to provide the desired coating to the tablets:

1. ***Film formers (polymers):*** A film former capable of producing smooth, thin films reproducible under conventional coating conditions and applicable to a variety of tablet shapes. Film former or polymer is

the chief ingredient of film coating formulation. Film formers can be classified as

(i) Enteric film formers

(ii) Non-enteric film formers

Enteric film formers: Enteric film formers are those which are used to produce enteric coated dosage forms. Enteric coated dosage forms are designed with an intention to show local action in the intestines without undergoing disintegration and drug release in the stomach. They are designed by considering the time required by them to pass through the stomach and reside in the intestine.

Objectives of enteric coating

a) Enteric coating prevents nausea or irritation caused by certain drugs like sodium salicylate.
b) It protects the acid sensitive drugs like antibiotics, enzymes and hormones from direct contact with the gastric acid.
c) Enteric coating helps in the absorption of drugs that have *absorption window* in the intestine.
d) Drugs which are intended for local action in the intestines can be administered in their concentrated form by providing them with an enteric coating.

Ideal characteristics of an enteric coating material

a) It should be non-toxic.
b) It should be easy to apply and should be inexpensive.
c) It should be compatible with the intestinal fluid and should allow its easy permeation.
d) It should be resistant to gastric acid.
e) It should form a good continuous film which should not change on ageing.
f) It should be soluble in the intestinal fluid and should not interfere with the bioavailability of drug.
g) It should be compatible with other components of the coating solution as well as drug.
h) It should be soluble in different solvents so that the film should have flexibility and appropriate mechanical strength.

i) It should allow printing of the mark or logo or brand name on the tablet surface.

Different variety of enteric polymers ranging from water resistant to pH-sensitive is available for coating tablets. These polymers are either emulsified, digested or swell and disintegrate in the intestinal fluid. These polymers possess free carboxylic acid groups in their structure and hence exhibit different pH solubility patterns. They are insoluble at low pH (acidic pH), but at higher pH (alkaline pH), they exhibit a sharp solubility profile.

The molecular weight of the polymer plays a significant role in its selection. It affects the viscosity of the coating formulation and also affects the flexibility and mechanical strength of the film. They are generally used in concentration of 7-18%. Since no commercially available polymer can fulfill all the characteristics of an ideal polymer, therefore a combination of selected polymers is used to achieve a film of desired proper. Various enteric polymers are given below:

a) *Cellulose derivatives*: Cellulose acetate phthalate (CAP), hydroxyl propyl methyl cellulose phthalate.
b) *Acrylic copolymers*; amino ethyl methacrylate
c) *Vinyl polymers*: polyvinyl acetate phthalate (PVP)

Cellulose derivatives (cellulose ethers)

(i) Cellulose acetate phthalate (CAP): It is the most extensively used polymer for enteric coating purpose. Though widely used. It has certain drawbacks. It dissolves only at pH 6 and retards drug absorption. It is hygroscopic, therefore allows permeation of moisture and gastric fluid. Its films are prone to removal of acetic and phthalic acids by hydrolysis. Hence, changes the film properties. It forms brittle films; therefore it is used in combination with other polymers to achieve the desired film characteristics.

(ii) Hydroxypropyl methyl cellulose phthalate: It is substituted ether of cellulose. It is soluble in water and forms a tackier and mechanically strong film, hence widely used.

Derivatives of these polymers *i.e.,* HP -50, HP-55 and HP-55-S are prepared by esterification with a phthalic anhydride. These derivatives are stable compared to cellulose acetate phthalate because of absence of acetyl groups. These are soluble at low pH 5-5.5, which helps in enhanced bioavailability of certain drugs.

Acrylic copolymers

The commercially available acrylic copolymers are Eudragit L and S respectively. These are copolymers of aminoethyl methacrylate.

(i) *Eudragit L* is soluble in intestinal fluid at pH 6. It is available as a solid, aqueous dispersion and as an organic solution.

(ii) *Eudragit S* is soluble at pH 7 and is available in the form of solid and organic solution. Both Eudragit L and S are resistant to gastric fluid.

Vinyl polymers: Polyvinyl acetate phthalate is the product of esterification of hydrolyzed polyvinyl acetate with a phthalic anhydride. Its solubility pattern and stability is analogous to HP-55.

Non-enteric film formers: Non-enteric film coating is done to provide the tablet with delayed or sustained release effects in the stomach. Non-enteric film-coated tablets release its contents slowly and prolong the drug effect. The various commercially available non-enteric polymers are discussed as follows:

(a) *Cellulose derivatives (cellulose ethers)*: Ethylcellulose, methyl hydroxyethyl cellulose, hydroxypropyl cellulose, hydroxypropyl methylcellulose (HPMC), sodium carboxymethylcellulose, hydroxyethyl cellulose, hydroxymethyl cellulose etc.

(b) *Acrylic polymers*: Eudragit L and S

(c) *Glycols*: polyethene glycols (PEG)

(d) *Vinyl polymers*: Polyvinylpyrrolidone (povidone)

Cellulose derivatives (cellulose ethers): Ethylcellulose: Ethyl cellulose as such insoluble in water and used in combination with water-soluble additive such as hydroxyl propyl methyl cellulose. This combination gives improved water solubility and also show a good sustained release effect.

Methyl hydroxyethyl cellulose: Its solubility is limited to few organic solvents hence not widely used.

Hydroxypropyl cellulose: Hydroxypropyl cellulose is soluble in water at a temperature below 40°C and insoluble above 45°C. It shows good solubility properties in gastric as well as intestinal fluids and also in various polar solvents. It forms a flexible film and it is suitable for sub-coating but not for colouring or glossing.

Hydroxypropyl methylcellulose: It is also known as hypromellose. It is prepared by reacting alkaline cellulose with methyl chloride followed by treating with propylene oxide. It is soluble in water, organic solvents and gastrointestinal fluids.

Sodium carboxymethylcellulose: This is sodium salt of carboxymethyl cellulose which is prepared by sodium cellulose with sodium salt of mono-chloro acetic acid. It forms a colloidal solution in water and insoluble in organic solvents. It forms tacky film and adheres well to the tablet surface.

Acrylic polymers: Acrylic polymers and copolymers are marketed under the trade name of Eudragit E, Eudragit RL and Eudragit RS. Eudragit E is a cationic copolymer synthesized from dimethyl aminoethyl methacrylate and other methacrylic acid esters. It is freely soluble in gastric fluid upto pH 5. Above pH 5, it expands allows the permeation of intestinal fluid. Eudragit RL and Eudragit RS are the copolymers prepared from acrylic and methacrylic acid esters. These are used to coat the tablets which are intended to produce delayed action.

Polyethylene glycols (PEG): Low molecular weight PEGs (200 to 600) are liquid at room temperature and are used as a plasticizer in coating solution but high molecular weight PEGs (900 to 8000) are solid waxes at room temperature and are used to modify the film properties.

Vinyl polymers: Polyvinylpyrrolidone (povidone) – It is soluble in water, gastrointestinal fluid and organic solvents. Povidone produces clear, smooth, glossy and hard films. It is commonly used as a binding agent and as a medium for dispersing colouring agents.

2. *Solvents*

Solvents play an important role in the formulation of coating solution. They serve as a vehicle to dissolve and disperse the components of coating solution and helps in the application of coating solution to the tablet surface. Examples for solvents are water, alcohol (methanol, ethanol, isopropanol) ketones (acetone, methyl ethyl ketone), chlorinated hydrocarbons (chloroform, trichloroethane, methylene chloride), esters (ethyl acetate, methyl acetate).

Ideal properties of solvents:

a) It should be environmental friendly.
b) It should be inert
c) It should be cost effective
d) It should be inert and non-explosive
e) It should have faster rate of drying

Water is universal solvent and it is readily available but some drugs undergo hydrolysis in such cases organic solvents are used.

3. *Plasticizers*

Plasticizers are used in film coating solution to modify the film quality. It actually modifies the physical properties of the polymers, thereby enhancing the flexibility of the coating. Various properties of the plasticizer to be considered before its selection are its viscosity, solubility, compatibility with other additives. The effective plasticizer is one which solubilises in selected solvent.

There are two types of plasticizers

(i) *Internal plasticizer*: These act by making chemical changes within the structure of the polymer itself and modify physical properties.
(ii) *External plasticizer*: These plasticizers are non-volatile liquids or polymers on combination with primary polymer results in changes in the adhesiveness, tensile strength and flexibility of the film.

Examples for plasticizers are:

(i) *Oils*: castor oil, mineral oil.
(ii) *Polyhydric alcohols:* Glycerine, propylene glycol, low molecular weight PEGs.
(iii) *Glycerides:* Acetylated monoglyceride.
(iv) *Organic acid esters:* Triethyl citrate, glyceryl triacetate, diethyl phthalate, acetyl triethyl citrate etc.
(v) Spans and tweens

4. *Colours*

Colourants are included in many film-coating formulations to improve the appearance and visual identification of the coated product. Various types of approved colourants exist that can be used in film coating. Some of the colourants are given below:

Water-soluble dyes (*e.g.,* FD&C Yellow #5 and FD&C Blue #2) Aluminum lakes (FD&C water-soluble dyes) Other lakes (*e.g.,* D&C Red #6) Inorganic pigments (*e.g.,* titanium dioxide, iron oxides. calcium sulfate, calcium carbonate) "Natural" colorants (*e.g.*, riboflavin, turmeric, oleoresin, carmine 40).

5. *Opacifiers*

These are finely inorganic substances which are added into the coating solution to mask the colour of the tablet core and colour of the other ingredients and to increase the film coverage. Examples: Titanium dioxide, magnesium carbonate, talc, aluminium silicate, calcium sulphate, aluminium hydroxide etc.

6. *Miscellaneous agents*

Includes favouring agents, sweetening agents, an antimicrobial agent, antioxidants, surfactants etc.

Methods of Coating

Different methods of coating are: pan coating, fluid bed coating, compression coating etc

A. *Pan coating:* In pan coating tablets are tumbled in a bowl or pan which rotates about an axis inclined about 30° to the horizontal. By correctly loading the pan a three-dimensional circulation is established and sufficient coating solution is added to wet the tablet surfaces. Internal baffles or hand manipulation of the wetted tablets ensures that the solution is evenly distributed and a satisfactory tumbling action maintained while the coating is dried by a stream of drying air coming into the chamber. Small amounts of dusting powder may be applied to reduce tackiness and cohesion of the tablets during the drying stage. The volume of coating solution for each application is critical; inadequate wetting leads to irregular coating, whereas with too large volume of tablets agglomerate and do not tumble well. The cycle of alternate wetting and drying is continued to build up a coating of the required properties. Initially, the tablets are subject to considerable abrasive action and for this reason, tablets should be more compressed than the corresponding uncoated tablets.

B. *Fluid-bed coating:* Wurster (1959) first described the application of sugar or film coatings to tablets suspended in an air stream. In this equipment, the coating solution is introduced into the fluidizing air stream at the base of a tall vertical tube in which tablets circulate as they are coated. Evaporated solvent and air are removed at the top of the chamber. The fluid-bed moist granulation equipment has now been modified by the makers for fluid-bed coating. As the tablets circulate in the air stream they are subjected to considerable abrasive action and for this reason, they are compressed with extra firmness on punches which give a well-rounded profile.

C. *Compression coating*: As noted earlier it is desirable on occasion to separate tablet ingredients to avoid incompatibilities, to facilitate manufacture or to produce a sustained action product. Layer tablets provide an acceptable means for ingredient separation but the protective effect of the coat enveloping the tablet is lacking. It is not an easy matter to ensure a sugar coat of the same thickness for all tablets in a batch by pan coating and although reasonable variation in coat thickness and weight is not significant in plain sugar coating such variation cannot be tolerated if the coat contains a potent medicament. The idea of applying granular coating materials to a performed core was conceived by Noyes in 1896 but could not be commercially exploited until the problem of core centration and the automatic rejection of coreless tablets had been solved. Some of the advantages of a compression coating process are:

(a) Chemically incompatible ingredients may be separated.
(b) Core tablets are not subjected to abrasive action and need not be hard.
(c) The process is 'anhydrous' and sealing coats are not required.
(d) Good control of coating weight can be achieved.
(e) The core and coat may be formulated for different properties *e.g.,* for a sustained action tablet the coating would provide the prompt dose and the core the sustained dose.
(f) The process is continuous, completely mechanized and removes much of the element of skill from tablet coating.

Coating Equipment

There are three types of coating equipments:

I. Standard coating pans
II. Perforated coating pans
III. Fluidized bed coating equipment

I. *Standard coating pans:* These are also called as conventional coating pans design of the conventional pharmaceutical coating pans are similar to the coating pans used earlier for coating confectioneries. They were available in different shapes like hexagonal, pear-shaped or spherical. Though these pans were simple in design and operation,

Standard coating pans showed certain drawbacks those are:

a) The poor mixing efficiency of tablets.
b) The improper balance between the introduced and exhausted air and increased the health hazards for the operator.
c) The drying efficiency was low because much of the drying took place on the surface of the tablet bed only.

Because of these above drawbacks, the use of conventional coating pans was discouraged and this paved the way for modification in the coating pans. A common feature of modified conventional coating pans is the presence of a large circular metal pan of about 8-60 inches in diameter, mounted angularly at an angle of 40°. The pan is rotated on its horizontal axis by means of a motor. Tablets are coated by spraying the coating tablet are dried by directing a stream of hot air (or drying air) into the pan. The exhausted air is removed through vents or ducts located either in front or rear portion of the pan. The additional feature of these modified coating pans is that the interior of the pan is accessible through the openings provided in the front and rear portions (Fig. 2.9).

(a) Pelligrini coating pan: Pelligrini coating pan is provided with an integral baffle system to ensure thorough proper mixing of the tablets being coated. Drying air is introduced through a duct located at back of the coating pan. The air is uniformly distributed over the tablet bed surface by means of an air diffuser. The moisture or solvent-laden air is exhausted through a duct which is attached to the back portion of the pan.

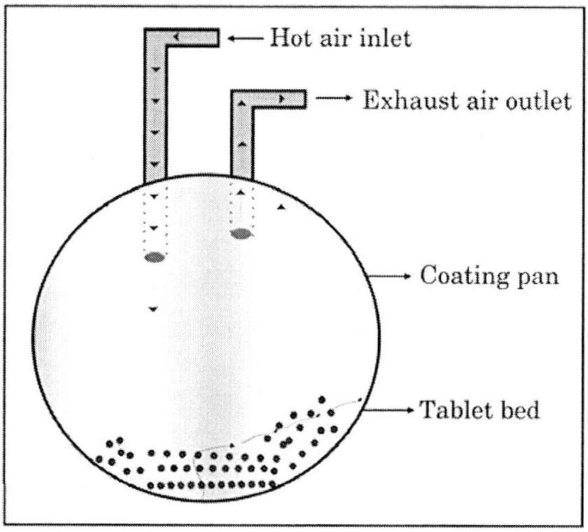

Fig. 2.9: Standard coating pan

The standard pelligrini pan is suitable only for sugar coating process but not for film coating due to its limitations in drying capabilities. This limitation was overcome by installing immersion sword air handling system to improve the drying efficiency.

(b) *Glatt immersion sword system:* Glatt immersion sword system consists of a stainless steel soundproof cabinet and in this system, the hot drying air is introduced into the pan through a sword like a device having perforations which are immersed into the tablet bed. When hot air is passed through the perforated sword, it flows out of the perforations in an upward direction and is in close contact with the tablets. This causes drying of the coated tablets. After drying the air is removed by means of an exhaust vent attached at the rear portion of the pan (Fig. 2.10).

(c) *Immersion tube coating pan:* The immersion tube system consists of a long tube with a spray nozzle at its tip. This tube is immersed in the tablet bed. Hot air gets passed through this tube into the tablet bed. Air flows in an upward direction through the tablet bed and escapes through the exhaust duct. During this operation, the coating material and the drying air are applied simultaneously (Fig. 2.11).

II. *Perforated coating pans:* Introduction of side-vented or perforated coating pans is an advancement in coating technology developed by Eli Lilly.

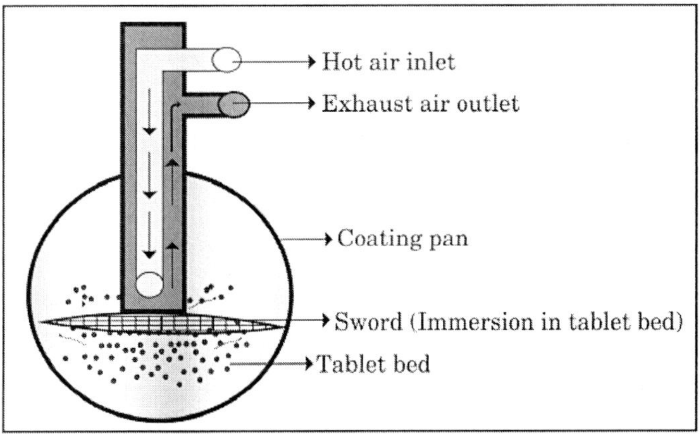

Fig. 2.10: Immersion sword system]

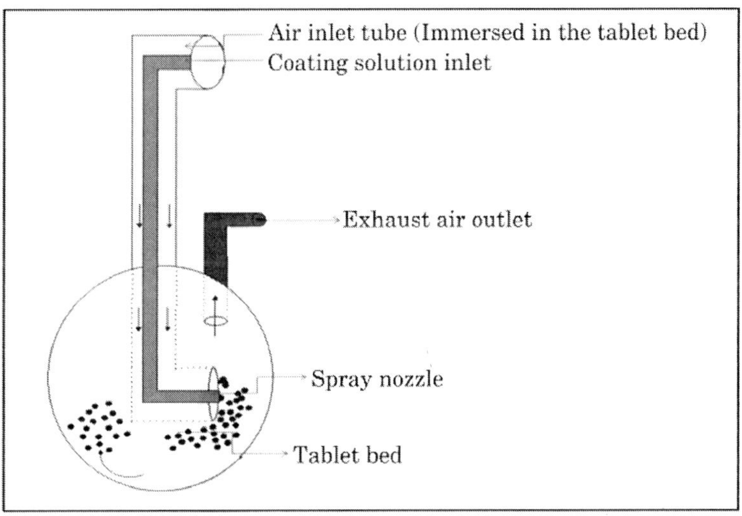

Fig. 2.11: Immersion tube coating pan

This type of coating pan consists of a perforated cylindrical pan which allows the drying air to be drawn through the rolling bed of tablets. The coating solution is sprayed by means of the spray nozzle which are located on the inside periphery of the pan. Finally, the exhausted air is vented out through the perforations.

Salient features of the perforated coating pans are:

1. Its design permits multi-directional air flow.

2. The equipment is in an enclosed system. Hence, provides high drying efficiency and rules out the possibilities of potential health hazards and explosion risks.
3. The system is completely automated and computerized. The pans are available in different batch capacities (3 – 40 kg).
4. The coating process is continuous *i.e.,* the uncoated material is introduced from one end and the coated material is retrieved from the other end.
5. They exhibit clean-in space systems that facilitate cleaning of the pans cabinets, ducts and vents. Hence are in compliance with GMP requirements.

Different types of perforated coating pans are accela cota, Hi-coater, Dria-coater, Glatt coater and Huttlin-butterfly coater.

In all these perforated coating pans the coating solution is applied through spraying nozzles located inside the pans. These type of coaters are suited for both sugar coating as well as film coating processes.

(a) *Accela cota pan:* In accela cota system, the drying air is directed into the perforated cylindrical pan through an inlet present at the top of the pan. It is then drawn into the tablet bed and is exhausted through a duct located at the bottom of the pan at a position immediately below the bed of tablets (Fig. 2.12).

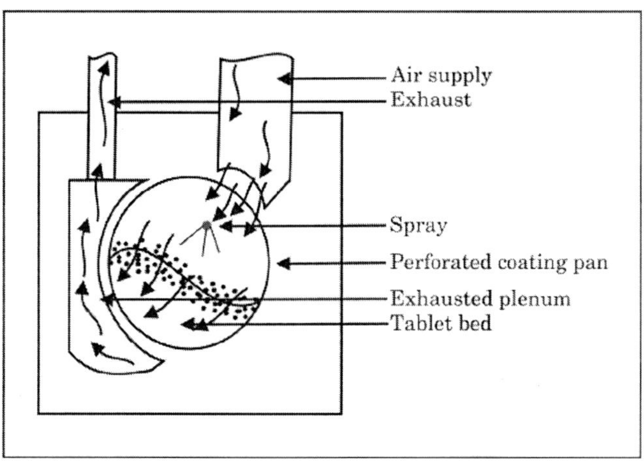

Fig. 2.12: Accela-cota system

(b) *Hi-coater pan:* Hi –coater consists of four perforated segments which are perpendicular to each other. Each of these perforations acts as an opening for exhaust air outlet which is fixed to the exterior of the pan surface. The exhaust outlet is so designed that it permits through any of the four perforations as the pan rotates. The drying air is introduced into the pan through an opening or duct located on the inside periphery of the top of the pan (Fig. 2.13).

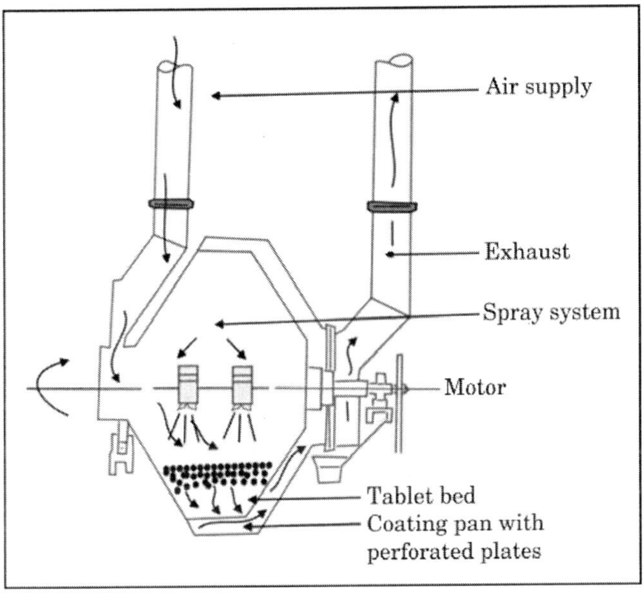

Fig. 2.13: Hi-Coater system

(c) *Dria-coater:* The Dria-coater works mainly by

i) The Dria-coater introduces drying air through the hollow perforated ribs located on the inside periphery of the drum.
ii) As the coating pan rotates, ribs dip into the tablet bed and drying air passes up through and fluidize the tablet bed.
iii) Exhaust is from the back of the pan (Fig. 2.14).

III. *Fluidized bed coating equipment:* Fluidized bed coating is also called as air suspension system is used for applying film coating to various pharmaceutical solid dosage forms such as tablets, pellets, granules and powders for producing modified release dosage forms. This is highly efficient drying systems.

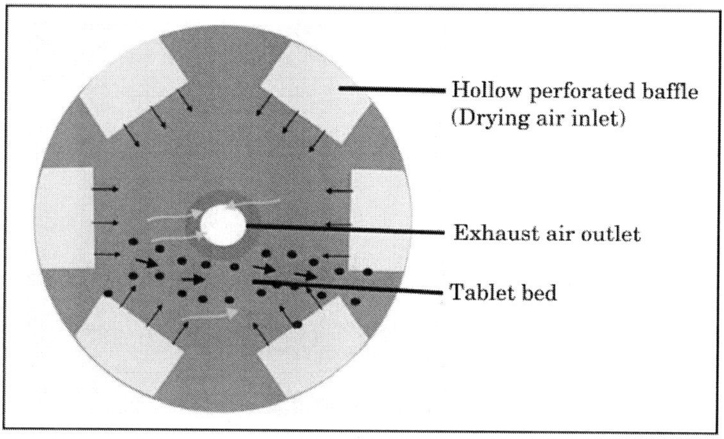

Fig. 2.14: Dria-Coater system

Considering the suitability of this process for applying film coating to various multi-particulates and also considering the purpose of coating (like taste masking, enteric-coating, modified release coating), three basic processing approaches have been developed.

1) *Bottom spray process (Wurster process):* This process is preferred for applying modified release coating to pellets, granules, powders and layered tablets. The coating solution is applied from a spray nozzle located at the bottom of the coating chamber.

2) Top-spray process (granulator process): This process is preferred for taste masking coating and hot melt coating. The coating solution is applied from a spray nozzle located in the upper region of the pan.

3) Tangential spray process (rotor process): This process is most suitable for preparing spheres. (spheronized granules) from powders. It also serves the purpose of applying modified release coating and drug layering. The spraying nozzles are located tangentially in the chamber.

Different type of fluidized bed coaters is Wurster fluid bed coating process, Glatt fluidized bed coater, automatic fluidized bed coater, vector-Freund coater, Huttlin-kugel coater.

The basic design of a fluidized bed coater is based on Wurster fluid-bed coating process or Wurster process. Different spray pattern is shown in Fig. 2.15.

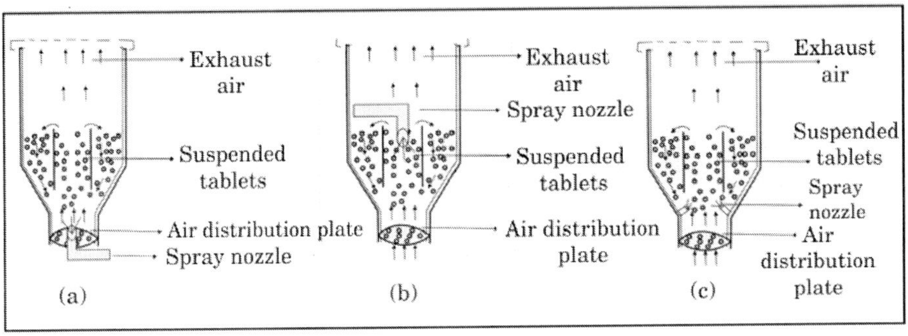

Fig. 2.15: Fluidized bed coating equipment a) Bottom spray b) Top spray and c) Tangential spray

Wurster fluid bed coating process: This method of coating was developed by Dale E Wurster. This is a highly efficient technique wherein coating of the tablets is carried out by suspending them in a stream of air (fluidization) and spraying them with the coating material. In this process, coating of the tablet core and drying takes place simultaneously.

Wurster process consists of a columnar coating chamber which is partitioned into two zones: the outer zone and the inner zone (coating zone). The diameter of the inner zone is approximately half of the outer zone. The bottom of the chamber consists of an air distribution plate with holes drilled into it for the passage of air. It also houses a centrally located spray nozzle for applying coating solution (film coating). The entire system is connected to a control unit which controls the process.

The coating process is carried out by taking the tablet cores in the coating chamber. A stream of air is passed through the air distribution plate which causes fluidization or suspension of the tablet core at the centre of the column. At the same time, coating material is sprayed through the nozzle to coat the suspended tablets. The inner partition wall causes deceleration of the suspended tablets. These suspended tablets fall towards the chamber wall and move downwards to re-enter the air stream at the bottom of the chamber. These are then fluidized again and the cycle is repeated several times until the tablet core is completely coated and the desired coating thickness is achieved. The supporting air stream serves as a medium for suspending the material and also facilitates drying of the coated tablets.

Though Wurster process possess excellent drying effects and produces a product with uniform coating and high gloss, certain tablets core which undergoes edge abrasion and chipping due to their friable nature are difficult to coat even under normal conditions.

Spray equipment (or spray guns): Spray equipment used to apply coating solutions or suspensions are of two types:

(a) Airless or hydraulic spray equipment: This type of sprayer consists of a spray gun having a nozzle with a small orifice of about 0.009 – 0.015 inch diameter. The coating solution is sprayed through the nozzle under a high pressure of 250 – 300 pounds per square inch (psi). This results in atomization of the liquid and it emerges as tiny droplets from the nozzle. The degree of atomization and the rate of application of the liquid are proportional to the orifice size, viscosity of the liquid and pressure. To prevent blocking of the orifice with suspended solid particles of the coating solution, the coating solution must be milled finely and filtered. This equipment is suitable for large-scale film coating process.

(b) Air spray equipment: In this type, the coating solution is sprayed at a low pressure of 5-100 pounds per square inch (psi) through a comparatively larger orifice of about 0.020 to 0.060 inches in diameter. Atomization of the liquid is achieved by bringing it in contact with a low pressure (compressed) air stream near the tip of the nozzle.

Air spray equipment is less expensive compared to airless spray equipment. It delivers coating liquids at low to high application rates. This type of equipment is suitable for small-scale operations and aqueous film coating process.

Facility and auxiliary equipment: The various facilities provide for the coating operation such as the premises, equipment, plant layout etc. should comply with the good manufacturing practices (GMP).

Adequate space should be provided for the coating equipment, preparation of coating formulation and for storage of the finished product. Facilities should be granted to process the exhaust air so as to retrieve the expensive organic solvents used in the formulation of coating solution.

Auxiliary equipment must be provided for each operation which is carried out during coating operation. For example: in the formulation of coating solution, various equipment like tanks filters, mills and mixer are required which should be provided to support the coating procedure.

Automated control system: In the initial days, tablet coating procedure was a completely manual operation. Addition of coating solution, mixing of tablets, drying of the coated tablets is done manually by the operator, such as process had many limitations like difficulty in achieving reproducible results, time management and keeping the records. These limitations paved way for automation of the process which has revolutionized the coating operation.

The various advantages of developing automated in product quality.

1. It has helped in attaining uniformity in product quality.
2. It had reduced the processing time.
3. The need of decisions making ability such as when to add the coating solution, when to apply drying air and for how long to carry on the operation are not necessary.
4. Automated process has fail-safe mechanism. It automatically shuts the process if anything goes wrong. Hence, it minimizes the chances of batch product from being getting ruined.
5. Hard copy documentation can be maintained.

Defects in Tablet Coating

1. Sticking and picking	Over-wetting or excessive film, tackiness causes tablet to stick to each other or to the coating pan. On drying, at the point of contact, a piece of the film may remain adhered to the pan or to another tablet, giving a picked appearance to the tablet surface and resulting in a small exposed area of the core. *Remedies* i) Reducing the liquid application rate ii) Increasing in the drying air temperature and air volume iii) Excessive tackiness may be an indication of poor formulation
2. Roughness	Rough or gritty surface is defect often observed when coating is applied by spray; some droplets may dry before reaching tablet bed and are deposited on the tablet core resulting in roughness of the surface.

Table *(Contd...)*

Table (*Contd...*)

	Remedies i) Moving nozzle closure to tablet bed ii) Reducing the degree of atomization can decrease the roughness
3. Orange peel effect	When coating solution is sprayed inadequately or improperly before drying causes a bumpy or orange peel effect on the coating. Spreading of the coating is hampered too rapid drying or by high solution viscosity. *Remedies* This can be solved by thinning coating solution with an additional solvent
4. Bridging	This defect is observed in tablets having monogram or bisection. During drying, the film may shrink and pull away from sharp corners (surface depression) resulting in bridging. *Remedies* i) This can be solved by increasing plasticizer content ii) Or by changing plasticizer
5. Filling	This defect is observed in tablets having monogram or bisection. Filling is caused when too much solution of coating is applied, which fills and narrows the monogram or bisect. If the solution is applied too fast, over wetting may cause the liquid to quickly fill and be retained in the monogram. *Remedies* i) Careful monitoring of liquid application rate ii) Thorough mixing of tablets in pan prevents filling
6. Blistering	When coated tablets require further drying in ovens, too rapid evaporation of solvent from tablet core and high temperature may affect the strength, elasticity and adhesion properties of the film. An unsmooth film surface shows number of uneven spots called blisters. (Entrapment of gases in or underneath the film due to overheating either during spraying or at the end of the coating run) *Remedies* This can be solved by employing milder drying condition
7. Hazing/dull film/blooming	It occurs when too high processing temperature is used for a particular formulation. It can also happen when the coated tablets are exposed to high humidity conditions and also due to migration of plasticiser to the surface of the coat.

Table (*Contd...*)

Table *(Contd...)*

	Remedies i) Reduce the processing temperature ii) Maintain optimum moisture content
8. Colour variation	A defect which involves variation in colour of the film. Reason is alteration of the frequency and duration of apppearance of tablets in the spray zone or the size/shape of the spray zone. And also improper mixing, uneven spray pattern, insufficient coating, migration of soluble dyes- plasticizers and other additives during drying. *Remedies* i) Use of lake dyes eliminates dye migration ii) Reformulation with different plasticizer
9. Cracking/ splitting	It is a defect in which the film either cracks across the crown of the tablet (cracking) or splits around the edges of the tablet (splitting). Reason: Internal stress in the film exceeds tensile strength of the film. Cause: Use of higher molecular weight polymers or polymeric blends. *Remedies* i) Use lower molecular weight polymers or polymeric blends ii) Adjust plasticizer type and concentration.
10. Cratering	It is a defect of film coating whereby volcanic-like craters appears exposing the tablet surface. Reason: The coating solution penetrates the surface of the tablet, often at the crown where the surface is more porous, causing localized disintegration of the core and disruption of the coating. Causes: Inefficient drying and higher rate of application of coating solution. *Remedies* i) Use efficient and optimum drying conditions. ii) Increase viscosity of coating solution to decrease spray application rate.
11. Pitting	It is a defect whereby pits occur in the surface of a tablet core without any visible disruption of the film coating. Reason: Temperature of the tablet core is greater than the melting point of the materials used in the tablet formulation. Cause: Inappropriate drying (inlet air) temperature. *Remedies* i) Dispensing with preheating procedures at the initiation of coating ii) And modifying the drying (inlet air) temperature such that the temperature of the tablet core is not greater than the melting point of the batch of additives used

QUALITY CONTROL TESTS FOR UNCOATED TABLETS

A. Un-Official Quality Control Tests

1) Tablet appearance
2) Organoleptic parameters
3) Size and shape of the tablet
4) Identification marking on tablet
5) Hardness and friability of tablet

Tablet appearance: Tablet appearance is one of the important parameter taken into consideration for the evaluation, based on consumer acceptance. It also ensures the uniformity among the batches of tablets produced, that may include surface texture, colour, odour, taste, identifying markings etc.

Organoleptic parameters: Organoleptic parameter includes colour, odour and taste. Colour distribution should be uniform within the tablet and batch to batch. Evaluation of colour in the tablet is done by Reflectance spectrophotometer, Tristimulus colorimeter and Microreflectance photometer. Non-uniform distribution of colour within the tablet is known as Mottling. Mottling should be avoided as it gives a bad impact on the patient's mind. The odour of the tablet helps to know whether the tablet is deteriorated, thereby indicating the stability of the tablet is affected (*e.g.*, instability of the aspirin tablet is indicated by acetic acid odour). Taste of the tablet is important criteria for patient's acceptance and taste of the tablet is important mainly in case of chewable tablets.

Size and shape of the tablet: For rapid production and good consumer acceptance the size and shape of the tablet is designed. It also enables identification of tablets.

Identification marking on tablet: Symbol of company, brand name, code of the product etc. are the identification markings on the tablet.

Hardness test: Hardness may be defined as force required to break the tablet when force is applied diametrically. Hardness is also termed as its crushing strength. Tablet requires a certain amount of strength or hardness and resistance to friability to withstand mechanical shocks during handling, packaging and shipping. Generally, used hardness testers are (1) Monsanto tester (2) Strong-Cobb tester (3) Pfizer tester (4) Erweka tester (5) Schleuniger tester.

Friability test: This test is applicable to compressed tablets and is intended to determine the physical strength of tablets.

Apparatus: It consists of a drum of transparent synthetic polymer with polished internal surfaces and subject to minimum static build-up. It has a diameter of 283-291 mm and a depth of 36-40 mm (see figure); one side of the drum is removable. A curved projection with an inner radius of 75.5 mm to 85.5 mm and extending from the middle of the drum to the outer wall enables the tumbling of the tablets at each turn of the drum. The outer diameter of the central ring is 24.5 mm to 25.5 mm. The drum is attached to the horizontal axis of a device that rotates at 25 ± 1 rpm. It should be ensured that with every turn of the drum the tablets roll or slide and fall onto the drum wall or onto each other (Fig. 2.16).

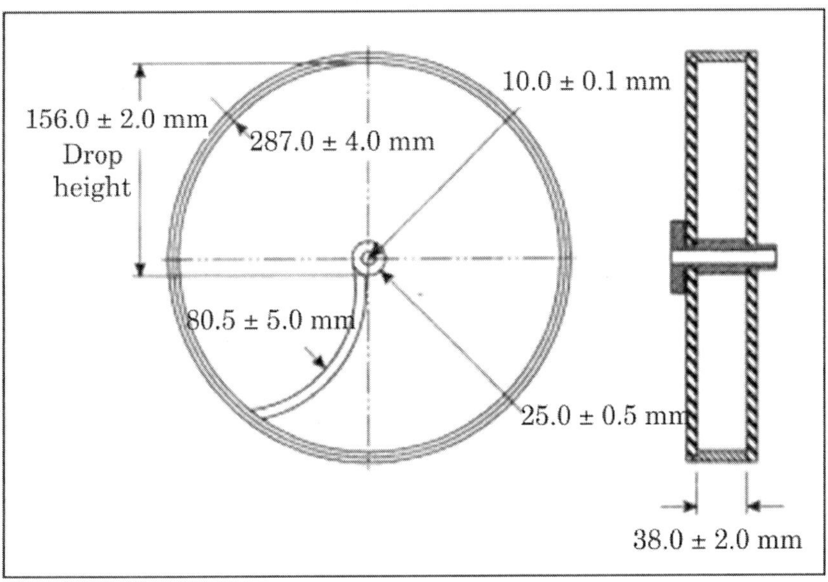

Fig. 2.16: Tablet friability apparatus

Friability of a tablet can determine in the laboratory by Roche's friabilator. This consists of a plastic chamber that revolves at 25 rpm, dropping the tablets of a distance of six inches in the friabilator, which is then operated for 100 revolutions. The tablets are reweighed and calculate the % friability. Compressed tablets that lose less than 1.0% of the tablet weight is consider acceptable. The friability issue of the tablet can be solved by addition of more tablet binder to granules and increasing the moisture content of granules.

B. Official Quality Control Tests

1) Weight variation test
2) Content uniformity test
3) Disintegration test
4) Dissolution test

Weight variation test (I.P. 2007): Weigh individually 20 tablets selected at random and calculate the average weight. Based on the average weight calculate upper limit and lower limit. Not more than two of the tablets deviate from the average weight by more than the percentage shown in the table and none deviates by more than twice that percentage. Percentage deviation allowed as per I.P. is given in Table 2.10.

Table 2.10: Percentage deviation allowed as per I.P.

Dosage form	*Average weight*	*Percentage deviation*
Uncoated Tablets	80 mg or less	10
	More than 80 mg but less than 250 mg	7.5
	250 mg or more	5

Content uniformity test (I.P. 2007): Tablets sample complies content uniformity test if each individual content is 85 to 115 per cent of the average content. The tablets sample fails to comply with the test if more than one individual content is outside these limits or if one individual content is outside the limits of 75 to 125 per cent of the average content.

If one individual content is outside the limits of 85 to 115 per cent of the average content but within the limits of 75 to 125per cent, repeat the determination using another 20 dosage units.

The preparation complies with the test if not more than one of the individual contents of the total sample of 30 dosage units is outside 85 to 115 per cent of the average content and none is outside the limits of 75 to 125 per cent of the average content.

Disintegration test (I.P. 2007)

Apparatus: The apparatus consists of a basket-rack assembly, a 1-litre beaker, a thermostatic arrangement for heating the fluid and a mechanical device for raising and lowering the basket in the immersion fluid at a constant frequency rate.

Basket-rack assembly: The basket-rack assembly is rigid and supports six cylindrical glass tubes, 77.5 ± 2.5 mm long, 21.5 mm in internal diameter and with a wall thickness of about 2 mm (Fig. 2.17). The tubes are held vertically by two superimposed transparent plastic plates, 90 ± 2 mm in diameter and 6.75 ± 1.75 mm thick perforated by six holes having the same diameter as the tubes. The holes are equidistant from the centre of the plate and are equally spaced from one another. Attached to the underside of the lower plate is a woven stainless steel wire cloth with a plain square weave with 2.0 ± 0.2 mm mesh apertures and with a wire diameter of 0.615 ± 0.045 mm. The upper plate is covered with a stainless steel disc perforated by six holes, each about 24 ± 2 mm in diameter, which fits over the tubes and holds them

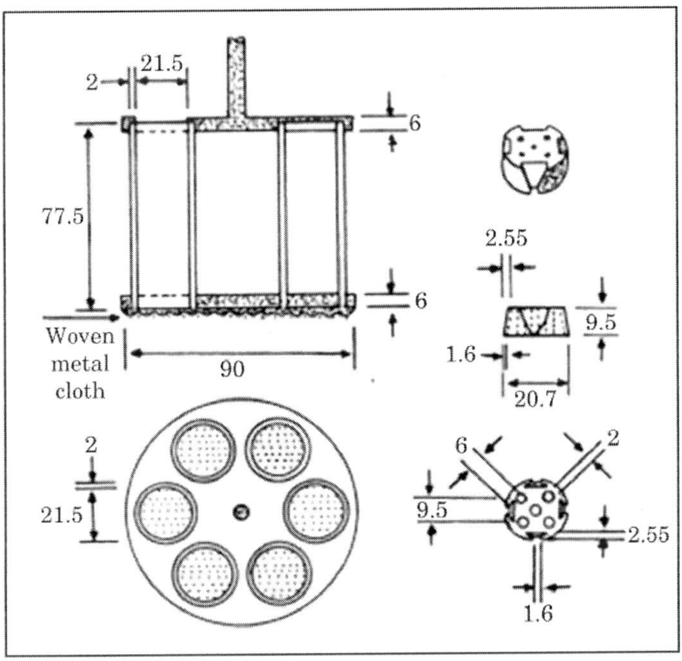

Fig. 2.17: Apparatus for disintegration test (all dimensions are given in mm)

between the plastic plates. The holes coincide with those of the upper plastic plate and the upper open ends of the glass tubes. A suitable means is provided to suspend the basket-rack assembly from the raising and lowering device using a point on its axis.

The plates are held rigidly in position and 77.5 mm apart by vertical metal rods at the periphery and a metal rod is also fixed to the centre of the upper plate to enable the assembly to be attached to the device for raising and lowering it smoothly at a constant frequency of between 28 and 32 cycles per minute through a distance of 50 to 60 mm. The time required for the upward stroke is equal to the time required for the downward stroke and the change in stroke direction should be smooth and not abrupt. There should be no appreciable horizontal motion or movement of the axis from the vertical.

Discs: A cylindrical disc for each tube, each 20.7 ± 0.15 mm thick in diameter and 9.5 ± 0.15 mm thick, made of transparent plastic with a relative density of 1.18 to 1.20, and pierced with five holes, each 2 mm in diameter, one in the centre and the other four spaced equally on a circle of radius 6 mm from the centre of the disc. Four equally-spaced grooves are cut in the lateral surface of the disc in such a way that at the upper surface of the disc they are 9.5 mm wide and 2.55 mm deep and at the lower surface 1.6 mm square.

Medium: The assembly is suspended in the liquid medium in a suitable vessel, preferably a 1-litre beaker. The volume of liquid is such that the wire mesh at its highest point is at least 25 mm below the surface of the liquid, and at its lower point is at least 25 mm above the bottom of the beaker. At no time should the top of the basket-rack assembly become submerged. There is a thermostatic arrangement for heating the liquid and maintaining the temperature at 37 ± 2° C.

Procedure: Unless otherwise stated in the individual monograph, introduce one tablet into each tube and, if directed in the appropriate general monograph, add a disc to each tube. Suspend the assembly in the beaker containing the specified liquid and operate the apparatus for the specified time. Remove the assembly from the liquid. The tablets pass the test if all of them have disintegrated.

If 1 or 2 tablets fail to disintegrate, repeat the test on 12 additional tablets; not less than 16 of the total of 18 tablets tested disintegrate.

If the tablets adhere to the disc and the preparation under examination fails to comply, repeat the test omitting the disc. The preparation complies with the test if all the tablets in the repeat test disintegrate.

Disintegration is considered to be complete when a) there is no residue on the perforated plate or b) if a residue remains, it consists only of a soft mass having no solid core which cannot be pressed with a glass rod.

The disintegration time of various types of tablet is as fallow:

- *Dispersible tablets*: Disintegrate within 3 minutes
- *Soluble tablets*: Disintegrate within 3 minutes
- *Effervescent tablets*: Disintegrate within 5 minutes
- *Sugar-coated tablets*: Disintegrate within 60 minutes
- *Film coated tablets*: Not disintegrate within 60 minutes
- *Delayed –release tablets*: Not disintegrate within 60 minutes
- *Gastroresistant tablets (Enteric coated)*: Not disintegrate in 0.1 N HCl within 1 h
- *Soft gelatin capsules*: 5-10 minutes

Dissolution test (I.P. 2007)

This test is designed to determine compliance with the dissolution requirements for solid dosage forms administered orally. The test is intended for a capsule or tablet using two types of apparatus: apparatus-1 and apparatus-2 these are described below.

Apparatus type-1: Use apparatus type 1 unless otherwise directed.

- All parts of the apparatus type 1 that may come into contact with the preparation under examination or with the dissolution medium must be made from materials which do not react or interfere with the study.
- No part of the assembly, including the environment in which the assembly is placed, contributes significant motion, agitation or vibration beyond that due to the smoothly rotating element.
- An apparatus that permits observation of the preparation under examination and the stirrer during the test is preferable.

Dissolution test apparatus type 1 is shown in Fig. 2.18, it consisting of the following:

- A cylindrical vessel (A) made of borosilicate glass or any other suitable transparent material, with a hemispherical bottom and with a nominal capacity of 1000 ml and an inside diameter of 98-106 mm.
- The vessel has a flanged upper rim and is fitted with a lid that has a number of openings, one of which is central.
- A motor with a speed regulator capable of maintaining the speed of rotation of the paddle within 4% of that specified in the individual monograph (as per USP it is 2%). The motor is fitted with a stirring element which consists of a drive shaft and blade forming a paddle (B).

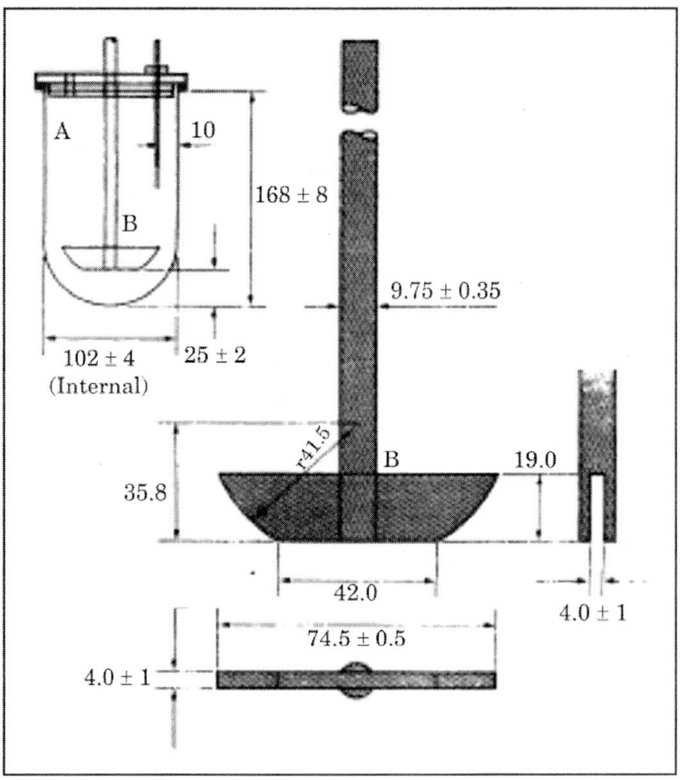

Fig. 2.18: Dissolution test apparatus type-1 (A: cylindrical vessel and B: paddle)

- The blade passes through the diameter of the shaft so that the bottom of the blade is flush with the bottom of the shaft. The shaft is positioned so that its axis is within 2 mm of the axis of the vessel and the lower edge of the blade is 23 to 27 mm from the inside bottom of the vessel.
- The apparatus operates in such a way that the paddle rotates smoothly and without significant wobble.
- A water-bath set to maintain the dissolution medium at 36.5 to 37.5° C. The bath liquid is kept in constant and smooth motion during the test.
- The vessel is securely clamped in the water bath in such a way that the displacement vibration from other equipment, including the water circulation device, is minimised.

Apparatus type-2:

- The assembly is the same as in apparatus type-1 except that in the stirring element the paddle is replaced by a basket (D), as shown in Fig. 2.19. The metallic shaft rotates smoothly and without significant wobble.
- The basket consists of two components:
  - The top part, with a vent, is attached to the shaft C, it is fitted with three spring clips, or other suitable means that allow removal of the lower part for introduction of the preparation under examination and that firmly hold the lower part of the basket concentric with the axis of the vessel during rotation.
  - The lower detachable part of the basket is made of welded-steam cloth, with a wire thickness of 0.254 mm diameter and with 0.381 mm square openings, formed into a cylinder with narrow rim of sheet metal around the top and the bottom.
- The basket may be plated with a 2.5 mm layer of gold for use with acidic media. The distance between the inside bottom of the vessel and the basket is maintained at 23 to 27 mm during the test.

Dissolution medium: Use the dissolution medium specified in the individual monograph. If the medium is a buffered solution, adjust the solution so that its pH is within 0.05 units of the pH specified in

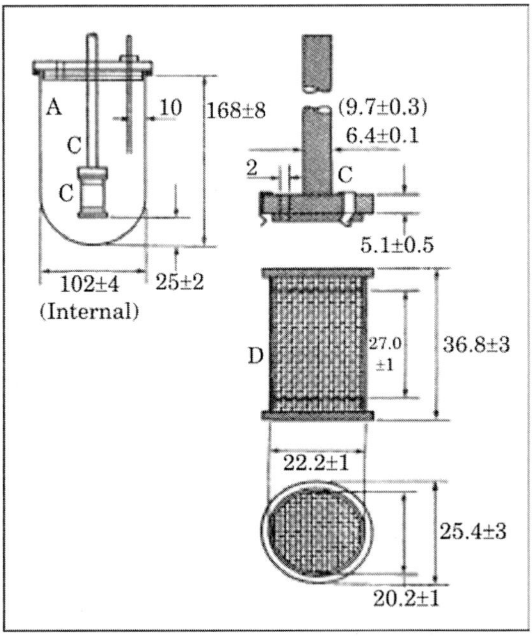

Fig. 2.19: Dissolution test apparatus type-2 (A: cylindrical vessel, C: shaft and D: basket).

the monograph. The dissolution medium should be deaerated prior to testing.

Time: Where a single time specification is given in the monograph, the test may be concluded in a shorter period if the requirement for the minimum amount dissolved is met. If two or more times are specified, specimen are to be withdrawn only at the stated times, within a tolerance of ± 2 per cent. Dissolution testing and interpretation can be done in three stages.

Method

- Place the stated volume of the dissolution medium into the vessel of the apparatus. Assemble the apparatus and warm the dissolution medium to 36.5°C to 37.5°C.
- Place a dosage unit in the apparatus, taking care to exclude air bubbles from the surface of the dosage unit.

- When apparatus type-1 is used, allow the tablet or capsule to sink to the bottom of the vessel prior to the rotation of the paddle.
- When apparatus type-2 is used, place the tablet or capsule in a dry basket at the beginning of each test. Lower the basket into position before rotation.
- Operate the apparatus immediately at the speed of rotation specified in the individual monograph. Within the time interval specified, or at each of the times stated, withdraw a specimen from a zone midway between the surface of the dissolution medium and the top of the rotating blade or basket, not less than 10 mm from the wall of the vessel.
- Except in the case of single sampling, add a volume of dissolution medium equal to the volume of the samples withdrawn. Perform the analysis as directed in the individual monograph.
- For each of the tablet or capsule tested, calculate the amount of dissolved active ingredient in solution as a percentage of the stated.

Acceptance Criteria

Conventional-release dosage forms

Stage 1(S1): Six tablets are tested and are acceptable each unit is not less than D* + 5 per cent**. If fail

Stage 2 (S2): Another six tablets are tested, test individually, Average of 12 units (S1 +S2) is equal to or greater than D, and no unit is less than D –15 per cent** if fail

Stage 3 (S3): Another 12 tablets are tested. The tablets are acceptable if the average of 24 units (S1+S2+S3) is equal to or greater than D, not, more than 2 units are less than D – 15 per cent** and no unit is less than D – 25 per cent**.

*D is the amount of dissolved active ingredient specified in the individual monograph, expressed as a percentage of the labelled content. **Percentages of the labelled content.

#Acceptance criteria for prolongedd release and modified release are different than acceptance criteria of conventional-release dosage forms. Those are not discussed here, for further details refer I.P. 2007.

QUALITY CONTROL TESTS FOR COATED TABLETS

Following IPQC and quality control test are performed for coated tablets

1. Uniformity in colour, shape, size and film texture is done by visual inspection.
2. The mechanical or tensile strength of the film tested using tensile strength testers. This test is performed to measure the force required to peel the film from the tablet surface. This test also optimizes and evaluates the concentration of plasticizers and additives used in the formulation.
3. *Tablet hardness:* Hardness test for the coated tablet is similar to that of uncoated tablets.
4. *Tablet thickness:* Thickness test for the coated tablet is similar to that of uncoated tablets.
5. Resistance to chipping and abrasion is evaluated by rubbing the coated tablets on a sheet of white paper. If all the films are soft they get easily abrased. If the films well adhere to the tablet surface, they will remain intact.
6. *Disintegration test:* Disintegration test for coated tablet is similar to that of uncoated tablets
7. *Dissolution test:* Dissolution test for coated tablet is similar to that of uncoated tablets
8. Weight variation test

Glossary

Elegant tablet	Attractive appearance of tablet
Excipients	Therapeutically inactive or non-drug components
Bioavailability	Availability of drug at the site of action
Maillard reaction	This is a type of chemical reaction which occurs between reactive carbonyl group of reducing sugar (such as lactose) and amine group of amino acid or drugs (such as aminophylline and amphetamine)
Diluents	Diluents are insert substances which add the necessary bulk to a formulation
Binders	Binders cause adhesion of powder particles to form granules
Disintegrants	Disintegrating agents are added to promote tablet breakup after administration

Super disintegrating agents:	These are the newer class of disintegrating agents which are required in less quantity compared to starch.
Lubricating agents	These are added to a tablet formulation to decreases the friction between the powders or granules or tablet and the die wall of tablet press
Glidants	These are the agents which are added to tablet formulation for easy flow of granules
Anti-adherents	These agents prevent the sticking of tablet material (powder or granules) to the faces of punches and to some extent to the die wall
Wetting agents	These agents are added to a tablet formulation containing the poorly soluble components and to enhance the dissolution rate of tablet
Colouring agents	These are the agents which impart colour to the tablet
Dyes	They are soluble colouring agents which becomes insoluble after application
Lakes	These are dyes in the form of dry powders adsorbed on hydrous oxide such as aluminium hydroxide
Pigments	They are insoluble colouring agents available as powders
Sweetening agents	These agents are added to a tablet formulation to impart sweet taste and to mask bitter taste
Flavouring agents	These agents are added to a tablet formulation to impart good flavour to the tablet
Granules	Small particles adhere together by forming bonds, resulting in the formation of large aggregates called granules
Direct compression	Direct compression is a dry process wherein the powdered material is compressed directly into the tablets
Dry granulation	The powder mixture is compacted in large pieces and subsequently broken down or sized into granules
Slugging	Powder mixture is compressed into large flat tablets or pellets about 1 inch in diameter
Wet granulation	Wet granulation method involves use of wetting/granulating agents for preparation of granules
Tablet tooling	A single punch press possess one die and one pair of punches that is a set of tabletting tools
Cams	One which controls the movement of upper and lower punches
Die table	The portion holding the dies is called the die table
Hopper	For holding and feeding granulation
Dies	That defines the size and shape of the tablet
Punches	Punches for compressing the powder/granulation within the dies
Cam tracks	Cam tracks for guiding the movement of the punches
Feed-frame	Which has several interconnected compartments helps to fill die cavity

Wipe -off blade	Which removes the excess granulation
Deformation	When stress is applied to a material, the material changes the form
Capping	When the upper or lower segment of the tablet separates horizontally, either partially or completely from the main body of a tablet
Lamination	Lamination is the separation of a tablet into two or more distinct horizontal layers
Chipping	Chipping is defined as the breaking of tablet edges
Cracking	Small, fine cracks observed on the upper and lower central surface of tablets, or very rarely on the sidewall are referred to as cracks
Sticking	Sticking refers to the tablet material adhering to the die wall
Picking	Picking is the term used when a small amount of material from a tablet is sticking to and being removed off from the tablet-surface by a punch face
Binding	Binding in the die is the term used when the tablets adhere, seize or tear in the die
Mottling	Mottling is the term used to describe an unequal distribution of colour on a tablet, with light or dark spots standing out in an otherwise uniform surface
Tablet coating	Applying a coating solution to the external surface of the tablet core
Sugar coating	Application of sugar (sucrose) based coating solution to the tablets
Sealing of tablets	Which is done to protect the tablet core from adverse effects of moisture
Grossing	Making tablets smooth and free from irregularities prior to application of the colour coat
Polishing	After colour coating, the tablets show a dull or mottoled appearance. Thus, they require polishing or finishing to impart the desired gloss and lustre
Printing:	Sugar-coated tablets are imprinted with manufacturers name, code or logo for identification purpose either before or after their polishing
Enteric coated tablets:	Enteric coated dosage forms are designed with an intention to show local action in the intestines without undergoing disintegration and drug release in the stomach
Plasticizers	Plasticizers are used in film coating solution to modify the film quality
Opacifiers	These are inorganic substances which are added into the coating solution to mask the colour of the tablet core and colour of the other ingredients and to increase the film coverage
Blistering	It is local detachment of film from the substrate forming blister

Cratering	It is defect of film coating whereby volcanic-like craters appears exposing the tablet surface
Picking	It is defect where isolated areas of film are pulled away from the surface when the tablet sticks together and then part
Pitting:	It is defect whereby pits occur in the surface of a tablet core without any visible disruption of the film coating
Blooming	It is defect where coating becomes dull immediately or after prolonged storage at high temperatures
Blushing	It is defect best described as whitish specks or haziness in the film
Colour variation	A defect which involves variation in colour of the film
Filling	It is defect that renders the intagliations indistinctness
Cracking/splitting	It is defect in which the film either cracks across the crown of the tablet (cracking) or splits around the edges of the tablet
Bridging	This occurs when the coating fills in the lettering or logo on the tablet and is typically caused by improper application of the solution

QUESTION BANK

Q. I: Multiple Choice Questions

1 In the process of sugar coating of tablets, the colourants are added in one of the following steps

a) Syrup coating c) Sub-coating
b) Polishing d) Seal coating

2 During compression of moisture critical granules a hygroscopic substance used to maintain moisture level is

a) Sorbitol c) Acacia
b) Talc d) Tragacanth

3 In tablet coating process inadequate spreading of the coating solution before drying causes.

a) Orange peel effect c) Blistering effect
b) Sticking effect d) Picking effect

4 The purpose of seal coating in sugar coating process for tablets is

a) To prevent moisture penetration into the tablet core c) To impart the desired colour to the tablet
b) To round the edges and build up tablet weight d) To give lustre to the tablet

5 The durability of a tablet to combined effect of shock and abrasion is evaluated by using

a) Hardness tester
b) Disintegration test apparatus
c) Friabilator
d) Screw gauge

6 In the preparation of multilayer tablets, one of the substances listed is used for hydrophilic matrix coating

a) C.M.C.
b) Shellac
c) Stearyl alcohol
d) Bees wax

7 Which filler cannot be used for the preparation of tablets for amine-containing basic drug to avoid discolouration of the tablets?

a) Dicalcium phosphate
b) Microcrystalline cellulose
c) Starch
d) Lactose

8 The first stage of wetting on addition of granulating agent to the powders is characterized by which one of the followings?

a) Capillary state
b) Pendular state
c) Funicular state
d) Droplet state

9 According to USP, the speed regulating devices of the dissolution apparatus should be capable of maintaining the speed within limits of what % of the selected speed?

a) 1%
b) 2%
c) 4%
d) 5%

10 What is primogel?

a) Substituted HPMC for direct compression
b) Modified microcrystalline cellulose for direct compression
c) Hydrogelling polymer for gel formation
d) Modified starch for disintegration

11 Which of the following is non-aqueous binder?

a) Ethyl cellulose
b) Starch
c) Veegum
d) Bentonite

12 When the angle of repose exceeds ____the powder flow is rarely acceptable for pharmaceutical manufacturing purpose?

a) 25
b) 30
c) 50
d) 60

13 Evaluation of colour in tablets is done by

a) Reflectance spectrophotometer
b) Microreflectance photometer
c) Tristimulus colorimeter
d) All of the above

14 Which of the following is not added to chewable tablet?

a) Glidant
b) Disintergrating agent
c) Lubricant
d) antiadhesive

15 The disintegration time of effervescent tablet is?

a) 2 min
b) 2.5 min
c) 3.5 min
d) 5 min

16 One of the following ingredients which improves the flow property of granule is

a) Glidant
b) Emollient
c) Lubricant
d) Surfactant

17 Which of the following is not used as enteric coating material?

a) Cellulose acetate phthalate
b) Pectin
c) Acrylate polymerase
d) Polyvinyl acetate phthalate

18 Slugs are prepared in which kind of granulation techniques?

a) Wet granulation
b) Dry granulation
c) Stem granulation
d) Melt granulation

19 The Wurster process can be used to

a) Coat tablets
b) Determine the disintegration time
c) Gas sterilize parenteral solutions
d) Automatic filling of capsules

20 Select the equation that gives the rate of drug dissolution from a tablet?

a) Ficks Law
b) Henderson Hasselbalch Equation
c) Noyes Whitney Equation
d) Michaelis Menten Equation

21 The diameter of mesh aperture in the I.P. disintegration test apparatus is given below choose the correct size

a) 2.00 mm
b) 4.00 mm
c) 1.00 mm
d) 1.50 mm

22 Choose the correct excipient for enhancing solubility in tablet manufacture

a) PEG
b) MCC
c) Talc
d) Lactose

23 If the car's index of powder is 10% then the type of powder flow is

a) Poor
b) Excellent
c) Very poor
d) Good

24 A super disintegrant in tablet formulation is

a) Sodium starch glycolate
b) Starch
c) PVP
d) Mg-Aluminium silicate

25 Sweetening agents commonly used in chewable tablet is

a) Sucrose
b) Cyclomate sodium
c) Saccharin sodium
d) Mannitol

26 Subcoating is given to tablets

a) To increase the bulk
b) To avoid deterioration due to microbial attack
c) To prevent the solubility in acidic medium
d) To avoid stickiness

27 Lamination is

a) Separation of tablet into two or more distinct layers
b) Partial and complete separation of the top and bottom crowns of a tablet
c) Process of sub-coating of tablets
d) None of the above

28 One of the following materials listed below is most commonly used in film coating of tablets identify.

a) Acacia
b) Simple syrup
c) Hydroxypropyl methyl cellulose
d) Beeswax

29 Disintegration time for sugar-coated tablets

a) 35 min
b) 45 min
c) 60 min
d) 75 min

30 Name of the equipment/s used to measure hardness of tablet

a) Pfizer tester
b) Strong Cobb tester
c) Erweka tester
d) All of the above

31 Excessive moisture can be responsible for _____ during tablet compression

a) Capping
b) Mottling
c) Picking
d) Sticking

32 Which of the following is opaquant extender?

a) Colloidal silica
b) Titanium dioxide
c) Guanidine
d) Magnesium stearate

33 Which is the test intended to determine, the phenomenon whereby tablet surface are damaged and/or show evidence of lamination or breakage when subjected to

a) Friability
b) Hardness
c) Dissolution
d) Disintegration

34 Which problem can arise if the material to be compressed into tablets tends to adhere to the die walls?

a) Picking
b) Sticking
c) Capping
d) Marbling

35 Eudragits are:

a) Phthalate polymers
b) Cellulose polymers
c) Acrylate polymers
d) Amide polymers

36 Enteric coated tablet is disintegrated in

a) Stomach
b) Mouth
c) Intestine
d) Liver

37 The first and most widely used diluents in tablet formulation is

a) Dextrose
b) Lactose
c) MCC
d) Starch

38 CAB-O-SIL is

a) Antiadherent
b) Lubricant
c) Disintegrant
d) Glidant

39 The enteric resin used for coating is

a) Cellulose acetate phthalate
b) Shellac
c) Zein
d) All of the above

40 Tablet within tablet is a technique is used for which type of coating?

a) Dip coating
b) Electrostatic
c) Vacuum film coating
d) Compressed coating

41 Which of the following tablet excipient has the lubricant, anti-adherants and glidant properties?

a) Cornstarch
b) Stearic acid
c) Talc
d) Colloidal silica

42 A synthetic sweetening agent which is nearly 200 times sweeter than sucrose and has no aftertaste is

a) Aspartame
b) Saccharin
c) Talc
d) Colloidal silica

43 Friability test is known as

a) LAL test
b) Swelling index
c) Brittle fracture index test
d) Sham test

44 Capping in tablet is mainly due to

a) Less upper punch pressure
b) Poor formulation of granules
c) Improper formulation design
d) Entrapment of air in tablet during compression

45 Modified starch is

a) Starch 1500 c) Starch 1000

b) Starch 1200 d) Starch 200

46 The concentration of PVP as a binder is

a) 1.0-5.0% w/v c) 0.5-3.0% w/v

b) 2.0-15% w/v d) 0.1-0.5% w/v

47 In weight variation of tablets maximum variation allowed for range 130-324mg tablets according to USP is

a) ±5% c) ±2.5%

b) ±10% d) ±7.5%

48 Angle of repose is directly proportional to

a) Horizontal plane constant c) Co-efficient of friction

b) Bulk density d) Weight of powder

Q. II: Very Short Answer Questions 2 Marks

1. Differentiate disintegrants and super disintegrants with examples.
2. What are disintegrants? Give two examples.
3. What are chewable tablets? Give their advantages
4. What are enteric coating polymers? Name any two examples.
5. What are lozenges?
6. List the lubricants used in tablets.
7. List in-process quality control tests for tablets.
8. What are anti adherents? Give examples.
9. List the manufacturing defects of tablets.
10. Write a note on sublingual tablets.
11. Role of lubricants and glidants used in tablets with examples.
12. Enlist the steps in sugar coating.
13. What are buccal tablets?
14. List non-enteric polymers used as film formers.
15. What is Maillard's reaction?
16. Why is friability test not required for coated tablets?
17. List out the coating equipment used.
18. List out the excipients used in formulation of tablets.
19. List out components of a film coating solution with its use.
20. Give ideal requirements of a tablets.
21. Brief note on effervescent tablets.

22. Give directly compressible additives for tablets.
23. Why disintegrants are used in tablet formulations?

Q. III: Short Answers Questions **5 Marks**

1. Define and classify tablets.
2. Differentiate diluents and directly compressible vehicles by giving examples.
3. Describe any two official quality control tests for tablets.
4. Describe the steps involved in sugar coating with suitable examples
5. Give the reasons for granulation
6. Add a note on tablet tooling
7. Add a note on rollar compactor
8. Give the mechanisms of disintegrating agents
9. Explain manufacturing defects found in tablets. How are they overcome?
10. Write a note friability test for tablets.
11. Explain the different excipients used in the preparation of tablets.
12. Give defects and remedies for coated tablets
13. Define mottling and weight variation. Give their causes and methods to overcome.
14. Explain direct compression technique of tablet manufacture with their merits and demerits.
15. What is the importance of coating? Explain compression coating.
16. Enumerate the various types of compressed tablets.
17. Explain how weight variation and content uniformity tests are performed?
18. Explain manufacturing defects of tablets.

Q. IV: Long Answers Questions **10 Marks**

1. (A) With a neat labelled diagram, explain rotary compression process of tablet manufacturing.

   (B) Describe the defects in film coating process.
2. A) Discuss the tablet compression cycle by multistation rotary press.

   B) Write the reasons and remedies for capping and lamination.
3. Describe dry granulation technique and list advantages and disadvantages.
4. What are granules? Describe the wet granulation and dry granulation techniques.
5. Give a detailed account of the different excipients and their functions used in the tablets.

6. Explain in detail about the in-process and final product quality control tests for uncoated tablets.
7. Explain in detail the working of single punch tablet machine with suitable diagram. Compare it with the working of rotary tablet machine.
8. Explain about sugar coating and film coating of tablets. Compare their merits and demerits.
9. Discuss different equipment used for tablet coating

CHAPTER 3

LIQUID ORALS

INTRODUCTION

Liquid orals are preparations comprising of solution, emulsion or suspension of one or more medicaments in a suitable vehicle. These are meant for oral administration either undiluted or diluted form. They may contain auxiliary substances such as suitable dispersing, emulsifying, suspending, wetting, solubilising, buffering, thickening, stabilising agents and antimicrobial preservatives. They may also contain permitted suitable colouring, sweetening and flavouring agents.

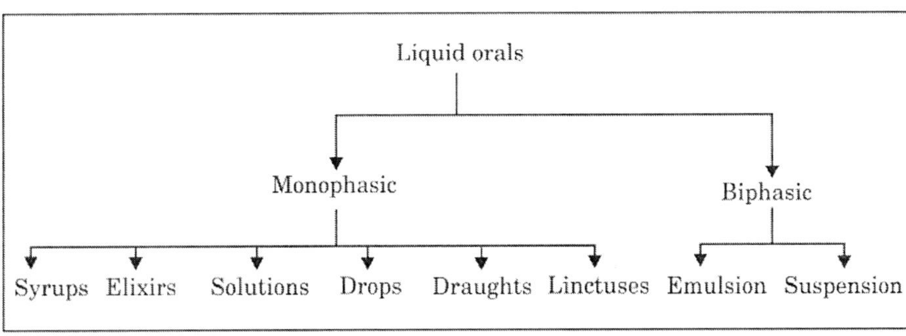

Syrups: Syrups are concentrated aqueous preparations of a sugar or sugar substitute with or without flavouring agents and medicinal substances.

Elixirs: Elixirs are clear, sweetened, aromatic, hydro-alcoholic, flavoured liquid preparations containing one or more active ingredients dissolved in a vehicle.

Solutions: Pharmaceutical solutions contain the drug dissolved in a solvent system. The solvent can be aqueous or oily. Solution is a homogeneous molecular mixture of two or more components.

Drops: Oral drops are solutions, emulsions or suspensions that are administered in small volumes, by means of a suitable device.

Draughts: Draughts are liquid oral preparations taken as single dose usual volume is 50 ml and, if several doses are prescribed they are dispensed in a separate container.

Linctuses: Linctuses are viscous, liquid and oral preparations that are generally, prescribed for the relief of cough. They contain medicaments which have demulcent, sedative, or expectorant action. Linctuses should be taken in small doses, sipped and swallowed slowly without diluting with water in order to have maximum and prolonged effect.

Emulsions: Emulsions are biphasic liquid dosage forms consisting of two immiscible liquids one of which is dispersed as minute globules into the other.

Suspensions: Suspensions are the biphasic liquid dosage form of medicament in which the finely divided solid particles dispersed in a liquid vehicle.

The liquid orals such as syrups, elixirs, suspensions and emulsions are discussed with reference to formulation considerations, formulae, method of preparations, evaluation and storage.

SYRUPS

Syrups are concentrated aqueous preparations of sugar or sugar substitute with or without flavouring agents and medicinal substances.

i) The concentrated aqueous preparations of sugar or sugar substitute without flavouring agents and medicinal substances are known as simple syrups. The concentration of sucrose in simple syrup is 66.7% w/w. The other sugars to which certain polyhydric alcohols may be added to inhibit crystallisation or to modify solubilisation, taste and other vehicle properties.
ii) Simple syrups containing flavouring agents but not medicinal substances are called non-medicated or flavoured syrups. The

simple and flavoured syrups are intended to serve as pleasant tasting vehicles for medicinal substances.

iii) Simple syrups containing medicinal substances (therapeutic agent) with or without flavouring agents are known as medicated syrup.

Sugarless syrups may contain sweetening agents and thickening agents. Syrups may contain ethanol (95%) as a preservative or as a solvent to incorporate flavouring agents. Antimicrobial agents may also be added to syrups.

Syrups provide a pleasant means of administering a liquid form of a disagreeable-tasting drug. They are particularly effective in the administration of drugs to youngsters, since their pleasant taste usually dissipates any reluctance on the part of the child to take the medicine.

Formulation considerations for syrup

In the preparation of medicated syrup, the water-soluble drug that is stable in aqueous solution may be added to the simple or flavoured syrup. However, care must be exercised to ensure compatibility between the drug substance and the other formulation components of the syrup. Also, certainly flavoured syrups have an acidic medium, whereas others may be neutral or slightly basic and the proper selection must be made to ensure the stability of any added medicinal agents.

Formulation of syrup

Most syrups contain the following components in addition to the purified water and medicinal agents (*a*) The sugar, usually sucrose, or sugar substitute used to provide sweetness and viscosity; (*b*) Antimicrobial preservatives; (*c*) Flavouring agents; and (*d*) Colourants.

1. *Vehicles:* Vehicle plays a significant role in the formulation of syrups. As mentioned above in medicated syrup the water-soluble drug is added to the simple or flavoured syrup. Simple or flavoured syrups are prepared by using the purified water as a vehicle. It is important to note that potable water should not be used for preparing the syrup because it contains both volatile and non-volatile impurities. Pharmacopoeial purified water is used as a vehicle for the preparation of syrup. Pharmacopoeial purified water is freshly boiled and cooled potable water. The process of boiling and cooling can be done by using reverse osmosis or distillation in order to kill all types of microorganisms.

2. *Sugar and sugar substitute:* Sucrose is the sugar, which is most frequently employed in syrups, although, in special circumstances, it may be replaced in whole or in part by other sugars or substances such as sorbitol, glycerin and propylene glycol. In some instances, all glycogenetic substances (materials converted to glucose in the body) are replaced by non-glycogenetic substances, such as methylcellulose or hydroxyethyl cellulose.

3. *Antimicrobial preservative:* The amount of a preservative required to protect syrup against microbial growth varies with the proportion of water available for growth, the nature and inherent preservative activity of some formulation materials (*e.g.,* many flavouring oils that are inherently sterile and possess antimicrobial activity) and the capability of the preservative itself. Among the preservatives commonly used in syrups with the usually effective concentrations are benzoic acid (0.1% to 0.2%), sodium benzoate (0.1% to 0.2%) and various combinations of methylparaben, propylparaben and butylparaben totalling about 0.1%.

4. *Flavouring agents:* Most syrups are flavoured with synthetic or naturally available flavouring agents, such as volatile oils (*e.g.*, orange oil, lemon oil etc), vanillin and others, to render good flavour to the syrup. Among all the flavoured syrups the raspberry syrup is excellent flavouring agent for bitter drugs in paediatric formulation. Since syrups are aqueous preparations, the flavouring agents must be water soluble. However, sometimes a small amount of alcohol is added to syrup to ensure the continued solution of poorly water-soluble flavouring agents.

5. *Colouring agents:* To enhance the appeal of the syrup, a colouring agent that correlates with the flavouring agents are added. Such as green with mint, brown with chocolate, etc. Generally, the colouring agent is water soluble, non-reactive with the other syrup components, colour should be stable at the pH range and under the intensity of light that the syrup is likely to encounter during its shelf life.

Methods of preparation of syrup

Depending on the physical and chemical characteristics of the ingredients used, syrups are prepared by one of four general methods, (1) solution of the ingredients with the aid of heat, (2) solution of the ingredients by agitation without the use of heat, or the simple admixture of liquid components, (3) addition of sucrose to a prepared medicated liquid or to a flavoured liquid and (4) percolation of either the source of the medicating substance or the sucrose. Sometimes syrup is prepared by more than one of these methods.

1. *Solution of the ingredients with the aid of heat*

i) This method is preferred when syrup are prepared quickly and syrup components are not damaged or volatilized by heat.

ii) In this method, the sugar is generally added to the purified water and heat is applied until the sugar is dissolved.

iii) Then, other heat-stable components are added to the hot syrup, the mixture is allowed to cool and its volume is adjusted to the required quantity by the addition of purified water.

iv) If heat-labile agents or volatile substances, such as volatile flavouring oils and alcohol are added, to the syrup after the sugar is dissolved by heat and the solution is rapidly cooled to room temperature.

2. *Solution by agitation without the aid of heat*

i) To avoid heat-induced inversion of sucrose, the syrup may be prepared without heat by agitation. On a small scale, sucrose and other formulating agents are dissolved in purified water by placing the ingredients in a vessel larger than the volume of syrup to be prepared, permitting thorough agitation of the mixture.

ii) This process is more time consuming than the use of heat, but the product has maximum stability. Huge glass lined or stainless steel tanks with mechanical stirrers or agitators are employed in the large-scale preparation of syrups.

iii) Sometimes simple syrup or some other non-medicated syrup, rather than sucrose, is employed as the sweetening agent and vehicle. In that case, other liquids that are soluble in the syrup or miscible with it may be added and thoroughly mixed to form a uniform product.

iv) When solid ingredients are to be added to syrup, it is best to dissolve them in a minimal amount of purified water and incorporate the resulting solution into the syrup.

3. *Addition of sucrose to a medicated or flavoured liquid*

i) When medicated liquid, such as a tincture or fluid extract, is employed as the source of medication in the preparation of syrup.

ii) The tincture or fluid extract is miscible with aqueous preparations, it may be added directly to simple syrup or to a flavoured syrup.

4. *Percolation method*

In the percolation method, either sucrose may be percolated to prepare the syrup or the source of the medicinal component may be percolated to form an extractive to which sucrose or syrup may be added. This latter method really is two separate procedures: first the preparation of the extractive of the drug and then the preparation of the syrup.

Examples of syrup

1. Prepare and dispense 100 ml of simple syrup I.P. Formula is given in below Table 3.1.

Table 3.1: Formula for simple syrup I.P.

Ingredients	*Quantity*
Sucrose	667 g
Purified water (Q.S)	1000 ml

Method of preparation sucrose to purified water and heat it to dissolve sucrose with occasional stirring. Cool it and add more of purified water to make the required quantity.

2. Prepare and dispense 100 ml of Tolu syrup I.P. Formula is given in Table 3.2

Table 3.2: Formula for Tolu syrup I.P.

Ingredients	*Quantity*
Tolu balsam	12.5 g
Sucrose	660 g
Purified water (Q.S)	1000 ml

Method of preparation

This syrup is prepared by percolation process. Initially add boiling purified water to the tared vessel containing Tolu balsam. Cover the vessel lightly and boil the contents gently for half an hour with continuous stirring. Add purified water to adjust the specified weight. Cool, filter the solution and add sucrose. Heat on a water bath to dissolve the sucrose. Finally, add a sufficient quantity of purified water to produce the required volume.

Quality control tests for syrups

1) *Visual inspection*: Syrup is carefully examined for appearance. The physical appearance of the products is critical for patient adherence and compliance. Therefore the product should be; clear and elegance in appearance.

2) *Light transmission matter/colour:* Light transmission matter is a newer tool - used to check syrup colour. Syrup sample is checked for colour by passing light through the sample. The % of light transmission – compared to light transmission rates set for different grades.

3) *pH measurement:* Measurement and maintenance of pH is also very important step in the quality control testing. Generally, pH of the preparation is measured by pH paper or pH meter. pH between 6.0 to 7.0 is ideal for syrup preparation.

4) *Physical stability:* Syrups must be stable physically *e.g.*, its appearance (no crystallization and microbial growth). Colour must be completely soluble with other ingredients. Odour and taste should be palatable and solid material is completely miscible in liquid.

5) *Sucrose concentration*: The determination of sucrose concentration is also very important in quality control test of syrups. If the concentration of sucrose in the syrup is very high it may crystallize and if less may favour the microbial growth. There is no specific method for the determination of sucrose in syrup; HPLC and UV-spectroscopy can be used.

6) *Refractive index:* The value of refractive index of syrups should be in the range of 1.4608 to 1.4630.

7) *Viscosity measurement:* Viscosity is a property of liquids that is directly related to the resistance to flow. Viscosity measurement is very important quality control test in case of syrups. Viscosity and consistency

directly relate with stability of syrups. Generally, viscosity is measured by Brookfield viscometers.

Container

Syrup preparation is usually packed in glass or plastic bottle, for this viscous preparations wide-mouthed bottle should be used. The products which require protection from light a light-resistant container is necessary.

Storage

The syrup should be stored in well dried and well-stoppered bottles in a cool and dark place. The syrup should be stored at a temperature not exceeding 25°C.

ELIXIRS

Elixirs are clear, sweetened, aromatic, hydro-alcoholic, flavoured liquid preparations containing one or more active ingredients dissolved in a vehicle. Non-medicated elixirs are employed as vehicles and medicated elixirs are used for the therapeutic effects.

Compared with syrups, elixirs are usually less sweet and less viscous because they contain a lower proportion of sugar and consequently are less effective than syrups in masking the taste of medicinal substances. However, because of their hydroalcoholic character, elixirs are better than aqueous syrups to maintain both water-soluble and alcohol-soluble components in solution. Also, because of their stable characteristics and the ease with which they are prepared (by simple solution), from a manufacturing standpoint, elixirs are preferred to syrups.

Formulation of elixirs

1. *Vehicles:* The main ingredients of the elixirs are ethyl alcohol (5-40%) and water. The proportion of alcohol in elixirs varies widely because the individual components of the elixirs have different water and alcohol solubility characteristics. Naturally, for elixirs containing agents with poor water solubility, the proportion of alcohol required is greater than for elixirs prepared from components having good water solubility. In addition to alcohol and water, other solvents, such as

glycerin and propylene glycol, are frequently employed in elixirs as adjunctive solvents.

2. *Preservatives:* Elixirs containing more than 10% to 12% of alcohol are usually self-preserving and do not require the addition of an antimicrobial agent. Some commonly used preservatives are benzoic acid (0.1% to 0.2%), sodium benzoate (0.1% to 0.2%) and various combinations of methylparaben, propylparaben and butylparaben totalling about 0.1%.

3. *Sweeteners:* Although many elixirs are sweetened with sucrose or with sucrose syrup, some use sorbitol, glycerin, and/or artificial sweeteners. Elixirs having a high alcoholic content usually use an artificial sweetener, such as saccharin, which is required only in small amounts, rather than sucrose, which is only slightly soluble in alcohol and requires greater quantities for equivalent sweetness.

4. *Flavouring and colouring agents:* All elixirs contain flavouring agents to increase their palatability and most elixirs have colouring agents to enhance their appearance.

Preparation of elixirs

Elixirs are usually prepared by a simple solution with agitation and/or by admixture of two or more liquid ingredients. Alcohol-soluble and water-soluble components are generally dissolved separately in alcohol and in purified water, respectively. Then the aqueous solution is added to the alcoholic solution, rather than the reverse, to maintain the highest possible alcoholic strength at all times so that minimal separation of the alcohol-soluble components occurs. When the two solutions are completely mixed, the mixture is made to the volume with the specified solvent or vehicle.

The presence of glycerin, syrup, sorbitol and propylene glycol in elixirs generally contributes to the solvent effect of the hydroalcoholic vehicle, assists in the dissolution of the solute, and enhances the stability of the preparation.

Example of elixir

1. Prepare and dispense 100 ml of piperzine citrate elixir I.P. Formula is given in Table 3.3

Table 3.3: Formula for piperzine citrate elixir I.P.

Ingredients	*Quantity*
Piperazine citrate	180 g
Glycerine	100 ml
Chloroform spirit	5 ml
Orange oil	0.25 ml
Syrup	500 ml
Purified water (Q.S.)	1000 ml

Method of preparation

Dissolve the piperazine in part of purified water add the orange oil, glycerine, syrup, chloroform spirit and sufficient quantity of purified water to produce the required volume.

Quality control test for elixirs

1) *pH measurement:* The measurement and maintenance of pH is important step in the quality control test. Generally, pH of the preparation is measured by pH paper or pH meter. pH between 6.0 to 7.0 is ideal for elixirs.

2) *Refractive index:* The value of refractive index of elixirs should be in the range of 1.4608-1.4630.

3) *Determination of alcohol concentration:* Elixir usually contains 5 to 40% alcohol. The determination of alcohol is performed unless otherwise specified in the individual monograph.

4) *Viscosity measurement:* Viscosity is a property of liquids that is directly related to the resistance to flow. Generally, viscosity is measured by Brookfield viscometers.

Container

Container for elixirs should be narrow-mouthed, screw-capped, colourless, plain bottle with a black coloured label.

Storage

Because of their usual content of volatile oils and alcohol, elixirs should be stored in tight, light-resistant containers and protected from excessive heat.

A disadvantage of elixirs for children and for adults who choose to avoid alcohol because of their alcoholic content.

EMULSION

Emulsions are biphasic liquid dosage forms consisting of two immiscible liquids one of which is dispersed as minute globules into the other.

The liquid which is converted into minute globules is called the 'dispersed phase' and the liquid in which the globules are dispersed is called continuous phase. Normally, two immiscible liquids cannot be dispersed for a longer period. So, an emulsifying agent is added to the system. It forms a film around the globules in order to scatter them indefinitely in the continuous phase so that a stable emulsion is obtained.

The emulsions having large globules in micrometer range are called macro or coarse emulsions. The emulsions having globule size in the range of 100-1000 A° (1-100 nm) are known as microemulsion. In contrast to macroemulsion, microemulsions are optically transparent, isotropic and thermodynamically stable. Microemulsion exhibits viscoelestic gel phase, when internal phase is added in excess.

Advantages

1. To mask the unpleasant taste of the drug.
2. Emulsions have enhanced bioavailability.
3. Sustained and controlled drug release can be achieved.
4. It is possible to include two incompatible ingredients, one in each phase of the emulsion.
5. Emulsions can be administered as a nutritional supplement.
6. Radio opaque emulsions are used as diagnostic agent in X- rays examinations.
7. Emulsions are used widely to formulate externally used products like lotions, creams, liniments

Disadvantages

1. Preparation needs to be shaken well before use.
2. Storage conditions may affect stability.

3. Emulsions are bulky and difficult to transport and prone to container breakages.
4. Liable to microbial contamination which can lead to cracking.

Types of emulsion

1. Based on the nature of the dispersed phase and a dispersion medium
   - Oil-in-water (*o/w*)
   - Water-in-oil (*w/o*)
2. Based on the globule size
   - *Macroemulsions*: The emulsions having globule size in micrometer range.
   - *Microemulsions*: The emulsions having globule size in the range of 100-1000 A° (1-100 nm).
3. Multiple emulsions: These are emulsion within emulsion and designated as o/w/o or w/o/w.

Test for identification of o/w or w/o type of emulsions

Dilution test: In this test, the emulsion is diluted either with oil or water. If the emulsion is o/w type and it is diluted with water, it will remain stable as water is the dispersion medium but if it is diluted with oil, the emulsion will break as oil and water are not miscible with each other. Oil in water emulsion can easily be diluted with an aqueous solvent whereas water in oil emulsion can be diluted with an oily liquid.

Conductivity test: This test is based on the basic principle that water is a good conductor of electricity. Therefore in case of o/w emulsion, this test will be positive as water is the external phase. In this test, an assembly consisting of a pair of electrodes connected to a lamp is dipped into an emulsion. If the emulsion is o/w type, the bulb glows.

Dye solubility test: In this test, when an emulsion is mixed with a water-soluble dye such as amaranth and observed under the microscope, if the continuous phase appears red, then it means that the emulsion is o/w type as water is the external phase and the dye will dissolve in it to give colour but if the scattered globules appear red and continuous phase colourless, then it is w/o type. Similarly, if an oil-soluble dye such as Scarlet red C or Sudan III is added to an emulsion and the continuous phase appears red, then it w/o emulsion.

Creaming test: The direction of the creaming precisely identifies the emulsion type, if the densities of the aqueous phase and oil phase are known. Water-in-oil emulsion normally creams downward as oil is usually less dense than water. In oil-in-water emulsions normally cream upwards.

Fluorescence test: Some fixed oils possess the physical property of fluorescing in the presence of UV radiations. On microscopic observation of emulsion under UV radiation, the whole field fluorescence indicates that oil is in the continuous phase (w/o type emulsion) and droplet fluorescence indicates that oil is present in dispersed phase (o/w type emulsions).

Formulation of emulsions

1. *Emulsifying agents*

These are substances added to an emulsion to prevent the coalescence of the globules of the dispersed phase. They are also known as emulgents or emulsifiers. These agents have both a hydrophilic and a lipophilic part in their chemical structure. All emulsifying agents concentrate at and are adsorbed onto the oil/water interface to provide a protective barrier around the dispersed droplets. In addition to this protective barrier, emulsifiers stabilize the emulsion by reducing the interfacial tension of the system. Some agents enhance stability by imparting a charge on the droplet surface thus reducing the physical contact between the droplets and decreasing the potential for coalescence. Thus these act in three ways:

i) Formation of a protective barrier
ii) Reduction of interfacial tension
iii) Decreasing the potential for coalescence by forming an electrical double layer.

Selection of emulsifying agents using HLB method

A system was developed in 1949 by William C. Griffin to assist in making systemic decisions about the amounts and types of surfactants needed in stable products. The system is called the HLB (hydrophile-lipophile balance) system and has an arbitrary scale. HLB numbers are experimentally determined for the different emulsifiers.

An emulsifier having a low HLB number indicates that the number of hydrophilic groups present in the molecule is less and it has a lipophilic character. For example, spans generally have low HLB number and they are also oil soluble. Because of their oil-soluble character, spans cause the oil phase to predominate and form a w/o emulsion. Applications of surfactants and HLB requirement are shown in Fig. 3.1.

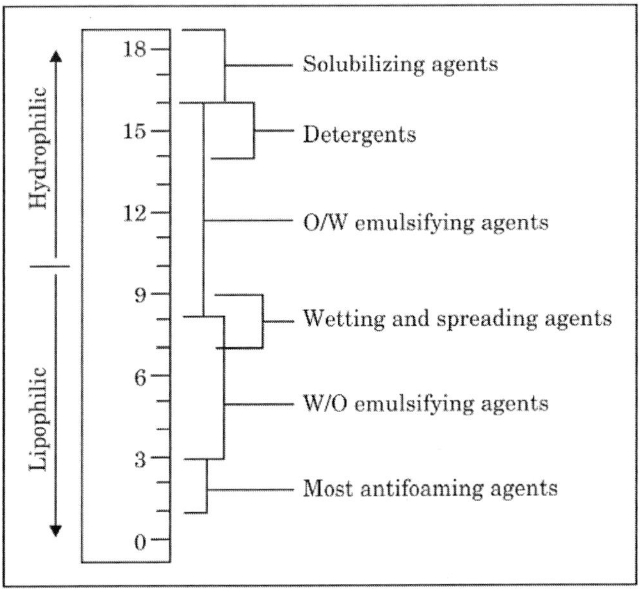

Fig. 3.1: Application of surfactants and their HLB requirements

A higher HLB number indicates that the emulsifier has a large number of hydrophilic groups on the molecule and therefore is more hydrophilic in character. Tweens have higher HLB numbers and they are also water soluble. Because of their water-soluble character, Tweens will cause the water phase to predominate and form an o/w emulsion. HLB values of different emulsifying agent and their applications are given in Table 3.4.

Classification of emulsifying agents

A) *Natural emulsifying agents*

1. *From vegetable sources*: These consist of agents which are carbohydrates and include gums and mucilaginous substances. Since

Table 3.4: HLB values of different emulsifying agent and their applications.

Emulsifying agent	*HLB value*	*Applications*
Glyceryl monostearate	3.8	Emulsifying agent w/o
Sorbitol monostearate	4.7	Emulsifying agent w/o
Acacia	8.0	Emulsifying agent o/w
Triethanolamine oleate	12.0	Emulsifying agent o/w
Tragacanth	13.2	Emulsifying agent o/w
Polysorbate 60	14.9	Detergent
Polysorbate 80	15.0	Solubilising agent
Polysorbate 20	16.7	Solubilising agent
Sodium oleate	18.0	Solubilising agent
Sodium lauryl sulphate	40.0	Emulsifying agent o/w

these substances are of variable chemical composition, these exhibit considerable variation in emulsifying properties. They are anionic in nature and produce o/w emulsions. They act as primary emulsifying agents as well as secondary emulsifying agents (emulsion stabilizers). Since carbohydrates act a good medium for the growth of a microorganism, therefore emulsions prepared using these emulsifying agents have to be suitably preserved in order to prevent microbial contamination. *e.g.,* tragacanth, acacia, agar, chondrus (Irish moss), pectin and starch.

Gum acacia: Gum acacia is generally, used in the concentration of 8-15% and gives a stable and palatable emulsion over the pH range of 2-10. Emulsions tend to cream using this as the viscosity is low. The other natural emulsifying agents from vegetable sources are tragacanth (1-2%), agar (2%), starch (2-5%) and pectin (1%). Tragacanth and starch are rarely used now because they form thick and coarse emulsions.

2. *From animal source:* The examples include gelatin (1%), egg yolk (12-15%) and wool fat (anhydrous lanolin). Type-A gelatin (cationic) is generally used for preparing o/w emulsion while type-B gelatin is used for o/w emulsions of pH 8 and above.

B) *Semi-synthetic polysaccharides*

Semi-synthetic polysaccharide includes mainly cellulose derivatives like sodium carboxymethyl cellulose, hydroxypropyl cellulose and methylcellulose. They are used for formulating o/w type of emulsions. They are nontoxic and are less subject to microbial growth. They primarily act by increasing the viscosity of the system. *e.g.,* Methylcellulose, hydroxypropyl cellulose and sodium carboxymethyl cellulose.

C) *Synthetic emulsifying agents*

This group contains surface active agents which act by getting adsorbed at the oil-water interface in such a way that the hydrophilic polar groups are oriented towards the water and lipophilic non-polar groups are oriented towards oil, thus forming a stable film. This film acts as a mechanical barrier and prevents coalescence of the globules of the dispersed phase. They are classified according to the ionic charge possessed by the molecules of the surfactant *e.g.,* anionic, cationic, non-ionic and ampholytic.

1. *Anionic surfactants*: The long anion chain on dissociation imparts surface activity, while the cation is inactive. These agents are primarily used for external preparations and not for internal use as they have an unpleasant bitter taste and irritant action on the intestinal mucosa. *e.g.,* alkali soaps, amine soaps, metallic soaps, alkyl sulphates and phosphates and alkyl sulphonates.

2. *Cationic surfactants*: The positive charge cations produced by dissociation are responsible for emulsifying properties. They are mainly used in external preparations such as lotions and creams. Quaternary ammonium compounds such as cetrimide, benzalkonium chloride and benzethonium chloride are examples of important cationic surfactants. These compounds besides having good antibacterial activity are also used in combination with secondary emulsifying agents to produce o/w emulsions for external application.

3. *Non-ionic surfactants*: They are the class of surfactants widely used as emulsifying agents. They are extensively used to produce both oil in water and water in oil emulsions for internal as well as external use. The emulsions prepared using these surfactants remain stable over a wide range of pH changes and are not affected by the addition of acids and electrolytes. They also show low irritancy as compared to other surfactants. *e.g.,* glyceryl esters such as glyceryl monostearate, propylene glycol monostearate, macrogol esters such as polyoxyl stearates and polyoxyl-castor oil derivatives, sorbitan fatty acid esters such as spans and their polyoxyethylene derivatives such as tweens (polysorbates 80 or polyoxyethylene sorbitan monooleate).

4. *Ampholytic surfactants*: These are the substances whose ionic charge depends on the pH of the system. Below a certain pH, these are cationic while above a defined pH, these are anionic. At intermediate pH, these behave as zwitterions. *e.g.,* lecithin.

D) *Finely divided solids*

This group consists of finely divided solids having balanced hydrophilic lipophilic properties. They accumulate at the oil/water interface and form a coherent interfacial film around the droplets of dispersed globules and prevent coalescence. If the solid particles are wetted by oil w/o emulsion is formed. If wetting is done by water then o/w emulsion is formed. The emulsions formed using finely divided solids are stable and less prone to microbial contamination. Examples: bentonite, aluminium magnesium stearate, attapulgite, colloidal anhydrous silica, hectorite etc.

E) *Auxiliary emulsifying agents*

A variety of fatty acids (stearic acid), fatty alcohols (stearyl or cetyl alcohol) and fatty esters (glyceryl monostearate) serve to stabilize creams through their ability to thicken the emulsion. Because these agents have only weak emulsifying properties, hence they are always used in combination with other emulsifiers.

2. *Preservatives*

The emulsions which are prepared by using an emulsifying agent, such as proteins, carbohydrates, sterol and non-ionic surfactants may lead to the growth of bacteria, fungi and moulds in the presence of water. The contamination of emulsion by these microorganisms may cause an unpleasant odour, taste and discolouration. Due to the breakdown of emulsifying agents, changes occur in the consistency of an emulsion which may lead to cracking of emulsion.

In order to preserve emulsion properly, it is desirable that along with maintaining precautions to avoid contamination, a suitable preservative is also included in the formulation of an emulsion. List of preservatives and their concentration is given in Table 3.5.

Table 3.5: List of preservatives and their concentration.

Preservatives	*Concentration (%)*
Benzoic acid	0.1 – 0.2
Methyl paraben and propyl paraben	0.1 – 0.2
Chloroform	0.25
Chlorocresol	0.1
Cetrimide	0.002 – 0.01
Phenyl mercuric nitrate	0.004 – 0.01

3. *Antioxidants*

During storage of emulsion the fats (obtained from vegetable and animal sources) and emulsifying agents (wool fat, wool alcohol) undergo oxidation by atmospheric oxygen. This can be avoided by using antioxidant, such as tocopherol, gallic acid, propyl gallate, ascorbic acid etc. Sometimes oxidation occurs due to enzymes produced by microorganisms. Such problems should be prevented by adding a suitable antimicrobial preservative.

4. *Flavours*

A combination of flavouring and sweetening agent provides greater palatability to emulsion. Vanillin is a good flavouring agent for liquid paraffin emulsion. Benzaldehyde is used as a flavouring agent for cod liver oil emulsion.

Method of preparation of the emulsion

Generally, the following methods are used for the preparation of emulsion on a small scale

1. Dry gum method
2. Wet gum method
3. Bottle method
4. Other methods

1. *Dry gum method:* In this method, the oil is first triturated with gum with a little amount of water to form the primary emulsion. The trituration is continued until a characteristic 'clicking' sound is heard and a thick white cream is formed. Once the primary emulsion is formed, the remaining quantity of water is slowly added to form the final emulsion. The ratio of oil: water: gum for preparation of primary emulsion is given in Table 3.6.

Example: Prepare and submit 100 ml of Arachis oil emulsion using a dry gum method. The formulation is given in Table 3.7.

Since Arachis oil is fixed oil so the ratio of oil: water: gum for preparing a primary emulsion is 4:2:1 so the formula for primary emulsion is given in Table 3.8.

Table 3.6: General formula for the preparation of the primary emulsion.

Type of oil	***Examples of oils***	***Oil: water: gum***
Mineral oil	Liquid paraffin	3: 2: 1
Fixed oil	Castor oil	4: 2: 1
	Almond oil	
	Arachis oil	
	Cod-liver oil	
Volatile oil	Turpentine oil	2: 2: 1
	Peppermint oil	
	Cinnamon oil	

Table 3.7: Formulation table for Arachis oil emulsion.

Ingredients	***Quantity***
Arachis oil	50 ml
Purified water add to	200 ml

Approximate volume of primary emulsion = 87. 5 ml and the total volume of emulsion = 200 ml. So the volume of water required is 200-87.5 = 112.5 ml.

Table 3.8: Formula for primary emulsion.

Ingredients	***Quantity***
Arachis oil	50 ml
water	25 ml
Acacia	12.5 g

Method: Measure the required quantity of Arachis oil in a dry measuring cylinder and transfer it into a dry mortar. Add calculated quantity gum acacia powder and triturate rapidly to form a uniform mixture. (The trituration should be either clockwise or anticlockwise if both the directions of triturations are followed that leads to breaking of emulsion). Add a required quantity of water and triturate vigorously until a clicking sound is produced and the product becomes white. Add remaining water intermittently to produce the required volume. Transfer the emulsion into a bottle, label and dispense.

2. *Wet gum method:* As the name implies, in this method first gum and water are triturated together to form a mucilage. The required quantity of oil is then added gradually in small proportions with thorough trituration to form the primary emulsion. Once the primary emulsion has been formed a remaining quantity of water is added to make the final emulsion. Example for castor oil emulsion is given in Table 3.9.

Table 3.9: Formula for castor oil emulsion.

Ingredients	*Quantity*
Castor oil	8 ml
Purified water	30 ml

Here, castor oil is a fixed oil. The proportion of oil: water: gum for preparing the primary emulsion is 4:2:1 and it is given in Table 3.10.

Table 3.10: Formula for primary emulsion.

Ingredients	*Quantity*
Castor oil	32 ml
Purified water	16 ml
Gum acacia powder	8 gm

Approximate volume of primary emulsion = 56 ml and total volume of emulsion = 120 ml. So the volume of water required is 120-56 = 64 ml.

Method: Powder the gum acacia in a mortar. Add water and triturate to form mucilage. Add the required quantity of castor oil in small portions with rapid trituration until a clicking sound is produced and the product became white. Add more of water in small portions to the primary emulsion with trituration to produce the required volume. Transfer the emulsion to a bottle, label and dispense.

3. ***Bottle method:*** This method is employed for preparing emulsions containing volatile and other non-viscous oils. Both dry gum and wet gum methods can be employed for the preparation. As volatile oils have a low viscosity as compared to fixed oils, they require a comparatively large quantity of gum for emulsification. In this method, oil or water is first shaken thoroughly and vigorously with the calculated amount of gum. Once this has emulsified completely, the second liquid (either oil or water) is then added all at once and the bottle is again shaken vigorously to form the primary emulsion. More of water is added in small portions with constant agitation after each addition to produce the final volume.

4. ***Other methods:*** Hand homogenizer: The homogenizer is hand operated and the coarse emulsion is passed through a fine orifice the emulsion is placed in the hopper of the homogenizer. The up and down movement of the handle causes course emulsion to draw in through inlet value and pass through homogenizing valve. In this way, the emulsion is forced to pass through the fine orifice the oil globules are broken into fine globules of uniform size.

Silverson mixer homogenizer: It consists of an emulsifier head which is covered with fine-meshed stainless steel sieve. The emulsifier head consists of a number of blades which rotate at a very high speed in order to produce a powerful shearing action. The blades are rotated by using an electric motor fitted at the top. The emulsifier head is placed in a vessel containing immiscible liquids, in such a way that it should get dipped into it. When the motor is started, the liquids are sucked through the fine holes and the oil is reduced into fine globules due to the rotation of the blades so a fine emulsion is produced which is then expelled out. The intake and expulsion of the mixture set up a pattern of circulation.

Stability of emulsions

An emulsion is a thermodynamically unstable preparation so care has to be taken that the chemical, as well as the physical stability of the preparation, remains intact throughout the shelf life. There should be no appreciable change in the mean particle size or the size distribution of the droplets of the dispersed phase and secondly droplets of the dispersed phase should remain uniformly distributed throughout the system. Instabilities seen in the emulsion can be grouped as:

1. *Flocculation:* In this case, neighbouring globules come closer to each other and form colonies in the external phase. This aggregation of globule is not clearly visible. This is probably the initial stage that leads to instability. Flocculation is due to interaction of attractive and repulsive forces whereas creaming is due to density difference in the two phases.

2. *Creaming:* An emulsion is said to cream when the oil or fat rises to the surface, but remains in the form of globules, which may be redistributed throughout the dispersion medium by shaking. An oil of low viscosity tends to cream more readily than one of high viscosity. Increasing the viscosity of the medium decreases the tendency to cream. Creaming is a reversible phenomenon which can be corrected by mild shaking. The factors affecting creaming are best described by Stoke's Law

$$V = \frac{2r^2 (d_1 - d_2)g}{9\eta}$$

Where, V = rate of creaming, r = radius of globules, d_1 = density of dispersed phase, d_2 = density of dispersion medium, g = gravitational constant and η = viscosity of the dispersion medium

The following approaches can be used for decreasing creaming

(i) Reduction of globule size: According to Stoke's law, the rate of creaming is directly proportional to the size of globules. Bigger is the size of the globules, more will be the creaming. Therefore in order to minimize creaming, globule size should be reduced by homogenization.

(ii) Increasing the viscosity of the continuous phase: Rate of creaming is inversely proportional to the viscosity of the continuous phase *i.e.*, more the viscosity of the continuous phase, less will the problem of creaming. Therefore to avoid creaming in emulsions, the viscosity of the continuous phase should be increased by adding suitable viscosity enhancers like gum acacia, tragacanth etc.

3. *Coalescence:* A few globules tend to fuse with each other and form bigger globules. In this process, the emulsifier film around the globule is destroyed to a certain extent. This step can be recognized by increased globule size and reduced number of globules. Coalescence is observed due to insufficient amount of emulsifying agent, incompatibilities between emulsifying agents and altered partitioning of the emulsifying agents.

4. ***Cracking or breaking:*** Cracking or breaking of emulsion is indicated by complete separation of oil and aqueous phases. It is an irreversible process *i.e.* simple mixing fails to resuspend the globules in to a uniform emulsion because the protective sheath around the globules is completely destroyed.

Cracking or breaking can be due to the addition of an incompatible emulsifying agent, chemical or microbial decomposition of an emulsifying agent, the addition of electrolytes, exposure to increased or reduced temperature or change in pH.

5. ***Phase inversion:*** In phase inversion o/w type emulsion changes into w/o type and vice versa. It is a physical instability. It may be brought about by the addition of an electrolyte or by changing the phase volume ratio or by temperature changes. Phase inversion can be minimized by using the proper emulsifying agent in adequate concentration, keeping the concentration of dispersed phase between 30 to 60 % and by storing the emulsion in a cool place.

Quality control and stability tests for emulsions

The physical parameters evaluated as quality control tests for emulsion are:

- Determination of globule size and globule distribution
- Determination of viscosity
- Determination of phase separation
- Determination of electrophoretic properties

1. ***Determination of globule size and globule distributuion:*** Determination of changes in the average globule size or the size distribution of globule is an important parameter used for the evaluation of emulsions. It is performed by optical microscopy, sedimentation by using Andreasen apparatus and Coulter counter apparatus.

2. ***Determination of viscosity:*** Determination of viscosity is carried out to assess the changes that might take place during ageing. Emulsions exhibit the non-newtonian type of flow characteristics. The viscometers which should be used include cone and plate viscometers.

Capillary and falling sphere type of viscometer should be avoided. For viscous emulsions, the use of penetrometer is recommended as it helps in the determination of viscosity with age. In case of o/w emulsions, flocculation of globules causes an immediate increase in viscosity. After this change, the consistency of the emulsion changes with time. In case of w/o emulsions, the dispersed phase globules flocculate quite rapidly resulting in a decrease in viscosity, which stabilizes after 5 to 15 days. As a rule, a decrease in viscosity with age reflects an increase in globule size due to coalescence.

3. ***Determination of phase separation:*** This is another parameter used for assessing the stability of the formulation. Phase separation may be observed visually or by measuring the volume of the separated phases.

4. ***Determination of electrophoretic properties:*** Determination of electrophoretic properties like zeta potential is useful for assessing flocculation since electrical charges on particles influence the rate of flocculation. Zeta potential or electrokinetic potential is the difference in potential between the surface of the tightly bound layer and the electroneutral region. The o/w emulsion having a fine particle size will exhibit low resistance but if the particle size increase, then it indicates a sign of oil droplet aggregation and instability.

Determination of instability in an emulsion

There is no quick and sensitive method for determining instability in emulsion. To speed up the stability testing the emulsion is subjected to various stress conditions such as:

- Temperature
- Centrifugation
- Agitation

After subjecting the emulsion to the stress conditions it is evaluated for above mentioned quality control tests. The recommendation for shelf life prediction in temperate (hot and humid) zone: The emulsion should be stable with no visible signs of separation for at least:

- 60 to 90 days at 45-50°C
- 5 to 6 months at 37°C

- 12 to 18 months at room temperature
- After one month storage at 40°C
- After 2 to 3 freeze-thaw cycles between –20 C to +20°C
- After 6 to 8 freeze thaw cycles between 4 to 45°C with storage at each temperature for not less than 48 hours.
- No deterioration by centrifuging at 2000 to 3000 rpm at room temperature. (Centrifugation at 3750 rpm in a 10 cm radius centrifuge for a period of 5 hours is equivalent to the effect of gravity for about one year)
- No deterioration by agitation for 24 to 48 hours on a reciprocating shaker (nearly 60 cycles per minute) at room temperature and at 45°C.

Containers

Depending on the use, emulsions should be packed in suitable containers. Emulsions meant for oral use are usually packed in well-filled bottles having an airtight closure. Light sensitive products are packed in amber coloured bottles. For viscous emulsions, wide mouth bottles should be used.

Labelling

A secondary label "Shake well before use" should be written on the label.

Storage

Emulsions should be stored in an airtight container protected from light, high temperature and emulsion should be stored in a cool place.

SUSPENSIONS

Suspensions are the biphasic liquid dosage form of medicament in which the finely divided solid particles ranging from 0.5 - 5 μ are dispersed in a liquid vehicle.

The solid particles act as dispersed phase whereas liquid vehicle acts as the continuous phase. In suspension particle size of the dispersed phase plays a very important role. The drugs which are not stable in solution form are suspended to maintain the chemical stability and its efficacy. The drugs which have bitter taste and solubility problems are formulated in the form of suspensions for oral use.

Advantages

1. *Stability*: Some drugs are not stable in solution form. In such cases, it is necessary to prepare an insoluble form of that drug. Therefore drugs are administered in the form of suspension. *e.g.,* Procaine penicillin G.

2. *Choice of solvent*: If the drug is not soluble in water and solvents other than water are not acceptable, the suspension is the only choice *e.g.,* parenteral corticosteroid.

3. *Mask the taste*: In some cases, drugs are made insoluble and dispensed in the form of suspension to mask the objectionable taste *e.g.,* chloramphenicol base is very bitter in taste, hence the insoluble chloramphenicol palmitate is used which does not have the bitter taste.

4. *Prolonged action*: Suspension has a sustaining effect, because, before absorption, the solid particles should be dissolved. The drug formulated as suspension follows zero order kinetics in which the concentration in solution depends on the drugs solubility. The drug in suspended particles acts as reservoir. As the drug from the solution depletes, more drug is released from the suspended particles so that the concentration remains constant. Ones the entire solid is exhausted, the system exhibits first order release rate.

5. *Bioavailability*: Drugs in suspension exhibit a higher bioavailability compared to other dosage forms (except solution) due to its large surface area, higher dissolution rate. *e.g.,* antacid suspensions provide immediate relief from hyperacidity than its chewable tablet form.

Disadvantages

1. Dose precision cannot be achieved unless suspensions are packed in unit dosage forms. Therefore, potent drugs cannot be administered as suspensions.
2. Sedimentation of solid particles is the major problem encountered during its shelf life.

3. Suspensions are being liquid dosage forms and relatively bulky, sufficient care must be taken during handling and transportation.
4. Suspensions are more prone to oxidation and hydrolysis.

Classification of suspensions

Depending upon the sedimentation rate of particles suspensions are classified into two types:

1. Flocculated suspension
2. Deflocculated suspension

1. *Flocculated suspension*

Flocculation is the formation of light, fluffy groups of particles held together by weak Van der Waal's forces. In flocculated suspension, the suspended particles are in open network or loose aggregation between them. Hence, flocculated particles are sediment together at a very high rate and as they are loosely held together, re-disperse very easily, just by shaking the container.

2. *Deflocculated suspension*

In this type of suspension, the dispersed particles exist as separate entities. The sedimentation rate is very slow but closed aggregation is formed and it is difficult to redistribute even after shaking the container. Difference between flocculated and deflocculated is given in Table 3.11

Formulation considerations

The following ingredients are used in the formulation of suspensions

i) Insoluble drug
ii) Vehicle (suspending medium)
iii) Wetting agents
iv) Compounds allowing control of stability and sedimentation (flocculating and suspending agent)
v) Preservatives
vi) Organoleptic additives (flavour, colour and taste)

Table 3.11: Difference between flocculated and deflocculated suspension.

Flocculated system	*Deflocculated system*
1. Particles form loose aggregation called flocs	1. Particles exist as separate entities
2. Formation of sediment is fast	2. Formation of sediment is slow
3. The rate of sedimentation is very high	3. The rate of sedimentation is very slow
4. No hard cake formation	4. The hard cake is formed
5. Sedimentation is redispersed by shaking the container	5. Redispersion is not possible even after shaking the container
6. Some flocs stick to the wall of the container	6. No such sticking is found
7. Supernatant is clear	7. The supernatant is not clear

1. ***Insoluble drug:*** The points to be considered related to the insoluble drug includes size of the particles, the size distribution of the powder, ease of wetting, the surface electric charge of the particles in suspension, chemical stability of the drug and possible interactions and incompatibilities with other suspension constituents.

2. ***Vehicle (suspending medium):*** Distilled water or deionized water, water-alcohol, a solution of glycerol are used as a vehicle in the preparation of oral suspension.

Structured vehicles: Structured vehicles are vehicles containing thixotropic compounds/polymers like acacia which are pseudoplastic or plastic in nature. Thixotropic compounds/polymers form a three-dimensional gel network structure which entraps the particles so that, ideally, no settling occurs. During shaking the gel network is completely destroyed (pseudoplastic and plastic in nature) so that administration is facilitated.

3. ***Wetting agents:*** It is difficult to disperse solid particles in a liquid vehicle due to the layer of adsorbed air on the surface. Thus, the particles, even high density, float on the surface of the liquid until the layer of air is displaced completely. The use of a wetting agent allows removing this air from the surface and easy penetration of the vehicle into the pores.

Powders, which are not easily wetted by water and accordingly show a large contact angle, such as sulfur, charcoal and magnesium stearate are called hydrophobic. Powders which are readily wetted by water are called hydrophilic *e.g.,* zinc oxide, talc. The wettability of a powder may be ascertained easily by observing the contact angle and spreading coefficient. Drave's test is commonly used to measure the efficiency of wetting agents.

Surfactants: They reduce the interfacial tension between the solid particles and a vehicle. As a result of the lowered interfacial tension, the spreading coefficient will be positive and the contact angle is lowered, air is displaced from the surface of the particles and wetting is promoted. Surfactants promote flocculation, hence surfactants with high HLB helps to stabilize suspensions. Disadvantages of surfactants are that they have foaming tendencies. All surfactants are bitter except pluronics and poloxamers. Polysorbate 80 is most widely used surfactant both for parenteral and oral suspension formulation.

Glycerin and similar hygroscopic substances: Alcohol, glycerin, polyethene glycol and polypropylene glycol flow into the voids between the particles to displace the air and reduce liquid air interfacial tension so that water can penetrate and wet the individual particles.

Hydrophilic colloids: Hydrophilic colloids coat hydrophobic drug particles in one or more than one layer. This will provide hydrophilicity to drug particles and facilitate wetting. As most of the hydrophilic colloids are negatively charged, they cause deflocculation of suspension because the force of attraction is declined. *e.g.,* acacia, tragacanth, alginates, guar gum, pectin, gelatin, wool fat, egg yolk, bentonite, veegum, methylcellulose etc.

4. *Compounds controlling stability and sedimentation*

A) *Thickening agents (suspending agents/viscosity modifier)*: Suspensions have the least physical stability amongst all dosage forms due to sedimentation and cake formation. As per the Stoke's law sedimentation can be minimized by increasing viscosity of suspensions. When the viscosity of the dispersion medium increases, the terminal settling velocity decreases thus the dispersed phase settle at a slower rate and they remain dispersed for a longer time yielding higher stability to the suspension. On the other hand as the viscosity of the suspension increases, it's pourability decreases and inconvenience to the patients for dosing increases. Certain suspensions with a high percentage of dispersed solids exhibit an increase in resistance to flow with increasing rates of shear. Such systems actually increase in volume when sheared and hence, they are termed as dilatant. There fore viscosity of suspension should be maintained within optimum range to yield stable (slow sedimentation) and easily pourable suspensions.

The viscosity of a pharmaceutical preparation may be determined through the use of a viscometer, such as a Brookfield viscometer, which measures viscosity by the force required to rotate a spindle in the fluid being tested.

Ideal thickening agent

- Should have a high viscosity at negligible shear, *i.e.,* during storage.
- Should have a low viscosity at a high shearing rate, *i.e.,* it should be free flowing during agitation, pouring, and spreading.

Pseudo-plastic substances such as tragacanth, sodium alginate, and sodium carboxymethylcellulose show these desirable qualities. A suspending agent which is thixotropic, as well as pseudo-plastic, are useful since it forms a gel on standing and becomes fluid when disturbed.

- Apart from above, suspending agents should also be inert, non-toxic and compatible with other excipients used in suspensions.
- They should be readily dissolved or dispersed in water without need of special technique.
- They should not influence the absorption or dissolution rate of the drugs.

The thickening agents are included in the formulation of suspension to improve the viscosity of vehicle thus stabilize the suspension. Thickening agents are categorised into polysaccharides and inorganic agents.

Polysaccharides:

The number of natural, semi-synthetic and synthetic polysaccharides is used as a thickening agent in the formulation of suspension.

a) Natural polysaccharides

Tragacanth: It is better thickening agent than acacia. It is used as compound tragacanth powder or tragacanth mucilage to suspend heavy in diffusible substances. Tragacanth mucilage is used when the vehicle is water or chloroform water.

Compound tragacanth powder contains starch 20%, tragacanth 15%, acacia 20% and sucrose. Compound tragacanth powder used in the concentration of 2 g per 100 ml of mixture. The compound tragacanth is always used when the vehicle is other than water or chloroform water.

Gum acacia: It is a good suspending agent and a protective colloid. It is more effective when it is used as compound tragacanth powder.

Sodium alginate: Sodium alginate forms viscous dispersion when added to water. Its 1% solution has the same suspending power as that of tragacanth mucilage.

Starch: Sometimes the starch is used in combination with some other suspending agent due to the high viscosity of its mucilage. It is one of the ingredients of compound tragacanth powder.

b) Semi-synthetic polysaccharides

The following cellulose derivatives are used as thickening agents such as methylcellulose (0.5-2%), sodium carboxymethylcellulose (0.25-1%), microcrystalline cellulose etc.

c) Synthetic polysaccharides

Carbomer (carboxy vinyl polymer): It is used in the concentration of 0.1 to 0.4%, it acts as a thickening agent

Colloidal silicon dioxide: It is white non-gritty powder acts as a suspending agent and used in the concentration of 1.5 to 4%.

Inorganic agents

Aluminium hydroxide: It is used as a suspending agent in the suspension containing barium sulphate, calamine and sulphonamide.

Clays: Aluminium magnesium silicate and bentonite are very commonly used as thickening agents. Aluminium magnesium silicate is a creamy white, colourless and tasteless powder. Bentonite is a very pale buff or creamy hygroscopic powder.

Co-solvents: Some solvents which themselves have high viscosity are used as cosolvents to enhance the viscosity of the dispersion medium: For example glycerin, propylene glycol, sorbitol. Glycerin viscosity is too high to pour easily and to spread on the skin. It shows the undesirable property of stickiness. It is too hygroscopic to use in the undiluted form.

B) Flocculating agents: Flocculating agents are added to enhance particle re-dispersibility in the dispersion medium. In contrast to deflocculated particles, flocculated suspensions can always be re-suspended with gentle agitation.

The best approach is to achieve a controlled flocculation of the particles, where they appear as floccules or like tufts of wool with a loose fibrous structure. Controlled flocculation of particles is obtained by adding flocculating agents, which are (1)-electrolytes (2)-surfactants (3)-polymers

Electrolytes act as flocculating agents by reducing the electrical barrier between the particles, thus, decrease the zeta potential, this leads to decrease in repulsion potential and makes the particle come together to form loosely arranged structure (floccules). *e.g.,* monobasic potassium phosphate

Optimum concentrations of surfactants bring down the surface free energy by reducing the surface tension between liquid medium and solid particles. The particles possessing less surface free energy are attracted towards each other by Van der-Waals forces and forms loose agglomerates. *e.g.,* Tween 80, sodium lauryl sulphate etc.

Polymers like starch, alginates, cellulose derivatives, carbomers, tragacanth are a long chain, high molecular weight compounds containing active groups spaced along their length. These agents act as flocculating agents because part of the chain is adsorbed on the particle surface with the remaining parts projecting out in the dispersion medium. Bridging between these portions leads to the formation of floccules.

5. *Preservatives*

The presence of suspending agent and medicaments may promote the growth of microorganisms due to their presence in the atmosphere.

Hence, to safeguard preparations it is necessary to incorporate preservatives in the suspension which inhibits or protect the preparation from microbial growth. Examples: methylparaben, propylparaben, benzoic acid, sodium benzoate etc.

6. *Organoleptic additives*

To have patient acceptance, the colour, flavour and taste of the preparation are improved by adding the suitable organoleptic additives. The bitter taste can be overcome by adding sweetening agent such as syrup or coating the particle suitable polymers and then suspending it. The fruit flavours can be used for suspension meant for internal use and cosmetic flavours for external preparations. The colouring agents are used so as to have better elegance and patient acceptance.

The general method of preparation of suspension

1. Weigh the required quantity of previously powdered drugs and excipients since particle size plays an important role in the stability of the suspension.
2. Mix all the additives along with drug in a mortar to have homogeneous mass. This is important specifically in case of potent drugs where the amount of drug to be incorporated is very small.
3. Add the vehicle slowly with proper trituration sufficient to form a smooth paste. This is required to have complete wettability and thorough mixing of all the ingredients.
4. Volatile materials or insoluble materials are mixed with or without a vehicle.
5. The paste is further diluted with the vehicle in geometric dilution until pourable.
6. Add other volatile substances, diluted previously if required preferably in the same vehicle.
7. Add any liquid ingredient if remaining and mix well.
8. Rinse the mortar and pestle with the vehicle and add to the preparation.
9. Make up the final volume as per the requirement and shake thoroughly.

Evaluation of suspension

Following are the evaluation parameters for suspension

1. Particle size
2. Rheological property
3. Electrokinetic property
4. Physical stability of the suspension
   - Sedimentation volume
   - Degree of flocculation

Particle size (Micromeritics): The stability of suspension depends on the particle size of the dispersed phase. Change in the particle size with reference to time will provide useful information regarding the stability of a suspension. A change in particle size distribution and crystal habit is studied by microscopy and Coulter counter method.

Rheological property: It provides information about settling behaviour of suspended particles in suspension and arrangement of the vehicle and the particle structural features. Brookfield viscometer is used to study the viscosity of the suspension. It is mounted on heli-path stand and using T-bar spindle. T-bar spindle is made to descend slowly into the suspension and the dial reading on the viscometer is then a measure of the resistance the spindle meets at various levels. This technique also indicates at which level of the suspension structure is greater owing to particle agglomeration. The dial reading is plotted against the number of turns of the spindle. The better suspension shows a lesser rate of increase of dial reading with spindle turns, *i.e.,* the curve is horizontal for long period.

Electrokinetic property: Electrokinetic property evaluation involves measurement of Zeta-potential on suspended particles using microelectrophoresis apparatus or Zeta meter. The determination of surface electric charge or zeta potential of suspension is helpful to find out the stability of suspension.

As mentioned above above, Zeta potential or electrokinetic potential is the difference in potential between the surface of the tightly bound layer and the electroneutral region.

Zeta potential governs the degree of repulsion between the adjacent ions of the like charges. Hence, it is used to predict the particle-particle interaction. Such information provides insights about the stability of the systems containing dispersed particles. An optimum zeta potential is desirable for the maximum stability.

Physical stability of suspension: Physical stability is defined as a condition in which particle remains uniformly distributed throughout the dispersion without any signs of sedimentation. It is difficult to achieve this condition. Hence, the definition can be restated as– if the particles settle, they should be easily re-suspendable by a moderate amount of shaking. Therefore the extent of sedimentation and ease of re-suspendability are evaluated by appropriate methods.

The extent of sedimentation is quantitatively expressed by two parameters. They give a gross picture of stability. These are applicable to flocculated suspension.

Sedimentation volume: Sedimentation volume is defined as

$$F = \frac{Vu}{Vo} = \frac{\text{Ultimate volume of sediment}}{\text{Initial volume of sediment}}$$

Where 'F' is sedimentation volume, it is a dimensionless number. Normally 'F' value is in between 0 to 1. In general higher, the sedimentation volume, the better is the physical stability. Sedimentation volume method is used as one of the common basic quality control tools because it is simple and easy to calculate.

The degree of flocculation: Degree of flocculation (β) is defined as

$$\beta = \frac{F}{F_\alpha} = \frac{\text{Sedimentation volume of flocculated system}}{\text{Sedimentation volume of deflocculated system}}$$

If the β value is near to one, then the suspension does not represent a flocculated suspension. It indicates that the system under study is a deflocculated system if β can assume any value greater than one. In general, the higher the value of β the greater physical stability of the suspension.

Containers

Suspensions should be packed in a container which is having adequate air space above the liquid to facilitate adequate shaking. The suspensions meant for oral administration should be packed in wide mouth bottles to permit easy removal with an accurate volume.

Labelling

The containers having liquid suspension must be labelled with the secondary label "shake well before use". In case of dry suspension powders the specified amount of vehicle to be mixed make be indicated clearly on the label.

Storage

The suspension should be stored in a cool and dry place but should not be kept in a refrigerator.

Dry Powders for Oral Suspension

A number of official and commercial preparations consist of dry powder mixtures or granules that are intended to be suspended in distilled water or some other vehicle prior to oral administration.

Most drugs prepared as a dry mix for oral suspension are antibiotics. The dry products are prepared commercially to contain the antibiotic drug, colourants (FD&C dyes), flavours, sweeteners (*e.g.,* sucrose or sodium saccharin), stabilizing agents (*e.g.,* citric acid, sodium citrate), suspending agents (*e.g.,* guar gum, xanthan gum, methylcellulose) and preserving agents (*e.g.,* methylparaben, sodium benzoate) that may be needed to enhance the stability of the dry powder or granule mixture or the liquid suspension.

When called on to reconstitute and dispense one of these products, the pharmacist loosens the powder at the bottom of the container by lightly tapping it against a hard surface and then adds the label-designated amount of purified water, usually in portions and shakes the slurry until all of the dry powder has been suspended.

It is important to add precisely the prescribed amount of purified water to the dry mixture if the proper drug concentration per dosage unit is to be achieved. Also, the use of purified water rather than tap water is needed to avoid the possibility of adding impurities that could adversely affect the stability of the resulting preparation. Generally, manufacturers provide the dry powder or granule mixture in a slightly oversized container to permit adequate shaking of the contents after the entire amount of purified water has been added. Pharmacists must realize that an oversized bottle is provided with each of these products, and they must carefully measure out the required amount of purified water.

Filling of suspension in containers

The method used for filling varies greatly depending on the characteristics of the liquid (example: viscosity, surface tension) foam producing qualities and compatibility with the materials used in the construction of the filling machine, the type of package into which the liquid is to be placed and the required production output. The mostly used filling methods are: gravimetric filling, volumetric filling and constant level filling

Gravimetric filling: In gravimetric filling, the containers are filled with liquids to a given weight. It is generally limited to large containers or to highly viscous products. It cannot be used in high speed, automatic equipment.

Volumetric filling: Volumetric filling is achieved by positive displacement piston action. The fill amount is measured by the stroke of the piston and cylinder assembly. In volumetric filling, problems may arise when containers which are not dimensionally uniform are used. An undersized package appears as full whereas oversized appears to be not completely filled.

Constant level filling: In constant level filling the fill amount is verified by adjusting the height to which the container is to be filled. Any variations in the dimensions of the container may result in the variations in the net fill per unit.

The techniques used for filling are:

Vacuum filling: In which the vacuum developed within the container causes the liquid to flow from the bulk liquid tank to the container and a seal is made between filling head and container. The excess liquid is drawn through a vacuum tube and is recycled.

Gravity vacuum filling: In which the bulk liquids are placed above the filling stem so that the driving force for liquid flow result from negative pressure in the container and the force of gravity.

Pressure vacuum filling: In which a positive pressure is applied to the bulk liquid and vacuum developed in the container results in pressure difference that allows for rapid filling of even high viscous liquids.

The common problem in all types of the process of filling and equipment is the formation of excessive foam. Foaming during filling operation can be decreased by using i) Filling equipment that minimizes product turbulence. ii) Closed system filling to limit the introduction of air that causes foam. iii) Mechanical defoaming devices and iv) Reduction in the speed of the filling line. The packaging materials should be checked for microorganisms before filling to ensure that microbial contamination is not introduced. The microbial contamination from the hands of operators should be avoided by using gloves that are sterilized or periodically disinfected.

Glossary

Syrups	The syrup is a concentrated or nearly saturated solution of sucrose in purified water
Purified water	This is freshly boiled and cooled potable water
Co-solvency	Co-solvency is a process of enhancing the solubility of poorly soluble drugs using co-solvents
Anti-oxidants	These protect the dosage form from degradation due to oxidation
Buffers	Buffers prevent any changes in the pH of the preparation which is important in the maintenance of activity, solubility and stability of the preparation
Chelating agents	Chelating agents complex with the traces of metal ions which may catalyse the undesirable chemical reactions and lead to degradation of the drug product
Preservatives	Preservatives prevent the microbial growth in preparations
Flavouring agents	Flavouring agents improve the palatability of the preparation by imparting a good flavour or masking the objectionable or unpleasant flavour of the drug and the additives
Elixirs	Elixirs are clear, sweetened, aromatic, hydro-alcoholic, flavoured liquid preparations containing one or more active ingredients dissolved in a vehicle
Emulsions	Emulsions are biphasic liquid dosage forms consisting of two immiscible liquids one of which is dispersed as minute globules into the other

HLB (Hydro-philiclipophilic balance)	To assist in making systemic decisions about the concentration and types of surfactants needed in stable products
Emulsifying agents	These are the substances added to an emulsion to prevent the coalescence of the globules of the dispersed phase
Creaming	An emulsion is said to cream when the oil or fat rises to the surface but remains in the form of globules, which may be redistributed throughout the dispersion medium by shaking
Cracking	The primary emulsion does not become white but acquires an oily translucent appearance
Phase inversion	In phase inversion o/w type emulsion changes into w/o type and vice versa
Flocculation	Neighbouring globules come closer to each other and form colonies in the external phase
Coalescence	Few globules tend to fuse with each other and form bigger globules
Suspension	Suspensions are the biphasic liquid dosage form of medicament in which the finely divided solid particles ranging from 0.5 – 5 μ are dispersed in a liquid vehicle
Wetting agents	These are the agents, which reduce the interfacial tension between the solid particles and a liquid medium, thus producing the suspension of the required quality
Stoke's law	The factors affecting creaming are best described by Stoke's Law

QUESTION BANK

Q. I: Multiple Choice Questions

1 Which of the following properties are characteristics of flocculated suspension?

P) Loosely packed sediment
R) Slow sedimentation rate
Q) Close packing of sediment to form
S) Rapid clearance of supernatant a cake

a) P and Q
c) R and S
b) P and S
d) P and R

2 A dilution test can be used for checking stability of

a) Suspension
c) Emulsion
b) Milk and magma
d) All of the above

3 ______ is needed for suspension, lotion, emulsion, creams and ointments to keep high container consistency and yet pour and spread easily when needed. It is also satisfactory for IM slow release yet easy to inject

a) Thixotropy
c) Rheology
b) Rheopexy
d) Newtonian flow

4 The concentration of sucrose in simple syrup BP is

a) 85 % w/w
b) 60.70 % w/w
c) 66.70 % w/w
d) 40.74 % w/w

5 HLB value of sodium lauryl sulphate is

a) 6.5
b) 13.8
c) 25.0
d) 40

6 Addition of sodium chloride to sodium oleate emulsion will:

a) Stabilize emulsion
b) Destabilize emulsion
c) Decrease the globule size of emulsion
d) None of the above

7 HLB system is used to classify

a) Surfactants
b) Preservative
c) Antioxidants
d) Sequestering agent

8 Benzyl peroxide is

a) An astringent
b) an emollient
c) A preservative
d) A keratolytic

9 Surfactants are characterized by the presence of

a) Water-soluble groups alone
b) Fat solubilizing groups alone
c) water and fat solubilizing groups in the same molecule
d) Groups with a positive charge

10 The distribution of globule is not uniform in an emulsion. This stage is called as

a) Creaming
b) Coalescence
c) Caking
d) Breaking

11 In the emulsion, which instability step can be prevented by an emulsifying agent?

a) Breaking
b) Coalescence
c) Creaming
d) Flocculation

12 In an emulsion, If the density of the dispersed phase is higher than the dispersion medium. As per Stokes' equation, the creaming is:

a) At the centre of the emulsion
b) In an upward direction
c) In downward direction
d) In both the direction

13 For an ideal suspension, sedimentation volume should be:

a) Zero
b) Less than one
c) Equal to one
d) More than one

14 Which of the following is used as a preservative in liquid orals?

a) Benzoic acid and its salts

b) Ascorbic acid

c) Alkyl esters of para hydroxybenzoic acid

d) All of the above

15 Elixirs are___________ solution

a) Aqueous

b) Alcoholic

c) Hydroalcoholic

d) None of the above

16 In an emulsion, the factors affecting creaming is explained by

a) Stoke's law

b) Rault's law

c) Henry's law

d) None of the above

17 According to Bancroft's rule, if the solubility of emulsifying agent is in water then what is type of emulsion produced?

a) Oil-in-water

b) Water-in-oil

c) Both a) and b)

d) None of the above

Q. II: Objective Type Questions **2 Marks**

1. Give examples of two anti-oxidants and preservatives used in liquid orals.
2. What is co-solvency? Give two examples of two co-solvents.
3. Define creaming and cracking.
4. What is the sedimentation volume?
5. Write on self-preservation of syrups.
6. What are syrups and elixirs?
7. Write the significance of viscosity in suspension.
8. How is the problem with foam formation minimized in liquid products?
9. Enlist the types of ingredients used for suspensions.
10. List the method of filling liquid orals.

Q. III: Short Answer Questions **5 Marks**

1. Write the method of preparation of suspension
2. Explain in detail various instability conditions of emulsions and its stabilisation methods.
3. Explain formulation of syrup
4. Write the various methods used for evaluation of emulsions.
5. Explain the evaluation and stabilization of suspensions.
6. Explain formulation of elixir.

7. Give the difference between flocculated and deflocculated suspensions
8. Write briefly on the preservation of liquid oral dosage forms.

Q. IV: Long Answer Questions **10 Marks**

1. Describe the different methods of filling orals liquid oral dosage forms
2. Discuss the stability of emulsion and suspension.
3. Write in detail formulation consideration for emulsion and suspensions.

UNIT-III

CHAPTER 4

CAPSULES

INTRODUCTION

The term capsule is derived from the Latin word capsula, meaning a small container. Capsules are solid dosage forms in which one or more medicinal and inert ingredients are enclosed in a small shell or container usually made of gelatin. Capsules are of two types, "hard gelatin capsules" and "soft gelatin capsules". Unpleasant taste and odour of drug can be masked by the tasteless gelatin shell. The administration of liquid and solid drugs enclosing in capsules is one of the most frequently utilized dosage forms.

(A) HARD GELATIN CAPSULE

Hard gelatin capsules are also known as dry-filled capsules or two – piece capsules. Hard gelatin capsules consist of two parts known as capsule body (the longer part) and the capsule cap (the shorter part). The drug substance is placed in the body and the cap is slid over it, hence enclosing the drug substance. They are often believed as the primary oral dosage form because of their simple manufacturing process compared to other oral dosage forms.

Advantages

1. Capsules mask the unpleasant taste and odour of drugs
2. Capsules serve as a convenient medium for dispensing solid, semisolid or liquid forms of drug substances.

3. Tightly sealed capsule shells provide protection to the enclosed drug from harsh conditions of the environment.
4. Capsules especially hard gelatin capsules, are best suitable for enclosing coated beads which help in sustained release action.
5. Capsules are best suited for all types of medicaments since they are available in various sizes.
6. Rectal and vaginal capsules are used as substitutes for suppositories based on oleaginous or water-soluble bases.
7. Improved and rapid bioavailability is provided by capsules.
8. As compared to tablets less excipients are required for capsules.
9. They are attractive in appearance, smooth in nature and can be easily administered.

Disadvantages

1. Hygroscopic drugs cannot be enclosed in a capsule shell as hygroscopic drugs absorb water from the capsule shell, which makes capsule shell brittle.
2. Reactions may occur between the contents of shell and fill materials, *e.g.,* powders which are deliquescent or efflorescent natured cannot be enclosed in capsules as they make the shell of the capsule moist.
3. Drugs which are highly acidic and alkaline in nature cannot be filled in capsules because acidic drugs lead to hydrolysis of gelatin, whereas alkaline drugs cause tanning effects which reduce the solubility of gelatin.
4. Compounds which are volatile or water-soluble or having low molecular weight cannot be filled in capsules as they get evaporated from the capsules shell.
5. Even liquid material such as water, glycerin or any solution of hydrocarbons cannot be filled in capsules, as they dissolve the capsules shell.
6. Even concentrated preparations cannot be enclosed in capsules as these preparations cause irritation in the stomach.
7. Large sized capsule shells or more than one capsule shell may be needed for filling large quantities of a single dose.
8. Capsules, when stored in low humid conditions, become brittle and tend to crack whereas when they are exposed to high humid

conditions the gelatin gets softened and sticks. This is due to the fact that 10-15% of water is present in capsules which accounts for its plasticizing property.

9. Exact filling of capsules is not easy and manufacturing process is costly.

Gelatin for Capsule Shells

Gelatin is a substance of natural origin that does not occur as such in nature. It is prepared by the partial hydrolysis of collagen, which is the main protein constituent of connective tissues. Animal skins and bones are the raw materials used for the manufacture of gelatin. There are two main types of gelatin: type A, which is produced by acid hydrolysis and type B, which is produced by basic hydrolysis.

Extraction of gelatin

Gelatin is a translucent brittle solid, colourless or slightly yellow, tasteless and odourless which is produced by prolonged boiling of animal skin, connective tissue or bones.

Gelatin is a protein product obtained by partial hydrolysis of collagen extracted from skin, bones, cartilage and ligaments. Gelatin melts when heated and solidifies when cooled. Gelatin is soluble only in hot water. Gelatin is industrially extracted from pork skin, calf skin and cattle bones (dry bones).

Extraction of gelatin from pork skin

- Pork skin is collected and hair is removed, it is cut down to get small pieces then washed with water and treated with 1-5% HCl for 10 to 30 h. The treatment with HCl causes hydrolysis of collagen into gelatin and separation of solid, liquid and fats.
- The above mixture is subjected to multiple hot water extraction by agitating with hot water. The gelatin is extracted into hot water and solution gets turbid.
- The obtained turbid solution is centrifuged at a warm temperature to remove fats and solid material. The turbid solution is filtered through ceramic microfilters at high pressure to get a clear solution. If still, turbidity appears in solution then it is passed through a column containing a synthetic resin which will adsorb some salt and absorbs some of the water content.

- The obtained clear solution is subjected to vacuum concentration or evaporation and all the solvent is removed by passing the solution through a series of evaporators to get a concentrate. Hot air is passed through the above concentrate and the solution is sterilized.
- The sterilized solution is cooled by passing the air, the gelatin solution starts gelling. When sufficient gel strength is achieved then it is passed through a perforated disc to get the noodles or ribbons of gelatin. This process is called an extrusion.

The ribbons are air dried to remove moisture and forms a solid which is then milled to get gelatin powder which is packed in the suitable container. Extraction of gelatin from different sources is shown in Fig. 4.1.

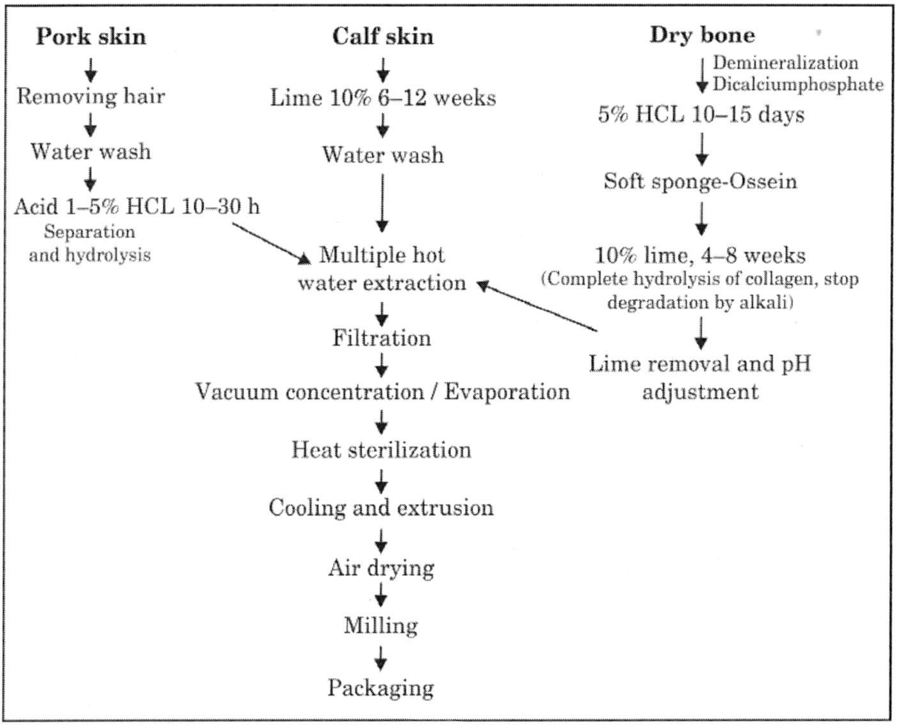

Fig. 4.1: Extraction of gelatin from different sources.

Extraction of gelatin from dry bone

- The bones of cattle is treated with 5% HCl for 10 to 15 days which causes demineralization and removes the dicalcium phosphate as a byproduct and get a soft sponge which is called as ossein.
- For complete hydrolysis of collagen, ossein is again treated with 10% lime for 4 to 8 weeks so that intermolecular bonds in collagen are broken down completely.
- Excessive line treatment will cause the degradation of gelatin so that lime has to be removed in time. pH is adjusted and multiple hot water extraction is carried out to extract gelatin. Further steps are similar to that of extraction of gelatin from pork skin.

Extraction of gelatin from calfskin

- Calfskin is collected and cut to get pieces which is then treated with 10% lime for 6-12 weeks.
- The lime-treated calfskin pieces washed with water for 10-30 h and then multiple hot water extraction is done and further steps are similar to that of pork skin.

Production of hard gelatin capsule shells

The capsule shells are made up of a mixture of gelatin, plasticizers, preservatives, solvents, flavours, thickening agents and water. Sometimes opacifying agents, colours and sugars are also added. The vegetable capsules are manufactured by using hydroxypropyl methylcellulose (hypromellose) and pullulan.

The raw materials used in the formulation of capsule shells are properly studied before selection. Their character, role and quality are taken into consideration as they have an effect on the finished capsules. The constituents used in the formulation of hard and soft gelatin capsules are same. They only differ in the concentration of water and plasticizer. Different constituents used in the formulation of hard and soft gelatin capsules are shown in Table 4.1.

1. *Gelatin*: Gelatin has unique physical, chemical and physiological properties which makes it the best possible ingredient in the manufacturing of capsule shells. Gelatin is non-toxic, good film-forming material produces a strong flexible film, readily soluble in biological

fluids at body temperature. Gelatin is the major component of the capsules and it has been the raw material of choice because of its ability of conversion of the solution to gel and to form a solid at a temperature just above ambient temperate conditions, which enables a homogeneous film to be formed rapidly on a mould pin.

Table 4.1: Different constituents used in the formulation of hard and soft gelatin capsules.

Sl. no.	*Raw materials*	*Examples*
1.	Gelatin	Type A gelatin and type B gelatin
2.	Plasticizers	Glycerine USP, polyhydric alcohol (sorbitol), triacetin
3.	Preservatives	Methyl paraben, propyl paraben and ascorbic acid (0.2%)
4.	Solvents	Oils
5.	Opacifying agents	Titanium dioxide (0.2-1.2%)
6.	Colours	Vegetable colours, FD&C, D&C, water-soluble dyes, pigments and certified lakes (q. s)
7.	Flavours	Ethyl Vanillin (0.1-2%) and Essential oils (upto 5%)
8.	Sugars	Sucrose (up to 5%)
9.	Acids	Fumaric acid (up to 1%)
10.	Thickening agents	Methylcellulose
11.	Water	–

Gelatin is obtained by the partial hydrolysis of collagen obtained from the skin, white connective tissue and bones of animals.

In commerce, gelatin is available in the form of a fine powder, a coarse powder, shreds, flakes, or sheets.

$$\text{Pork skin} \xrightarrow{\text{Acid hydrolysis}} \text{Type -A gelatin}$$

$$\text{Bones or animal skin} \xrightarrow{\text{Alkaline hydrolysis}} \text{Type -B gelatin}$$

Preparation gelatin from animal skin and bones

Capsule shells can be prepared by using either of the two types of gelatin, but the use of a mixture of both the types is in practices. Pork skin is responsible for plasticity while gelatin from bones is responsible for firmness of the gelatin capsules. The isoelectric point of type-A gelatin lies around pH 9 while that of type-B gelatin lies around pH 4.7.

2. *Plasticizers*: Plasticizers are used to impart softness, elasticity and thickness to the capsules shell. The accurate amount of plasticizer to be added depends upon the use and storage conditions of capsules. Plasticizers are used as single or in a combination of two or more. Examples: Glycerine, polyhydric alcohol like sorbitol.

3. *Preservatives:* Preservatives are used to retard the growth of microorganisms. They are usually added to maintain the stability of the shell for a desired period of time. Examples: Methylparaben, propylparaben and ascorbic acid (0.2%).

4. *Solvents:* Solvents are used to make the capsule shells elegant and easily swallowable. Example: Oils

5. *Opacifying agents:* They are used to minimize the transparency and make the capsule shells characteristic (opaque). Example: Titanium dioxide (0.2-1.2%).

6. *Colours*: The addition of colours gives a pleasant appearance to the shells. Single or a combination of two or more colours can be added when desired, provided that they should not impart colour to the enclosed medicaments. Examples: Vegetable colours, F, D &C, D & C water-soluble dyes, pigments and certified lakes (q. s).

7. *Flavours*: These are added to impart good flavour to the capsule shell. They also neutralize the undesirable odour of other ingredients. Examples: Ethyl Vanillin (0.1-2%) and essential oils (up to 5%).

8. *Sugars*: Sugars are used to impart a sweet taste to chewable gelatin capsules and to mask the objectionable taste of the other ingredients. They are used very rarely. Example: Sucrose (up to 5%).

9. *Acids*: These are used for lessening the aldehydic tannings of gelatin. Example: Fumaric acid (up to 1%).

10. *Thickening agents:* These are added to adjust the viscosity of gelatin. Example: Methylcellulose.

11. *Water:* Water content varies in the capsule shells depending upon the storage conditions. Hard gelatin capsules contain 12-16% of water.

For hard gelatin capsules shells, if moisture content below 10% shells become brittle and above 16% moisture content may cause filling problem and loss of mechanical strength.

Steps of hard gelatin capsule shells production

Capsule shells are manufactured by an automatic machine which consists of pins or pegs made up of stainless steel to produce capsules shells of desired shapes and sizes. The mould pins (approximately 50, 000 mould pins) per machine are attached to the plates which are movable. Both caps and bodies are manufactured simultaneously. Capsule shells are manufactured using the automatic machine in five steps (Fig. 4.2) include:

1. ***Dipping*:** The gelatin solution of required viscosity is taken in a reservoir. The plate holding pins are dipped into gelatin solution carefully to the suitable depth for the required period of time. This helps in achieving the proper length and thickness of shells.

2. ***Spinning*:** The pins are slowly withdrawn from the solution and then rotated during their transfer to the upper level of the machine, in order to form a uniform film thickness over pins.

3. ***Drying*:** The plate holding the pins is slowly raised from the gelatin solution and is subjected to blow drying with air having controlled temperature and humidity. During this period the gelatin sets or gels over the pins.

4. ***Stripping and Trimming:*** The pins are moved through a series of controlled air drying kilns for the gradual and precisely controlled removal of water. The capsules are stripped from the pins by bronze jaws and trimmed to length by stationary knives while the capsule halves are being spun in chunks or collets.

5. ***Joining of caps and bodies:*** The trimmed caps and body parts are joined and released from the machine.

During the manufacturing, the capsules the pins used for making bodies of capsules have the diameter smaller than those used for making caps. This helps in perfect compressing of caps over the bodies. Hence, in the manufacturing of capsule shells, all the above 5 steps are carried out one after the other with extreme care.

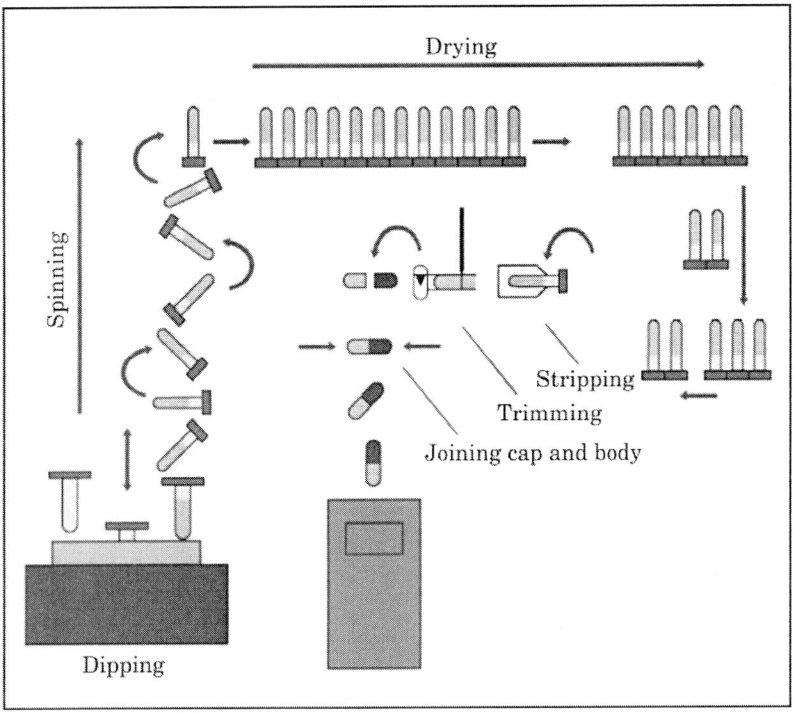

Fig. 4.2: Various steps involved in production of hard gelatin capsule shells.

Size of hard gelatin capsules

For human use, gelatin capsule shells are available in eight different sizes varying in lengths, diameters and capacities. They are numbered from 000 (largest size) to 5 (smallest size).

Capsules are usually used for placing a single dose of drugs but when the dose to be administered is quite large and cannot be placed in a single capsule shell, then two or more capsule shells may be used. On the other hand, when the available dosage of medicament is insufficient to fulfil the capacity of capsule body, then any suitable diluents are incorporated.

The largest powdered drug which can be placed in hard gelatin capsules is about 1000 mg and the minimum dose is 65 mg. depending upon the nature of powdered drug, 65 mg may be placed in capsule size 5 and 1000 mg in capsule size 000. Different size of capsule and powder fill capacity is shown in Table 4.2.

Table 4.2: Different size of capsule and their fill capacity.

Capsule size	*Height (cm)*	*Diameter (cm)*	*Volume (ml)*	*Fill weight (mg) powder Having density 0.70 g/ml*	*Fill weight of Aspirin (mg)*
000	2.61	0.99	1.37	960	1040
00	2.33	0.85	0.95	665	650
0	2.17	0.76	0.68	475	520
1	1.94	0.69	0.50	350	325
2	1.80	0.63	0.37	260	260
3	1.59	0.58	0.30	210	195
4	1.43	0.53	0.21	145	162
5	1.11	0.49	0.13	90	97

For human use, empty capsules ranging in size from 000 the largest to 5 the smallest is as shown in Fig. 4.3.

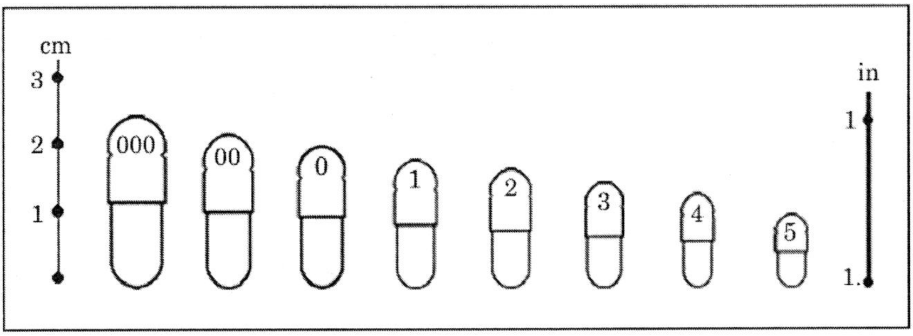

Fig. 4.3: Actual sizes of hard gelatin capsules. From left to right, sizes 000, 00, 0, 1, 2, 3, 4, and 5.

Larger sizes of numbers 10, 11 and 12 are also available which approximately contain 7.5, 15 and 30 g of drug substance respectively. These capsules are used for veterinary purpose.

Capsule size selection

The selection of the capsule size is determined by the dose of the drug, density and compaction characteristic of drug and other excipients. If the dose of the drug is inadequate to fill the volume of the capsule body, diluents are added. Information on the density and compaction characteristics of the material to be filled can serve as a guide in proper selection of the capsule size. A properly filled capsule should have its body filled with drug mixture, not cap. The cap is intended to fit snugly over the body to retain the contents.

Size selection of capsule is based on the tapped density of formulation and capsule volume; these can be calculated by formula:

$$\text{Tapped density} = \frac{\text{Weight of formulation}}{\text{Tapped volume}} \text{ g/ml}$$

$$\text{Capsule volume} = \frac{\text{Capsule fill weight of formulation}}{\text{Tapped density}}$$

Formulation of hard gelatin capsules

The main objective of formulating a capsule is to have a capsule with good stability, accurate dose, elegance, ease in filling and better bioavailability. The hard gelatin capsules are filled with active ingredient (therapeutic agent) along with certain additives. The substances other than the drug used in the preparation of a dosage form (here capsules) are known as additives (or excipients or adjuncts). The additives used in capsules for three main reasons:

- To prevent the microbial degradation of capsules
- To make the process of preparation of capsules easy
- To maintain the stability of the drug

The difference in proportion of additives in two different capsules having the same therapeutically active compound may alter their bioavailabilities, which consecutively alters the desired therapeutic effect of the drug. Some of the additives used in capsules include diluents, disintegrants, glidants, surfactants, protective sorbents, anti-dusting agents and lubricants etc.

(a) Diluents (fillers): When the bulk of the dose of a particular drug substance is too small to completely fill the smallest available capsule shell, diluents are added to the drug substance to produce the proper capsule fill volume. Other than providing bulk, diluents also provide cohesion to the powdered drug. This is helpful while transferring the

blend of the drug into the capsule shell. The amount of diluents to be added depends upon the amount of drug substance and the capacity of capsule shell. Both organic and inorganic substances are used as diluents in the capsules.

Lactose and starch are the widely used diluents in the manufacturing of capsules. The flowability and compactibility of the diluents get enhanced when they are modified. These modified diluents can be conveniently used for filling capsules in fully automatic machines. Diluents with coarse and medium particle size are regarded as the well suitable additives of capsules. They also play an important role in the disintegration of capsules. Examples of organic, inorganic and chemically modified diluents are shown in Table 4.3.

Table 4.3: Organic, inorganic and chemically modified diluents.

Organic diluents	*Inorganic diluents*	*Chemically modified diluents*
Lactose	Calcium carbonate	Pre-gelatinized starch
Mannitol	Calcium phosphate	Spray processed lactose
Microcrystalline cellulose	Magnesium carbonate	Un-milled dicalcium phosphate dihydrates
Starch		
Sorbitol		

(b) Disintegrants: They promote breaking up of the capsule contents in the stomach, hence helps in provoking faster therapeutic effect. The disintegrants having superior properties of swelling or/and absorption of moisture are known as super disintegrants. Some of the examples of super disintegrants are croscarmellose, sodium starch glycolate, crospovidone and pregelatinized starch.

(c) *Glidants (lubricants):* They are used when the powdered drug is to be filled in the capsule shells by automatic machines. They help in enhancing the flow property of powdered drug by either one or more of the following ways:

(i) Alteration of surface charges.

(ii) Imparting of easy movement of the formulation particles

(iii) Prevention of moisture.

(iv) Reduction of coarseness by stuffing the surface irregularities.

(v) Reduction of attractive forces between the particles of formulation.

The commonly used glidants include corn starch, calcium stearate, colloidal silica, magnesium stearate, stearic acid and talcum. The best flow of powder requires an optimum concentration of glidants. This optimum concentration differs with every glidant and it may be the concentration needed to cover all the drug particles. Glidants exceeding this concentration may produce variation in the flow. The powdered drug having good flow properties need no addition of glidants but those powders lacking this property need the addition of a suitable amount of glidants.

(d) *Surfactants*: These agents minimize the waterproofing properties of certain water-insoluble agents filled in the capsules. Hence, after dissolution of the capsule shell in the stomach (GI fluid), these agents displace the air surrounding the drug thereby enhance the dissolution and absorption of drug. Both hydrophilic and lipophilic surfactants are used in capsule formulation *e.g.,* sodium lauryl sulphate, sodium-lauroyl sarcosinate, sodium docusate, sodium stearate, sodium stearoyl -2 lactylate, cetylpyridinium chloride, glyceryl monostearate (lipophilic surfactants).

(e) Protective sorbents: These agents are added to retard the moisture absorption by hygroscopic agents and also for physical separation of incompatible or eutectic agents. Inert substances are used as protective sorbents. The commonly used protective sorbents are calcium carbonate, magnesium carbonate, calcium oxide and magnesium oxide.

(f) Anti-dusting agents: Dust is considered to be the major problem in large-scale operations of capsule filling technique. If dust of potent drugs is inhaled by the operators it may lead to severe health problems. To prevent such circumstances, the additives are mixed with some anti-dusting agents. The ratio of anti-dusting agents to the drug substance has to be strictly monitored as its excess quantities may lead to cohesion of drug particles. The commonly used anti-dusting agents are edible oils.

(g) *Lubricants*: These agents are added to the formulation because they (i) reduce the friction between the sliding surfaces and the powder plug; (ii) prevent the adhesion of powders over pistons and metal surfaces; (ii) facilitate the ejection of plugs from dosator and dosing – disc type machines. The commonly used lubricants are calcium stearate, magnesium stearate and stearic acid. All these lubricants are hydrophobic stearates and among them, magnesium stearate is the most commonly used. Several lubricants which are less hydrophobic lubricants are polyethylene glycols, sodium stearyl fumarate and hydrogenated vegetable oils. High concentration of magnesium stearate may retard the release of medicaments from the capsule shell.

Ideal properties of additives used in the capsule formulation

- It should be of good quality and not impart any impurities to the dosage form
- It should not react with other additives of the preparation
- It should be stable throughout the shelf-life of the product
- It should not alter the therapeutic activity of the drug
- It should be odourless and tasteless to the maximum extent possible

***Preparation of formulation*:** Hard gelatin capsules are commonly filled with dry formulation but when needed, suitable liquids or wet formulation can also be filled.

A. Dry formulation

For preparation of dry formulations, the therapeutically active constituents are thoroughly mixed with suitable additives. The uniform mixture so obtained is filled into the capsule shells. Drugs in very low doses are to be strictly monitored while blending for uniformity, lack of which may alter the desired therapeutic effect. The pre-formulation examination is carried out to know whether all the active and inactive constituents may be mixed as such or need to undergo various operations like particle size reduction, drying etc. to attain uniformity. Powders, pellets, capsules and tablets can be formulated as capsules in dry formulation.

(i) Powders: The filling of powders into capsules in known as Accofil or Elancofil. For filling powdered drug in the capsule shell, the density and the particle size of both, the drug and the additives should be alike for uniform mixing. When the reduction of particle size is required; the ingredients can be milled to obtain particles of 50-1000 um and then blended. Micronization may be performed to produce particles of 1-20 um when the dose of the drug is very low.

(ii) *Pellets*: The filling of pellets into capsules is known as Rotofil. The drug substances which are designed for modified release are moulded in the form of pellets and are coated with suitable coating agents. These coated pellets are then filled in the empty capsule shells.

(iii) Capsules or tablets: Small capsules or tablets are sometimes placed in the capsules shells and the remaining capsule body is filled with weighed inert materials. This may help to isolate the chemically incompatible substances or to add the already weighted potent drugs. Instead of weighing the powdered potent drugs; the same drug available in tablet form can be placed in the capsule shell.

B. *Wet formulation*

The latest developments in the fields of formulation science and technology offer new opportunities for filling liquid and semi-solid formulations in hard gelatin capsules. The formulation in liquid dosage form enhances the bioavailability of several barely-soluble drug actives to achieve a solid oral dosage form. Also, controlled release characteristics can be developed using semisolid formulation.

The filling of liquids into capsules is known as Qualiseal. Though usually powders are filled, but sometimes liquids like fixed oils or volatile oils which do not permeate through the gelatin walls are also filled in the hard capsule shells. The liquids may also be mixed with inert powders and made into pastes or dough mass before filling.

The drug substances which are eutectic or possess the property of liquefying in the presence of other ingredients are to be mixed with absorbents or diluents like kaolin, magnesium carbonate or light magnesium oxide. These agents help to separate the interacting drug substances and absorb the liquids produced.

Methods of Capsule Filling

The moisture content of capsules is directly related to the relative humidity of air to which they are exposed. Capsules are removed from their packaging and exposed during the filling process. The ideal conditions for a filling area are a temperature between 20° C and 25° C and a relative humidity between 35% and 55% which will maintain the moisture content of the capsules within the desired range of 12.0% to 16.0%. Capsules can be filled outside these conditions if sufficient care is taken. The capsules are filled by either of the following methods.

(i) Manual filling
(ii) Hand filling or semi-automatic machines
(iii) Fully automatic capsule filling machines

Manual filling

The manual filling can be opted when very few numbers of capsules are to be filled.

Principle: Manual filling involves separation of caps and bodies, filling of bodies and finally joining of caps and bodies to produce accurately filled capsules.

Method: The ingredients to be encapsulated are triturated to obtain uniform sized particles and placed on a sheet of clean paper. With the help of a spatula, the triturated ingredients are made into a cake such that the height of the cake is almost one third the height of the capsule.

The required numbers of empty capsules are taken and their caps are separated from the bodies. A single body of the capsule is held in between the thumb and the forefinger and is punched into the cake of powdered drug repeatedly until filled. Finally, the cap is placed over the filled body.

This procedure is repeated for the rest of the capsules and they are punched in the same way. This is because; the quantity of powdered drug packed in the capsules depends upon the degree of compression. After capping, the capsules are to be weighed periodically to examine the invariability of the process to avoid improper filling.

Hand filling machine or semi-automatic machine

Principle: The principle of hand filling machine is similar to that of manual filling, except that the rate of capsule filling process is enhanced.

The hand filling machine consists of a fixed lower plate and a movable top plate. Both the plates have grooves for placing capsule bodies and caps. The lower plate has clamps which can carry bodies and helps in removal and replacement of caps. It has the capacity of filling 24 capsules simultaneously. When properly handled, it can produce about 2000 capsules in a day.

Working: The capsule shells are placed in the lower plate manually with the caps facing up. The top plate is placed over this lower plate, a slight pressure is applied and the plate is lifted. It results in separation of caps and bodies (caps in top plate and bodies in the lower plate). The measured amount of powdered drug is spread evenly in all the bodies. Finally, the top plate is replaced over the lower plate so that the caps are placed on the filled capsules bodies *i.e.,* the capsules are sealed and locked simultaneously.

The degree of accuracy lies on the size of capsules and the compression force applied while packing. Finally, the filled and sealed capsules are picked with the hands and are preceded for polishing, finishing, packing etc.

Fully automatic capsule filling machine

Nowadays fully automatic capsule filling machines are being manufactured by a number of companies in the world. A few of them are Eli Lilly and company, Formatic SNC, Hofliger and Karg, Macofer SAS, mG2 SPA, Osaka, parke-Davis and company, perry Industies and Zanasi Nigris. *The principles involved in the filling of hard gelatin capsules are discussed at the end of this chapter.

Capsule Sealing

After filling some manufacturers make tamper-evident capsules by sealing the joint between the two capsule parts. One manufacturer makes distinctive-looking capsules by sealing them with a coloured band of gelatin (Kapseals, Parke-Davis). If removed, the band cannot be restored without expert resealing with gelatin. Capsules may also be sealed through a heat-welding process that fuses the capsule cap to the body through the double wall thickness at their juncture. The process results in a distinctive ring around the capsule where heat welded. Still another process uses a liquid wetting agent that lowers the melting point in the contact areas of the capsule's cap and body and then thermally bonds the two parts using low temperatures (40–45°C). Industrial capsule-sealing machines are capable of producing 60,000 to 150,000 gelatin-banded, heat-welded, or thermally coupled capsules per hour.

Although it is difficult and tedious, extemporaneously prepared capsules may be sealed by lightly coating the inner surface of the cap with a warm gelatin solution immediately prior to placement on the filled capsule body.

Sorting and finishing filled hard gelatin capsule

Sorting: This operation is needed to separate the imperfect and the damaged capsules. Although on a large scale it is done manually, some automatic equipment like Rotosort is also available. Rotosort mechanically sorts the improperly joined caps and bodies, unfilled bodies, dust and the excess powder. It can deal with about 150000 capsules per hour.

The commonly used steps for finishing filled hard gelatin capsule include:

1. Cloth dusting
2. Polishing
3. Brushing

Cloth dusting: It is a manual method in which a small number of capsules is rubbed with a cloth or gauze which may or may not contain inert oil. It helps in removing the adhering material from the surface of the capsule. It also imparts shine to the capsules.

Polishing: A special pan is used for polishing the filled capsules. These pans are lined with cheese or a polyurethane cloth which captures the dust and other powder adhering to the capsules leaving them clean and shiny. Polishing of capsules can also be done by placing the filled capsules in the rotating pans containing salt like sodium chloride granules. After polishing, these granules are separated from the capsules. Nevertheless, this type of polishing must be performed before imprinting the capsules as the print may be affected by sodium chloride.

Brushing: In this method, capsules are projected under soft rotating brushes which remove the dust from the capsule automatic shells. This process is supplemented by exposure of capsules to vacuum.

Automatic equipment like Erweka KEA can also be used for dusting and polishing hard gelatin capsules. It works under vacuum by shaking the capsules between its tassels made up of soft plastic against the punctured plastic sleeves. Any extraneous matter from the capsules is removed by the vacuum.

Difficulties and trouble shooting in hard gelatin capsule filling

(i) Deliquescent or hygroscopic powders: A gelatin capsule contain water which is extracted or taken up by a hygroscopic drug and renders the capsule very brittle which leads to cracking of the capsule. The addition of an adsorbent like magnesium carbonate, heavy magnesium oxide or light magnesium oxide overcomes this difficulty provided the capsules are packed in tightly closed glass capsule vials.

(ii) Eutectic mixtures: Certain substances when mixed together tend to liquefy and form a pasty mass due to the formation of a mixture which has a lower melting point than room temperature. For filling this type of substances each troublesome ingredient is mixed with an absorbent separately then mixed together and filled in capsules. The absorbents used are magnesium oxide and kaolin. Another method in dealing with such type of difficulty is that the substances are mixed together so as to form a eutectic mixture, then an absorbent like magnesium carbonate or kaolin is added.

(iii) Addition of inert powders: When the quantity of the drug to be filled in capsules is very small and it is not possible to fill this much small amount in capsules then inert substance or diluents are added so as to increase the bulk of the powder, which can be filled easily in capsules.

(iv) Use of two capsules: Some of the manufacturers separate the incompatible ingredients of the formulation by placing one of the ingredients in smaller capsule, and then placing this smaller capsule in a larger capsule containing the other ingredients of the formulation.

(v) Filling of granular powder: Some powders which lack adhesiveness and most granular powders are difficult to fill in the capsules by punch method because they are not compressible and flow out of the capsule as soon as they are lifted from the pile of powder into which they are punched. To overcome this difficulty the non-adhesive powders should be moistened with alcohol and the granular powders should be reduced to powder before filling into capsules.

Manufacturing Defects of Hard Gelatin Capsules

Manufacturing defects of hard gelatin capsules (Table 4.4 and Fig 4.4) are classified according to the following definitions:

Major A: Affects the performance of capsule as package for the final product or could contribute to a major filling problem.

Major B: Would cause a problem on capsule filling machine.

Minor: Has no effect on the performance of a capsule as a package, it is slight blemish that makes the capsule visually imperfect.

Table 4.4: Manufacturing defects of hard gelatin capsules.

Major A defects	
Hole	An irregular opening in the cap or body
Split	A split in the film starting from the cap or body edge
Cracked	A cap or body with many splits
Uncut cap/body	An untrimmed cap or body
Failure to separate	Cap and body may not be separated properly
Trimming	A piece or the whole trimmed end of a cap or body inside a closed capsule
Double dip	Extra thick cap due to being dipped twice
Short cap	Cap length is 1 mm less than specified length
Short body	Body length is 0.4 mm less than specified length
Joined in lock	Capsule is in locked position
Double cap	A capsule with an additional cap covering the body end
Unjoined	A single cap or body
Thin spot (cap shoulder)	A thin area in the cap shoulder which may rupture when the capsule is filled
Mashed	A mechanically damaged capsule that has been squashed flat
Long cap/body	Length of cap or body is 1 mm more than specified length
Pinched	Cap or body is damaged in collets. Pinches> 3 mm are classified as a Major A defect
Telescope	A closed capsule with a protruding piece of either cap or body produced by a double split
Major B defects	
Long joined	Capsule not closed sufficiently to engage the pre-lock
Dye speck	A coloured spot of pigment aggregate different from the colour of cap or body
Inverted end	A cap or body with the end pushed inwards
Damaged edgelarge	The edge of the cap is roughly trimmed. The imperfection is V-shaped and >1 mm into the specified length
Small pinched	Cap or body is damaged in collets. Pinches < 3 mm are classified as a Major B defect.
Turned edge	Folded over the edge on body cut line
Thin spot	A thin area in the cap or body wall which may rupture when the capsule is filled
Grease	Mould release aid spots on the inside of capsule

Minor defects

Scrape	A scratch mark on the surface of a cap or body
Crimp	Cap or body is damaged in collets outside of the capsule > 3 mm
Grease light	Small marks of grease
Dent	A depression formed in the end of cap or body. The dent is less than half of the diameter of the capsule part
Damaged edge small	The edge of the cap is roughly trimmed. The imperfection is V-shaped and <1 mm into the specified length
Bubble	An air bubble in the cap or body wall which has a diameter greater than 0.4 mm
Starred end	Multiple small imperfections located at the ends of the cap or body
Chips, tails, string	Small fragments of gelatin still attached or free within the capsule from different colour than cap or body
Dye speck	A small pigment aggregate from the components of the cap or body
Black speck	A non-contaminant black spot

In Process and Final Quality Control Tests for Capsules

1. *Raw material*

The gelatin of capsule shell should be assayed for various physical properties like bloom strength, viscosity, iron content, microbial test etc.

(a) *Bloom strength*: Bloom strength is defined as an assessment of cohesive strength of the cross-linking between the molecules of gelatin. It is also known as gel strength or gel rigidity of gelatin and depends upon its molecular weight. The harder the gelatin, the higher is its bloom strength.

Determination of bloom strength: A gelatin solution having a concentration, of 6.66% w/v is kept for 17 hours at a temperature of 10°C. A plastic plunger of 0.5-inch diameter is taken. The weight (in gram) required to move the plastic plunger 4 mm into the stored gelatin solution determines the bloom strength of gelatin. Depending upon the requirements of capsules manufacturers, bloom strength lies in between 150-250 g. The gelatin used in hard capsule manufacture is of a higher bloom strength (200-250 g) than that used for soft capsules (150 g) because a more rigid film is required for the manufacturing process.

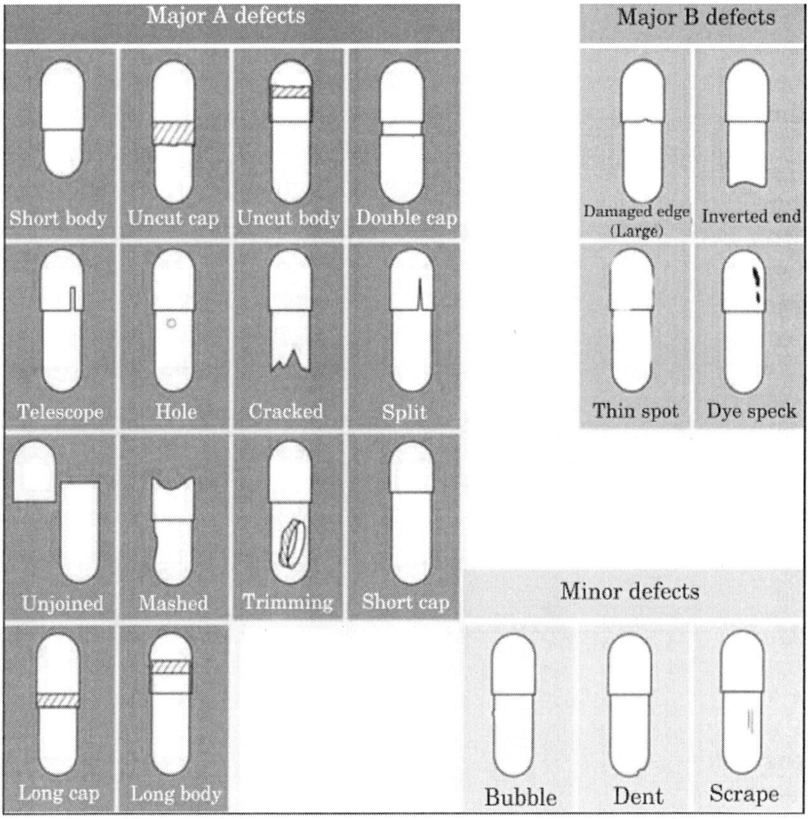

Fig. 4.4: Manufacturing defects of hard gelatin capsules.

Physical stability of capsules is directly proportional to bloom strength of gelatin *i.e.,* on increasing the bloom strength the physical stability of capsules increases. Also, the cost of gelatin capsules shells largely depends upon their bloom strength. More the bloom strength, the higher is the cost because of this reason, the capsules of higher bloom strength are rarely used or used only when capsules of high physical stability are needed.

(b) *Viscosity*: It is defined as the assessment of chain length of gelatin molecules in 6.66% w/v concentrated gelatin solution in warm water at 60°C. It decides the manufacturing aspects of gelatin sheet. The quality of the required gelatin sheet depends upon the standard gelatin formulation. Accordingly, manufacturing is carried out at an appropriate drying condition on a fixed sealing temperature. The gelatin sheets so produced are pharmaceutically elegant, hard non-viscous and are easy to cut. The required viscosity of gelatin lies in between 25-45 millipoise.

(c) *Iron content*: Iron is present in the raw gelatin as well as in the water used for manufacturing of gelatin capsules shells. Excess quantity of iron in the soft gelatin capsules can affect the FD and C (Food, Drugs and Cosmetics) certified dyes and may also react with the other organic compounds. Because of this reason iron is not used in concentration of more than 15 ppm in their manufacturing.

Manufacturing of gelatin sheets for storing, hygroscopic drug substances needs the following adjustments in their properties: adjustment of bloom strength between 180-250 g, adjustment of viscosity between 25-32 millipoise and adjustment of amount of water (reduced to half) for satisfactory working of copulating machine and also to prevent the uptake of moisture from capsule shells.

2. *Moisture permeation test (I.P. 2007)*

The degree and rate of moisture penetration is determined by packaging the dosage unit together with colour revealing desiccant pellet the expose the packaged unit to known relative humidity over a specified time. After some time observe the desiccant pellet for colour change, any change in colour indicates absorption of moisture and by measuring pre-weight and post-weight of pellet, the amount of moisture absorption can be calculated. The standard moisture content specification for hard gelatin capsule is 12–16% w/w.

3. *Content uniformity test (I.P. 2007)*

Determine the content of active ingredient in each of 10 capsules taken at random using the method given in the monograph or by any other suitable analytical method of equivalent accuracy and precision. The capsules comply with the test if not more than one of the individual values thus obtained is outside the limits 85 to 115 per cent of the average value and none is outside the limits 75 to 125 per cent. If two or three individual values are outside the limits 85 to 115 per cent of the average values repeat the determination using another 20 capsules. The capsules comply with the test if in the total sample of 30 capsules not more than three individual values are outside the limits 85 to 115 per cent and none is outside the limits 75 to 125 per cent of the average value.

4. *Weight variation test (I.P. 2007)*

Weigh an intact capsule. Open it without losing any part of the shell and remove the contents as completely as possible. Weigh the shell. The difference between the weighings gives the weight of the contents. Repeat the procedure with another 19 capsules.

Calculate the average weight. Based on the average weight calculate upper limit and lower limit. Not more than two of the capsule content weight deviates from the average weight by more than the percentage shown in the table and none deviates by more than twice that percentage. Percentage deviation allowed as per I.P. is given in Table 4.5.

Table 4.5: Percentage deviation criteria (I.P. 2007)

Average weight of capsule contents	*Percentage deviation allowed*
Less than 300 mg	10%
300 mg or more	7.5%

5. *Disintegration test (I.P. 2007)*

Disintegration test is a method to evaluate the rate of disintegration of solid dosage forms (capsules or tablets). Disintegration is defined as the breakdown of solid dosage form into small particles after it is ingested.

Method: Unless otherwise stated in the individual monograph, introduce one capsule into each tube and, if directed in the appropriate general monograph, add a disc to each tube. Suspend the assembly in the beaker containing the specified liquid and operate the apparatus for the specified time. Remove the assembly from the liquid. The capsules pass the test if all of them have disintegrated.

If 1 or 2 capsules fail to disintegrate, repeat the test on 12 additional capsules; not less than 16 of the total of 18 capsules tested disintegrate.

If the capsules adhere to the disc and the preparation under examination fails to comply, repeat the test omitting the disc. The preparation complies with the test if all the capsules in the repeat test disintegrate. Disintegration is considered to be complete when a) there is no residue on the perforated plate or b) if a residue remains, it consists only of a soft mass having no solid core which cannot be pressed with a glass rod.

6. *Dissolution test (I.P. 2007)*

Apparatus type-1: The capsule sample is allowed to sink to the bottom of the flask before stirring. The paddle is immersed in a dissolution medium. The flask is maintained at 37 ± 0.5°C by a constant temperature bath. For dissolution test, I.P. specifies the dissolution test medium and volume, type of apparatus to be used, rpm of the shaft, time limit of the test and assay procedure. The test tolerance is expressed as % of labelled amount of drug dissolved in the time limit.

Apparatus type-2: A single capsule is placed in a small wire mesh basket attached to the bottom of the shaft connected to a variable speed motor. The basket is immersed in a dissolution medium (as specified in monograph) contained in the flask. The flask is cylindrical with a hemispherical bottom. The flask is maintained at 37 ± 0.5°C by a constant temperature bath. The motor is adjusted to turn at the specified speed and sample of the fluid are withdrawn at intervals to determine the amount of drug in solutions

Dissolution testing and interpretation can be done in three stages:

Stage 1 (S1): Six capsules are tested and are acceptable each unit is not less than D* + 5 per cent**. If fail

Stage 2 (S2): Another six capsules are tested, test individually, Average of 12 units (S1 + S2) is equal to or greater than D, and no unit is less than D –15 per cent**. If fail

Stage 3 (S3): Another 12 capsules are tested. The capsules are acceptable if the Average of 24 units (S1 + S2 + S3) is equal to or greater than D, not more than 2 units are less than D – 15 per cent** and no unit is less than D – 25 per cent**.

*D is the amount of dissolved active ingredient specified in the individual monograph, expressed as a percentage of the labelled content and **Percentages of the labelled content.

Principles of Hard Gelatin Capsule Filling Machines

Hard gelatin capsule filling machines work on following principles

1. *Auger fill principle*

The capsule filling machines like Lilly and Parke Davis and Type 8 capsule filling machines work on this principle.

The empty hard gelatin capsules are taken from the feed hopper into the rectifying unit. The rectifier descends the capsules such that the caps are turned up and the bodies down. This turning is based on the outer dimensional differences of cap and the body. When vacuum is applied, the capsules from the rectifying unit are placed one by one in the filling ring kept on the rotating mode. This ring consists of two parts, the upper ring and the lower ring. Both the parts of the rings have cavities, holes for placing the capsule shells. The bodies, due to vacuum are pulled into the lower ring (vacuum is applied from the underside of the lower ring) and cap part remains in the upper ring. When all the cavities in the ring assembly are filled, the ring is kept aside and the body halves in the lower ring are ready for filling. The lower ring is rotated with a suitable speed and the hopper containing powdered drug is held over this ring. The auger drives the powdered drug into the capsule bodies. After the bodies are completely filled, the hopper is set aside and the rotating ring is stopped. Now the ring holding the caps is placed over the ring holding the bodies which are then joined together. The constant flow of powder mix depends upon its flow properties which in turn depends upon the concentration of individual additives.

The average fill weight using auger fill principle depends upon the size of the capsule, speed of filling machine and the specific volume of the formulation. However, the weight variation depends upon the speed of filling machine, specific volume of the formulation, presence of glidants and flowability of fill material but it is independent of the size of the capsule.

2. *Vibratory fill principle*

The vibratory fill machines like Osaka machine works on the vibratory fill principle. In this type of machine, the feed is placed in the feed hopper and the capsule bodies are passed under it. A perforated resin plate (connected to a vibrator) is placed in the feed hopper. Due to vibrations of the resin plate, the powder flows freely through the pores into the capsule bodies. The weight of the feed to be filled depends upon two criteria *i.e.,* i) The frequency of vibration of the resin plate and ii) The position of the capsule body under the feed hopper

Pins are present below the capsule bodies for their support. Capsule bodies are filled when the pins are pulled down (below the level of discs). But whenever there is an overfilling. The capsule bodies are pushed up to reach the level of the disc plate and the excess of the powder is forced out by scrapping with the hanging edge of the hopper.

In this process, there may be a slight compression of the powder which helps in altering the fill weight of capsule bodies. Weight variation depends upon the characteristics of the powder. However, several lubricants like stearates may be used to prevent the adherence of powder to the equipment.

3. *Piston-tamp principle*

Fully automatic capsule filling machine works on piston-tamp principle by using piston or tamping pins. This piston tamps alter the shape of powder by compressing the powder to form plugs (slugs). These plugs are transferred into the empty capsule bodies with the application of slight pressure. Finally, the bodies are ejected from the machine. The tamping is done with very little compression force, normally in the range of 50-200 N. Hence, the formed plugs are very soft and cannot be removed from the bodies in one piece. Piston tamp principle can be explained by two types of machines (i) Dosing disc type machines and (ii) Dosator type machines.

***(i) Dosing disc type machines*:** Examples of dosing disc type machines are:

a. Hofliger-Karg (bosh GKF models)
b. Harro-Hofliger KFM models

a) *Hofliger-Karg (bosh GKF models):* The dosing disc placed at the bottom of the filling chamber has many cavities bored in it. A stopper plate is present below this disc. It is slidable and works as a stopper of powder. The powder to be filled in the capsules is filled in the cavities of dosing disc. The disc is rotated and the 5 sets of pistons tamp (compress) the powder to form plugs. The pistons tamp every plug five times in every cycle. After five tamps, the extra powder is scraped off by the scrapper. Finally, the plugs are ejected with the help of transferring piston and are placed in the capsule bodies.

The dose of the powder depends upon:

- Depth of the powder
- Cavity depth or thickness of the dosing disc
- Compression pressure

Auger helps to control the flow of powdered feed. In case, the level of the powder is below the required level, the capacitance probe automatically activates the auger to fill the remaining cavity. The powder is spread by centrifugal action of rotation in the dosing disc and the baffles are used to maintain a uniform level of powder. The weight variations in the fill depend upon the angle of repose of the powder. Higher the angle of repose the powder is not freely flowing and lower angle of repose the powder flows too freely.

Carr's compressibility index (CCI): According to the scientist Heda, the carr's compressibility index values must lie in between 18 and 30 to have low weight variations. The powders with CCI values more than 30 (poorly flowing powders) adhere to the ejecting medium. Hence, CCI is inversely proportional to the flowability of the powder. It is calculated for loose bulk density and tapped (compressed/compact) density as follows:

$$\text{CCI }\% = \frac{\text{Tapped density} - \text{Bulk density}}{\text{Tapped density}} \times 100$$

These machines usually need appropriate lubrication so that they are helpful in the easy ejection of powder. Decrease the friction between the sliding components and to prevent adhesion of powder over pistons.

b) *Harro-Hofliger KFM model:* This machine is similar to Hofliger–Karg (Bosh GKF models). The minor differences are Harro-Hofliger

KFM Model consists of three tamping (compression) stations, powder is tamped two times in every cavity and powder mixture in hopper is continuously agitated to have a uniform flow:

(ii) *Dosator type machines*: Examples of dosator type machine

1. Zanasi
2. MG2
3. Farmatic

A dosator type machine is made up of an open-ended cylinder known as dosator. A piston is fitted on its upper end, whose position is set to a determined height known as piston height. The dosator is placed over a powder bed of determined height by agitators and scrapers. The height of the bed is greater than the piston height. The powder enters the open end of dosator and the piston gives a slight tamping blow to compress it thereby, converting the powder into a plug. Now the dosator containing the plug is withdrawn from the powdered bed, passed onto an empty capsule body into which the plug is ejected.

The under/overfill weight of the capsules depends upon the piston height and then upon the height of the powder bed.

Features essential for perfect filling of capsules in dosator machines:

(a) *Slight compactibility:* It helps in formation of plugs and also prevents the loss of powder during transfer from dosator to the capsule body.

(b) *Fluidity*: It helps in flowing of powders from reservoir to the powder bed. It is also helpful in filling up the space formed in the powder bed due to the placement of dosator.

(c) *Bulk density*: Moderate bulk density is needed. Powders with low bulk density or entrapped air may face problems during compression.

(d) *Lubricity:* It helps in the smooth and complete ejection of plug from dosator.

Carr's Compressibility index (CCI): According to Heda, the carr's compressibililty index (CCI) values must lie in between 25 and 35 (for Zanasi LZ 64 machines) to have low weight variations. The powders with CCI values less than 20 (free-flowing powders) may need higher compression forces *i.e.,* in between 150 and 200 N to improve powder retention in the dosator. The powders with high CCI values (more than 30) can produce plugs with low weight variation and good strength.

4. *Vacuum fill principle*

Machine working on vacuum fill principle is Perry Accofil machine. This machine consists of an open-ended cylinder. The upper end of this cylinder is fitted with a piston. The open end (lower end) is placed in the bulk powder. Vacuum is applied and the piston is moved upward by sucking the predetermined amount of powder. This results in filling of the cylinder. The powder is filled up to the piston height and the vacuum is held until the piis positioned over an empty capsule body. Now, the vacuum is broken and pressure in the form of compressed air is applied just to expel the powder into the capsule body. This principle is not commonly employed as it is a lengthy process.

B) SOFT GELATIN CAPSULES

Soft gelatin capsules are also known as soft elastic capsules or softgel. Soft gelatin capsules are one piece, hermetically sealed, soft gelatin shells enclosed with liquid, suspension, semisolid, powder and sometimes prepared tablets. The capsule shell is made up of gelatin, plasticizers, preservatives, solvents, opacifying agents, water and colours. The constituents of soft and hard gelatin capsule shells are similar. The difference lie only in the concentrations of plasticizers and water, the shells of soft gelatin capsules contain more plasticizers and more water than the shells of hard gelatin capsules.

It is estimated that more than 40% of new chemical entities (NCEs) coming out of the current drug discovery process have poor biopharmaceutical properties, such as low aqueous solubility and/or permeability. These suboptimal properties pose significant challenges for the oral absorption of the compounds and for the development of orally bioavailable dosage forms. Development of soft gelatin capsule (softgel) dosage form is of growing interest for the oral delivery of poorly water-soluble compounds (BCS class II or class IV).

Advantages

The softgel dosage form offers several advantages over other oral dosage forms include:

1. As delivering a liquid matrix designed to solubilize and improve the oral bioavailability of a poorly soluble compound as a solid unit dosage form.
2. Delivering low and ultra-low doses of a compound.
3. Delivering a low melting compound and minimizing potential generation of dust during manufacturing and thereby improving the safety of production personnel.
4. Soft gelatin capsule provides ease of use - easy to swallow, no taste, unit dose delivery, and tamper proof.
5. Soft gelatin capsules can hold an exactly measured quantity of medicaments in all the batches.
6. Available in a wide variety of colours, shapes and sizes.
7. Preparation is easier; hence quality control tests can be carried out without any difficulty.
8. Can be easily modified for their biopharmaceutical features.
9. Soft gelatin capsules accommodate a wide variety of compounds filled as a semisolid, liquid, gel or paste.

Disadvantages

1. There may be interactions between filling materials and shell.
2. Choices for filling equipment are very few.
3. Manufacturing requires complicated machinery and it is expensive.
4. Limited choices of excipients/carriers compatible with the gelatin.
5. Drugs from the oily vehicle may pass into the shell.
6. Stability concerns with highly water-soluble compounds and compounds susceptible to hydrolysis.

Nature of Soft Gelatin Capsule Shell

The shell of soft gelatin capsule is composed of gelatin, plasticizer or combination of plasticizers and water. In addition, it may contain preservatives, colouring and opacifying agents, flavourings and sweeteners, possibly sugars to impart chewable characteristics to the shell, gastro-resistant substances and in special cases even active compounds.

The water serves as a solvent to make molten gelatin mass with a pourable viscosity at 60-70°C. The ratio by weight of water to dry gelatin (w/g) can vary from 0.7 to 1.3, depending on the viscosity of the gelatin being used. After capsule formation, most of the water is removed by drying, leading to finished capsules with a moisture content of 4-10%.

Gelatin

The gelatin used for pharmaceutical or health and nutrition soft capsule products are described by the official pharmacopoeias such as USP (United States Pharmacopoeia), PhEur (European Pharmacopoeia) etc., or approved by local authorities, with additional physicochemical specifications. The specifications and controls for gelatins are discussed in a hard gelatin capsule.

A perfect soft capsule gelatin should have the following specifications:

- Gel strength: 150-200 Bloom, depending on the gelatin type
- Viscosity (60°C/6-23 % w/w in water): 2.8-4.5 mPas, depending on the gelatin type
- The well-controlled degree of viscosity breakdown
- Well-defined particle size to allow fast dissolution and de-aeration of the molten mass, even at high gelatin concentrations
- A broad molecular weight distribution to provide a fast setting and the fusion temperature being well below the melting temperature of the plasticized wet film.

Plasticizers

The formation of a soft capsule requires the use of a non-volatile plasticizer in addition to water to guarantee the mechanical stability, *i.e.,* the elasticity of the capsule shells during and after the drying process. The additional plasticizer has to counterbalance the stresses that are induced in the shrinking capsule shells, as the plasticizing effect of water in the shells decreases upon drying.

Practically, only a few plasticizers are in use, namely polyalcohols, which are approved by the official pharmacopoeias or by local regulatory authorities. Glycerol (85% and 98% w/w), special grades of non-crystallising aqueous sorbitol and sorbitol/sorbitan solutions and combinations of these are the most used. In addition, propylene glycol and low molecular weight polyethylene glycol (PEG 200) have been used.

The type and concentration of plasticizer(s) in the shell is related to the composition of the fill, *i.e.,* the possible interactions with the fill, the capsule size and shape, the end use of the product and the anticipated storage conditions. The ratio by weight of dry plasticizer to dry gelatin (P/G) determines the strength of the shell and usually varies between 0.3 and 1.0. The choice of the proper shell formula with respect to the gelatin/plasticizer combination is crucial to the physical stability of the capsules, during manufacture and on storage.

An ideal plasticizer should interact with the gelatin molecules in such a way as to reduce effectively the glass transition temperature (Tg) of the gelatin shell without inhibiting the formation of crystallites that stabilise the three-dimensional gel network structure. In addition, if present in concentrations higher than saturation, it should be physically embedded in the sol phase of the gel network to avoid bleeding out.

Glycerol, the most frequently used soft gelatin capsule plasticizer, combines these advantages of high plasticizer effectively, a sufficient compatibility and a low volatility with the ability to interact specifically with the gelatin allowing for the formation of a stable thermo-reversible gel network. Its plasticizing capability is mainly resulting from direct interactions with the gelatin and only slightly from its hygroscopicity allowing for an additional indirect moisturising effect.

Other additives

Soft gelatin capsules, which contain more moisture than hard capsules, may have a preservative, such as methylparaben and/or propylparaben, to retard microbial growth. In addition to gelatin, the plasticizer(s), water and preservative optional components in the capsule shell are limited in their use. For economic reasons, the addition of active ingredients in the shell is usually not recommended and limited to inexpensive compounds in chewable capsules. The use of water-insoluble polymers to impart sustained- release characteristics to the capsules have failed owing to their limited compatibility with the gelatin mass. Formulations with gastro-resistant enteric soluble polymers are under development.

Colouring and opacifying agents are used frequently to give the shells the desired colour and a proper finish, *i.e.,* to allow the shell to protect the fill from light and to mask the unpleasant look of the fill. As a general rule, the colour of the capsule shell is chosen to be darker than the colour of the fill. Before a colour is chosen, mixtures should be checked to ascertain that fading or darkening of the capsule shells does not occur on storage, as a result of reactions between the colouring agent and other components of the shell or fill.

Size of soft gelatin capsules

The soft gelatin capsules are made from gelatin and water but with the addition of a polyhydric alcohol, such as glycerol or sorbitol, to make them flexible. Sorbitol is less hygroscopic than glycerol. They usually contain a preservative, such as beta-naphthol. They are available in a variety of shapes and sizes as given in Table 4.6.

Table 4.6: Different shapes of soft gelatine capsules.

Shape	*Capacity*
Round	0.05 – 5 ml
Oval	0.05 – 7 ml
Oblong	0.15 – 25 ml
Tubes	0.5 – 10 ml
Miscellaneous	–

They are most suitable for liquids and semisolids and are widely used, in spherical and ovoid forms for vitamin preparations such as cod liver oil, vitamin A and D and multiple vitamins.

Base adsorption

Base adsorption can be defined as weight of the liquid base in gram required so that its capsulatable mix can be prepared with 1 g of a solid or a mixture of solids. Base adsorption parameters help in selecting the appropriate size of soft gelatin capsules for filling medicaments. Base adsorption of a solid depends upon its:

(a) Density
(b) Hydrophobicity or hydrophilicity
(c) Moisture content
(d) Particle shape and size
(e) Physical state like amorphous, crystalline and fibrous

Determination of base adsorption

Determination of base adsorption involves judging the fluidity of the liquid base. The procedure for determination of base adsorption is as follows:

1. A small amount of weighed solid is taken in a 150 ml beaker of known weight. For ease in processing, the weight of the solid is taken is 40 g.
2. About 100 g of liquid base (wetting agent) is taken in another 150 ml beaker of known weight.
3. A small proportion of liquid base is added to the solid with continuous mixing by using a stirrer. Mixing is done to ensure uniform and complete wetting of the solid with the liquid base. For non-ionic or glycol type of bases, wetting agents are rarely needed. But for bases like vegetable oils they are essential. Presently the best suited naturally occurring wetting agent known as soy lecithin is used in a concentration of 2-3% by weight of vegetable oil. It is commonly used in the preparation of food and drugs and has no extra benefit beyond 3%.
4. The addition of liquid base with stirring is continued until the mixture gains a consistency of ointment and flows steadily from the spatula held at an angle of 45° above the mixture.
5. When the mixture stops flowing, the stream of the flow is cut off rapidly near the stirrer rather than stretching out in between the flow.
6. Base adsorption is calculated by formula:

$$\text{Base adsorption} = \frac{\text{Weight of liquid base (g)}}{\text{Weight of solid (g)}}$$

It is defined as the volume (in minims) of 1 g of solid weight of liquid base (in g) required producing a capsulatable mixture. It is calculated by using base adsorption values by formula.

$$\text{Minim per gram (M/g)} = \frac{(\text{Based adsorption } + \text{ 1 g of solid}) \times \text{Volume}}{\text{Weight of mixture}}$$

Smaller capsules are produced when the base adsorption of solids is low and density of blend (mix) is high.

Soft gelatin capsule content

Soft gelatin capsules can be used to dispense active compounds that are formulated as a liquid or semi-solid solution, suspension or microemulsion pre-concentrate. The proper choice of the shell composition therefore only depends on the stability of the active ingredient, the capsule size, shape and end use and the anticipated storage conditions. The formulation of the fill is individually developed to fulfil the following requirements:

- To optimize the chemical stability of the active compound
- To improve bioavailability of the active compound
- To allow for an efficient and safe filling process
- To achieve a physically stable capsule product.

The various types of content that may be encapsulated into soft gelatin capsules include:

1. *Lipophilic liquids (oils):* Lipophilic liquids like triglyceride oils (soya bean oil) are commonly used as filling matrix. The drugs like steroids (*e.g.,* oestradiol) or vitamin D analogues (*e.g.,* hydro-xycholecalciferol) are mixed with these oils and encapsulated in the soft gelatin shells. Other examples of lipophilic liquids used as filling matrices are isopropyl alcohol and aromatic oils.

2. *Hydrophilic nonvolatile liquids:* Hydrophilic liquids like polyethylene glycol 400 having high molecular weight are frequently used. Less amounts (below 10% by weight) of water, glycerine or ethanol can also be used as liquid matrices.

Liquids that can easily migrate through the capsule shell are not suitable for soft gelatin capsules. These materials include water above 5% and low–molecular-weight water-soluble and volatile organic compounds such as alcohols, ketones, acids, amines and esters.

3. *Microemulsion system:* Microemulsion consists of an oil–surfactant–water system having droplet size in sub-micrometre range. For the preparation of microemulsions, a blend of oil and surfactant together with the active ingredient is filled into the soft gelatin shells. Once the capsule disintegrates into the GI fluid, the liquid matrix forms microemulsions with the aqueous GI fluids. Due to the high surface area of the droplets, the drug is rapidly diffused from the oil phase into the aqueous GI fluids. Thus, the drug is readily solubilized as well as retained in solution form after its dilution in the GI fluid.

4. *Nanoemulsion system*: The properties and functions of this system are similar to that of microemulsion system. The only difference is that the size of the droplets of emulsions is about 100 nm.

5. *Emulsifying oils:* A mixture of pharmaceutical oil and a non-ionic surfactant like polyoxyethylene sorbitan monooleate serves as a self-emulsifying oil matrix. They quickly disperse in the GI fluid to give oil-surfactant droplets. These droplets help in the transfer of drugs through the lipophilic membranes and facilitate drug absorption.

6. *Suspensions*: The drugs which are insoluble in the liquid matrices of soft gelatin capsules and which are poorly soluble in the GI fluids can be formulated as suspensions using a suitable vehicle. These suspensions, when encapsulated in the soft gelatin capsules along with suitable excipients, have better bioavailability.

Factors affecting the contents of soft gelatin capsules

1. *Temperature*: The contents to be encapsulated must have same consistency. At the time of encapsulating, they should be able to flow by gravity at a temperature of 35°C or less. This is because the temperature at which the gelatin is sealed is maintained between 37-40°C.

2. *Viscosity*: The contents varying in viscosities from 0.22 to more than 3000 cp can be encapsulated without any problem, except for a few liquids like glycerin, which sticks to the side valves and pumps of the capsule filling equipment.

3. *pH:* The contents to be encapsulated should be neither strongly acidic nor basic. Their pH should be in between 2.5 to 7.5. This is because the strongly acidic liquids may cause leakage and hydrolysis of capsule

shell and the strongly basic liquids may cause tanning which in turn affects the solubility of capsule shell.

4. *Water miscibility and volatile nature*: Contents like water, ethyl alcohol, emulsions etc., pose certain problems on encapsulation because of their volatile nature and water solubility. This type of liquids leak through the capsule shell and volatilize leaving it brittle and damaged.

Formulation Strategies

Soft gelatin capsule formulation strategies have to consider the specific shell/fill interactions that may occur during manufacture, drying and on storage and control their rate and extent to achieve a stable product.

Two major types of interactions have to be distinguished:

- Chemical reactions of fill components with the gelatin and the plasticizer
- Physical interactions, *i.e.,* migration of fill components in or through the shell and vice versa.

Cross-linking of gelatin leading to solubility problems of the shell is a well-known problem associated with the encapsulation of drugs containing reactive groups such as the aldehyde group. It can be successfully reduced by the use of succinylated gelatin, an approach that is often used for health and nutrition products, and in some countries even for pharmaceutical products. Esterification and trans-esterification of drugs with polyols present another unwanted chemical reaction that may occur. Since glycerol is more reactive than other polyols, glycerol-free shell formulations and/or the addition of polyvinyl pyrrolidone to the fill are preferred to reduce this problem.

Methods of Preparation of Soft Gelatin Capsules

Soft gelatin capsules are prepared and filled on a large scale. The various methods available for preparation of soft gelatin capsules are:

1. Rotary die process
2. Plate process
3. Accogel process
4. Bubble method

Rotary die process: It works on the principle developed by R.P. Sherer in 1933. The capsules prepared by this process have uniformly filled medicaments with accurate doses. The Rotary die process is as shown in Fig. 4.5.

It is a fully automatic continuous process in which the liquid gelatin is made to flow from an overhead tank to form two gelatin sheets on two different rotating drums. These gelatin sheets are conveyed between two rotating dies from opposite directions. As the sheets come in between the dies, the metered filling material is injected which creates pockets in the sheets. Simultaneously, these formed pockets are sealed by pressure and heat and are cut off from the sheets as capsules.

The capsules so formed are adhered with mineral lubricants applied on gelatin sheets for ease in movement. These lubricants can be removed by passing the capsules through naphtha bath. The capsules are then passed through air dryers under pressure to rinse off the excess moisture. Finally, they proceed for packaging.

Advantages:

- Heavy materials like pastes and ointments are easily encapsulated.

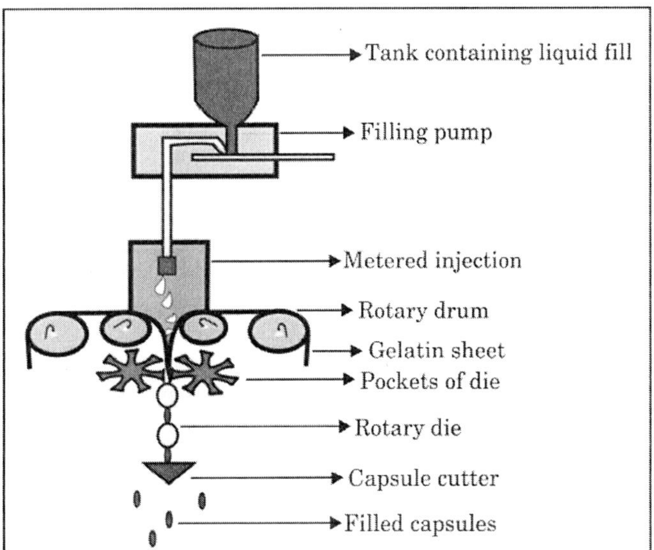

Fig. 4.5: Rotary die process

- Solid medicaments are easily processed with suitable vehicles and encapsulated.
- Capsules are filled with accurately measured medicaments and tightly sealed.
- Bicoloured capsules are formed when different coloured gelatin sheets are used.

Plate process: It is a semi-automatic method in which a warm sheet of soft gelatin is laid over a plate having die pockets. Vacuum is applied from underside of this plate to pull the gelatin sheet into the pockets. The liquid medicament is evenly poured into these dies and another sheet of soft gelatin of similar or a different colour is laid over it. Finally, a die press is laid over the assembly of these sheets which upon application of pressure seals and cuts off the capsules simultaneously.

The capsules are removed and washed with a volatile solvent. Washing is done to remove the adhering oil from the capsules.

Accogel process: It works on the principle developed by Lederle Laboratories in 1949. It is a unique machine in which powdered dry solids, liquids or a combination of liquids and powdered dry solids can be accurately filled into the soft gelatin capsules.

The machine consists of mainly 3 parts:

- Measuring roll
- Die roll
- Sealing roll

As the measuring roll and die rolls rotate, the measured doses are transferred to the gelatin-linked pockets of the die roll. The continued rotation of the filled die converges with the rotating sealing roll where a second gelatin sheet is applied to form the other half of the capsule. Pressure developed between the die roll and sealing roll seals and cuts out the capsules. The soft gelatin capsules so prepared may be of various colours, shapes and sizes.

Bubble method: Truly seamless, one-piece soft gelatine capsules can be made by a bubble method. A concentric tube dispenser simultaneously discharges the molten gelatin from the outer annulus and the liquid content from the inner tube. The liquids are discharged into chilled oil as droplets which consists of a liquid medicament core within a molten gelatin envelope. The droplets assume a spherical shape under surface tension forces, and the gelatin congeals on cooling. The finished capsules then must be degreased and dried.

Finishing of Soft Gelatin Capsules

Inspection of capsules

Capsules produced on a small or a large scale should be uniform in appearance. The visual or electronic inspection should be undertaken to detect any flaws in the integrity and appearance of the capsules. Defective capsules should be rejected. In commercial manufacture, Current Good Manufacturing Practice regulations require that if the number of production flaws is excessive, the cause must be investigated and documented and steps undertaken to correct the problem.

Soft gelatin capsules may be post-treated after production or coated to improve product stability, to modify the dissolution rate and to enable enteric capsules to be produced.

1. The low surface roughness of soft capsule shells and the intrinsic insolubility of the shell components in organic solvents means that coatings applied as an organic solution usually do not adhere properly to the capsules, resulting in onion-like coatings of layers peeling off immediately after drying or on storage. Aqueous coatings, on the other hand, may result in capsule swelling, softening and/or sticking together, since water is acting as a plasticizer for the gelatin capsule shells.
2. Capsules with modified dissolution characteristics, such as gastro-resistant enteric soft gelatin capsules, have been described in the scientific and patent literature and can be achieved by adding gastro-resistant, enteric-soluble polymers to the gelatin mass prior to capsule formation, or by aldehyde post-treatment or enteric coating of the dried capsules. All three attempts have their specific difficulties. For soft gelatin capsules produced by the rotary die process, the last two approaches are in practical use.
3. Aldehyde post-treatment of soft gelatin capsules has been known for many years as a popular means to reduce their dissolution rate, *i.e.,* the capsules take a long time to dissolve and have left the stomach before this occurs. Formaldehyde has been described

to cross-link effectively soft capsules to render them gastro-resistant.

4. An alternative to aldehyde, soft gelatin capsules may be coated with a gastro-resistant, enteric-soluble polymer. Owing to the aforementioned difficulties associated with organic and aqueous soft capsule coating, a protective subcoat is usually applied as an alcoholic solution prior to the application of the gastro-resistant, enteric polymer layer.

In Process and Final Quality Control Tests

1. *Raw material analysis:* All the ingredients of soft gelatin capsules are controlled and tested to ensure compliance with pharmacopoeial specification.
2. *Excipient test:* In order to ensure the manufacture of a high-quality soft gel products *e.g.,* it is important to limit certain trace impurities such as aldehydes and peroxides that may be present in PEGs. The presence of high levels of these impurities gives rise to cross-linking of gelatin polymer, leading to in-solubilisation through polymerisation.
3. Soft gel seal thickness at the time of encapsulation is controlled and tested to ensure proper sealing.
4. Fill material weight and capsule shell weight are tested and maintained as per the requirement.
5. Soft gel shell moisture level and soft gel hardness at the end of the drying is tested.

   Bloom strength, viscosity and iron content of prepared gelatin solution is checked and maintained within the limits of specifications. Procedures for determination of these parameters are explained in quality control tests of hard gelatin capsules.
6. *Weight variation test:* Weigh an intact capsule. Open the capsule without losing any part of the shell and remove the contents as completely as possible. To remove the contents of a soft capsule the shell may be washed with ether or other suitable solvent and the shell allowed to stand until the odour of the solvent is no longer detectable. Weigh the empty shell. The weight of the contents is the difference between the weighings. Repeat the procedure with a further 19 capsules. Determine the average weight. Calculate the upper limit and lower limit based on the

average weight of capsule. Not more than two of the individual weights deviate from the average weight by more than the percentage deviation shown in the below Table 4.7 and none deviates by more than twice that percentage.

Table 4.7: Percentage deviations as per I.P.

Average weight of capsule contents	*Percentage deviation*
Less than 300 mg	10
300 mg or more	7.5

7. *Uniformity of content:* Determine the content of active ingredient in each of 10 capsules taken at random using the method given in the monograph or by any other suitable analytical method of equivalent accuracy and precision. The capsules comply with the test if not more than one of the individual values thus obtained is outside the limits 85 to 115 per cent of the average value and none is outside the limits 75 to 125 per cent. If two or three individual values are outside the limits 85 to 115 per cent of the average value, repeat the determination using another 20 capsules. The capsules comply with the test if in the total sample of 30 capsules not more than three individual values are outside the limits 85 to 115 per cent and none is outside the limits 75 to 125 per cent of the average value.
8. *Disintegration test:* Disintegration is defined as the breakdown of solid dosage form into small particles after it is ingested. Disintegration test is a method to evaluate the rate of disintegration of solid dosage forms (capsules or tablets).

   Method: A capsule is placed in every glass tube and the basket containing these glass tubes is positioned in the beaker containing the required fluid such that all the capsules dip properly. The apparatus is then operated for a specified time. The capsule passes the disintegration test when the drug particles must pass through the mesh/wire screen *i.e.,* the capsule must disintegrate and all the particles must pass through the mesh within the time specified in the monograph. However, the insoluble coating particles or the soft mass without palpable core are exempted.

   Note: if one or two capsules does not disintegrate in the specified time, then the test is repeated with another 12 capsules. The net result of 18 capsules tested for disintegration should prove that at least 16 are disintegrated within the specified time. According to U.S. Pharmacopoeia, the disintegration time of capsules is 45 min.

9. *Dissolution test:* Dissolution test for soft gelatin capsule is performed same as mentioned in hard gelatin capsule.

The Package, Storage and Stability of Soft Gelatine Capsules

The main aim in packaging of filled capsules is to prevent contamination and moisture gain or loss during long-term storage. They are plastic blister packed or aluminium foil strip packed or packed in glass or plastic bottles with screw caps.

The containers are designed in such a way that they prevent exposure of capsules to excessive humidity. In some containers, dehydrating powder (desiccants) is placed which retards the excess moisture absorption by capsules.

Long-term storing of capsule shells requires proper maintenance of temperature and humidity these are as shown in Table 4.8.

Table 4.8: Storage conditions for capsules

Storage conditions	*Relative humidity (%)*	*Temperature °C*
Minimum	35	15
Best possible	50	20
Maximum	65	25

Storage of capsules in areas other than the above mentioned conditions may evoke the following response which is given in Table 4.9.

Table 4.9: Storage conditions and responses of capsules.

Condition	*Effect on soft gelatin capsule*
Very high humidity	Capsules soften, stick together and lose shape
Very low humidity	Capsules contract in size and become fragile
High or fluctuated Temperatures	Capsules form lumps and condensation in seen on the surface of containers

Some important points to be attended during capsules storage:

(1) Never store capsules near sources of water

(2) Never freeze capsules

(3) Never store uncovered capsules on the ground.

Stability tests of capsule include

(a) Shell integrity test

(b) Determination of shelf life

a) Shell integrity test: This test is performed to find out the integrity of capsule shell. Specifications test for the capsule shell integrity is given in Table 4.10.

Table 4.10: Specifications for the test

Relative humidity	***Temperature***	***Type of container***
80%	Room Temperature	Open
–	40°C	Open
–	40°C	Tightly closed

Method: The capsules which are to be tested and the standard capsules are placed in one of the above conditions for two weeks with periodic examination. The gross and the net changes occurring in them are as follows:

1. The standard capsule shells kept at the room temperature and 80% RH becomes more soft, sticky and swollen.
2. The test capsules kept under the same conditions undergo the following changes:
   (i) Gross changes include colour fading, discolouration, disintegration, leaking and turning brittle or soft.
   (ii) Net changes include loss of volatile ingredients, grooves growing darker and wider and a little change in colour of the shell.

Many times due to slower drying, soft spots appear over the test capsules which touch the container or the other capsules. These types of spots are not developed in the standard capsules. Later on, these spots turn harder and are not considered as defects of the capsule shell. In case they do not turn harder (due to capsule ingredients) physical stability problems may arise. So such flaws must be corrected as soon as possible by altering the ingredients of the shell or the fill materials.

b) Determination of shelf life: Shelf life or the expiry date of packed capsules is determined under normal storage conditions.

- The capsule manufacturers routinely conduct accelerated physical stability tests on all new capsule products as an integral part of the product development program.
- Stability tests have proved adequate for determining the effect of the capsule shell content on the gelatin shell.
- The tests are strictly relevant to the integrity of the gelatin shell and should not be confused as stability tests for the active ingredients in the capsule content.
- Stability tests results are used as a guide for the re-formulation of the capsule content or the capsule shell, or for the selection of the proper retail package.

Applications of soft gelatin capsules

The soft gelatin capsules have a wide range of application in pharmaceutical field. Among them, few are mentioned below.

- *Ophthalmic soft gelatin capsules*: Now a day's soft gelatin capsules are very commonly used for filling ophthalmic ointments. These capsules are meant for a single application to the eye. Just before application, the capsule is punctured with a sterile needle, the contents instilled into the eye and the shell discarded.
- *Chewable soft gelatin capsules:* The chewable gelatin dosage form offers excellent mouthfeel and chewing experience as compared with other chewable dosage forms. Chewable soft gels are particularly suitable for pediatric populations, where swallowing whole tablets or capsules is often a problem and chewable tablets are often rejected.
- *Controlled release soft gelatin capsules*: Banner's scientists have developed a controlled release technology that is able to achieve a large variety of release patterns. The controlled release softgel can be applied to a wide range of active molecules. Banner's controlled release softgel technology uses a lipid matrix in a standard softgel shell.
- *Enteric coated soft gelatin capsules*: The enteric softgels were prepared by coating with enteric polymers using traditional

coating technology and mode of working as same as enteric coated dosage.

- *Gelatin-free soft gelatin capsules*: Gelatin-free soft capsules are made from vegetable ingredients. They have all the advantages of standard softgels, but do not contain gelatin. Gelatin free soft capsules are particularly suitable for vegetarians or other populations that prefer non-animal products.
- *Suckable soft gelatin capsules*: It consists of a gelatin shell containing the flavoured medicament to be sucked and a liquid matrix inside the capsule. The drug may be present in both the shell and fill matrix
- *Twist-off soft gelatin capsules*: These are designed with a tag to be twisted or snipped off, thereby allowing access to the fill material. It can be very useful for unit dosing of topical medication, inhalations, or indeed for oral dosing of a pediatric product.

Comparison between hard and soft gelatin capsules is given in Table 4.11.

Table 4.11: Comparison between hard and soft gelatin capsules.

Hard gelatin capsules	***Soft gelatin capsules***
1. Hard gelatin capsules shell consists of two parts namely a body and a cap.	1. Soft gelatin capsules, are sealed hermetically as one piece capsule.
2. Hard gelatin capsules contain 12-16% moisture	2. Soft gelatin capsules contain 4-10% moisture.
3. Hard gelatin capsules are cylindrical in shape	3. Soft gelatin capsules are available in round, oval and tube-like shapes
4. The ratio of plasticizer and gelatin is 0.4:1 in hard gelatin capsule	4. The ratio of plasticizer and gelatin is 0.8:1 in soft gelatin capsule
5. Hard gelatin capsules are sealed after they are filled to ensure that the medicines do not come out of the capsule due to handling	5. Filling and sealing of soft gelatin capsules are done in a combined operation on machines.
6. Hard gelatin capsules are firm and rigid	6. Soft gelatin capsules are soft and flexible
7. High bloom strength gelatin is used	7. Low bloom strength gelatin is used
8. Hard gelatin capsule shell is thin	8. Soft gelatin capsule shell is relatively thick

Glossary

Capsules	Capsules are solid dosage forms in which one or more medicinal and inert ingredients are enclosed in a small shell or container usually made of gelatin
Gelatin	Gelatin is obtained by the partial hydrolysis of collagen obtained from the skin, white connective tissue, and bones of animals.
Bloom strength	Bloom strength is defined as an assessment of cohesive strength of the cross-linking between the molecules of gelatin
Viscosity	It is defined as the assessment of chain length of gelatin molecules in 6.66% w/v concentrated gelatin solution in warm water at 60°C
Plasticizers	Plasticizers are used to impart softness, elasticity and thickness to the capsules shell
Preservatives	Preservatives are used to retard the growth of microorganisms
Opacifying-agents	They are used to minimize the transparency and make the capsule shells characteristic
Thickening agents	These are added to adjust the viscosity of gelatin
Glidants	They are used when the powdered drug is to be filled in the capsule shells by automatic machines
Protective sorbents	These agents are added to retard the moisture absorption by hygroscopic agents
Sorting	Sorting means to separate the imperfect and the damaged capsules
Cloth dusting	It is a manual method in which small number of capsules are rubbed with a cloth or a gauze which may or may not contain an inert oil
Brushing	Capsule are projected under soft rotating brushes which removes the dust from the capsule shells

QUESTION BANK

Q. I: Multiple Choice Questions

1 Which one of the following drying methods is commonly used in pharma industry for drying of soft shell capsules?

a) Truck drying
c) Fluid bed drying
b) Vaccum drying
d) Microwave drying

2 By addition of which of the following the shells of soft gelatin capsule may be made elastic?

a) Polyethylene glycol
c) Sorbitol
b) Propylene glycol
d) Dibutyl phthalate

3 Bloom strength is used to check the quality of

a) Lactose
b) Ampoules
c) Hardness of tablets
d) Gelatin

4 Which of the following statements is not true?

a) Capsules are more straight forward to manufacture than tablets
b) Capsules are formulated to increase bioavailability of poorly soluble drugs
c) Capsules may coloured to aid identification
d) The stability of the drug, when formulated as a capsule, is always greater than that of tablets

5 Which of the following are suitable as liquid fills for hard gelatin capsules?

a) Polyethylene glycols
b) Arachis oil
c) Fatty acid ester
d) All of the above

6 Ideally, solid fills for HGCs should exhibit which the following properties?

a) Homogeneity of mix
b) Low angle of repose
c) Low shearing stresses during powder flow
d) All of the above

7 Which of the following excipients are common components of the fill of SGCs?

a) Lipophillic liquids
b) Water miscible liquids
c) Both A and B
d) None of above

8 Capsule shell of SGC and HGC are made up of

a) Gelatin
b) CMC
c) Butenol
d) Propylene glycol

9 Type A gelatin exhibits an isoelectric point in the pH of ______

a) 4.4
b) 9
c) 5
d) 7

10 ________is always present in raw gelatin

a) Potassium
b) Sodium
c) Iron
d) Nickel

11 The viscosity of gelatin range from

a) 10-20 millipoise
b) 50-60 millipoise
c) 25-45 millipoise
d) 15-35 millipoise

12 Non gelatin capsules made from______

a) Starch
b) HPMC
c) Pullulan
d) All of above

13 Green bones are used for the preparation of gelatin of type

a) A
b) B
c) C
d) A and B

14 In capsules, ROTOFIL is used for filling

a) Powders
b) Pellets
c) Lipids
d) Corrosive liquids

15 Gelatin and glycerin are used for the preparation of Lamellae in a specified ratio. Identify the correct ratio

a) 5:1
b) 1:1
c) 9:1
d) 10:1

16 ______is the assessment of cohesive strength of cross-linking of gelatin molecules

a) Bloom volume
b) Bloom strength
c) Viscosity
d) None of the above

17 The iron content in gelatin solution should not be more than

a) 5 ppm
b) 1 ppm
c) 10 ppm
d) 15 ppm

18 The standard moisture content specification for HGC is ________% w/w

a) 13-16
b) 50-60
c) 90
d) 5-10

19 Which of the following is principle of filling of capsules?

a) Augur fill
b) Vibratory fill
c) Piston tamp fill
d) All of the above

20 Drugs which are highly acidic in nature causes_____ of gelatin

a) Hydrolysis of gelatin
b) Tanning of gelatin
c) Non-tanning effect on gelatin
d) None of the above

21 Drugs which are highly basic in nature causes

a) Tanning effect on gelatin
b) Hydrolysis of gelatin
c) Both a and b
d) None of the above

22 ______is the largest capsule size

a) 000
b) 1
c) 0
d) 5

23 Which of the following is not a component of gelatin solution

a) Plasticizer
b) Granulating agent
c) Opacifying agent
d) Thickening agent

24 The following are major defects of capsule EXCEPT

a) Capsules are not uniform in colour

b) Capsules are not free from foreign matter

c) Capsules having surface spots

d) Small marks of grease

25 What is the % deviation allowed (as per I.P.) for capsule weighing less than 300 mg?

a) 5

b) 7.5

c) 10

d) 15

26 What is the % deviation allowed (as per I.P.) for capsule weighing more than 300 mg?

a) 10

b) 5

c) 7.5

d) 15

27 Physical stability of capsule is directly proportional to ______

a) Weight of gelatin

b) Bloom strength

c) Viscosity of gelatin

d) None of the above

28 Osaka machines follows______ principle.

a) Vibratory fill

b) Auger fill

c) Piston tamp

d) Vaccum fill

29 Compression force required in piston tamp is

a) 50-200 N

b) 100-150 N

c) 30-300 N

d) 500-600 N

30 Machine working on vacuum fill principle is

a) Accofil machine

b) Osaka machine

c) Dosator type machine

d) Dosing disc machine

31 Efflorescent materials may cause the capsules to _____

a) Soften

b) Harden

c) Brittle

d) Viscous

32 The liquid fill capacity of capsules is restricted and should not exceed _____% of the capsule body volume

a) 80

b) 70

c) 50

d) 90

33 Rotosort is new filled capsule sorting machine sold by

a) Eli lilly and company

b) Erweka

c) Hartnett company

d) None of the above

34 Method used for finishing the capsules

a) Pan polishing
c) Brushing
b) Cloth dusting
d) All of these

35 _____ is the most successful method for the sealing of capsules to prevent leakage

a) Gelatin closing
c) Gelatin packing
b) Gelatin banding
d) All of the above

36 Succinylated gelatin is used to reduce

a) Discolouration of gelatin
c) Cross-linking of gelatin with aldehyde functional group drugs
b) Softening of capsule
d) Migration of dyes

37 The moisture content of capsules ranges between _____% w/w.

a) 12-16
c) 50-60
b) 20-25
d) 30-40

38 Selection of capsule size depends upon

a) Density
c) Both a and b
b) Fill weight of formulation
d) None of the above

39 _____is the only equipment that accurately fills powdered dry solids into SGC

a) Impingement machine
b) Accogel machine
b) Roto weigh machine
d) None of the above

40 Base adsorption phenomenon involves

a) Judging the fluidity of liquid base
c) Makes decision on filled materials
b) Judging the fluidity of solid base
d) None of the above

41 Soft gelatin capsule is _____piece capsule shell

a) Two
c) Three
b) One
d) Five

42 For hard gelatin capsules, the ratio of dry glycerin to dry gelatin is

a) 0.4/1
c) 0.2/1
b) 0.6/1
d) 0.8/1

43 For soft gelatin capsules, the ratio of dry glycerin to dry gelatin is

a) 0.8/1
c) 1/1
b) 0.4/1
d) 2/1

44 Deliquescent powders may______ the capsules

a) Soft
b) Dry
c) Degrade
d) All of the above

45 Which of the following step involved in manufacturing of capsule shell?

a) Spinning
b) Dipping
c) Stripping
d) All of the above

Q. II: Very Short Answer Questions **2 Marks**

1. Give the storage conditions for capsules.
2. List out the finishing techniques of hard gelatin capsules.
3. Write the advantages of soft gelatin capsules.
4. Define base adsorption and minim per gram factor.
5. Give examples of plasticizers.
6. What is the role of humidity in the storage of hard gelatin capsules?
7. Mention the difference between type A and type B gelatin.
8. Name the quality control tests for capsules.
9. Give the different sizes of hard gelatin capsules.
10. Define bloom strength and write its importance.
11. Writing the importance of plasticizers in making capsules.
12. Write the pharmaceutical applications of soft gelatin capsules.
13. Write the role of viscosity in the manufacturing of soft gelatin capsules.
14. Write the effect and limit of iron content in soft gelatin capsules shell.
15. Name four different shapes of soft gelatin capsules.
16. Name four machines used to fill hard gelatin capsules.
17. Write on the viscosity of liquids to be encapsulated in soft gelatin capsules.
18. List out the components of hard gelatin capsule shell with their use.

Q. III: Short Answer Questions **5 Marks**

1. Differentiate between hard gelatin and soft gelatin capsules.
2. Give the quality control tests for hard gelatin capsules.
3. Write a note on manufacturing defects of hard gelatin capsules.
4. Explain the formulation of hard gelatin capsules.
5. Explain the working of rotary die machine with a neat labelled diagram.
6. Explain the different steps involved in the production of hard gelatin capsule shell.
7. Explain in detail extraction of gelatin.

8. Describe briefly the manufacturing of soft gelatin capsules.
9. Write a note on the nature of capsule content of soft gelatin capsules.
10. Write a note on formulation of powder in manufacturing of hard gelatin capsules.
11. Explain the nature of the soft gelatin capsule shell.
12. Write a note on stability of capsules.
13. Write on the nature of hard gelatin capsule shell.
14. Explain one method used for manufacture of soft gelatin capsules.
15. Discuss the importance of base adsorption and minim/gram factors.
16. Explain the formulation of soft gelatin capsules.

Q. IV: Long Answer Questions **10 Marks**

1. Mention the equipment used in the manufacture of hard gelatin capsules and write in detail the method of filling of capsules.
2. Write a brief note on soft gelatine capsules. Explain the construction and working of rotary die machine used in the manufacture of soft gelatin capsules.
3. Explain in detail in-process and final quality control test for hard gelatin capsules.
4. Explain in detail in-process and final quality control test of a soft gelatin capsule.
5. Discuss in detail about materials to be filled, filling, finishing, sealing and locking aspects of hard gelatin capsules.

CHAPTER 5

PELLETS

INTRODUCTION

Pellets are small, free-flowing, spherical particulates prepared by the agglomeration of fine powders or granules of drug substances and excipients. Pellets are generally produced *via* a pelletization process whereby a powder blend consisting of a drug and excipient is agglomerated into spherical granules. After being processed, pellets are usually filled into hard gelatin capsules or compressed into tablets. Furthermore, they can be formulated as an immediate release or sustained release dosage forms. Pellets can be coated to deliver a drug to a specific site of action in the gastrointestinal tract. Pellets provide the development scientist with a high degree of flexibility during the design and development of oral dosage forms. They can be divided into desired dose strengths without formulation or process changes and also be blended to deliver incompatible bioactive agents simultaneously or particles with different release profiles at the same or different sites within the gastrointestinal tract.

Advantages

1. Pellets are of small size and have good flow properties.
2. They can be divided into desired dosage strength without process or formulation changes.
3. Ease of handling, such as filling into capsules
4. Incorporation of incompatible ingredients in a single dosage form

5. Drugs with different release profiles and absorb at different sites in the gastrointestinal tract can be formulated as pellets.
6. Protection against degradation of active ingredients by oxidation or moisture by providing a film coating
7. High degree of patient acceptance when filled in capsules due to their elegance as compared to tablets
8. High drug loading capacity without producing large particles
9. Pellets are less susceptible to dose dumping effect and decrease the side effect
10. Due to their small size reduction in gastrointestinal irritation compare to a tablet
11. Pellets reduce variation in gastric emptying rate and intestinal transit time thus reduce inter and intrapatient variability
12. Less sensitive to food ingestion compared to single unit dosage forms because the small pellets can pass the pylorus even in the closed state.
13. They can be formulated as sustained, controlled, or site-specific delivery of the drug from coated pellets.

Disadvantages

1. Tabletting of pellets destroys film coating on the pellets.
2. The size of the pellets may vary from formulation to formulation *i.e.,* 0.05 mm to 2 mm.

Desirable Properties

1. ***Uncoated pellets:***

   Uniform spherical size
   Narrow particle size distribution
   Good flow property
   Low friability
   Even surface
   Low dust formation
   Reproducible packing
   Ease of coating

2. ***Coated pellets:***
   Maintain all the above properties
   Desirable drug release characteristics

Reasons for Pelletization

The reasons for pelletization of a pharmaceutical compound are listed as follows:

- To increase the uniformity of drug distribution in the product
- To reduce dust formation, resulting in an improvement of the process safety, as fine powders can cause dust explosions and the inhalation of fines can cause health problems.
- To densify the material and facilitate metering or volumetric dispensing
- To enhance the flow rates and dose uniformity.
- To improve the appearance of the product.
- To improve the hardness and friability.
- Controlled release application of pellets due to the ideal low surface area-to-volume ratio that provides an ideal shape for the application of film coatings.

Formulation

Active pharmaceutical ingredient: The different drugs can be used to develop immediate release, sustained release pellets with diversified applications in different areas. Pellets can be formulated with the drugs that can be delivered even subcutaneously and intramuscularly depending on the size variations where the size range is maintained below 600 µ and are called as micropellets. Pellets technology is widely used to delivery GIT drugs at a specific site to release the drug in a controlled manner.

Binder: These are adhesive materials that can be incorporated into pellet formulations to bind powders and maintain the integrity of pellet formation and addition of the binder may be as a solution than dry form, which is considered to be more efficient than dry mixing followed by liquid addition. When applied as solution form, binders are dissolved or dispersed in the organic or aqueous solvent; the latter is most preferred and commonly used system in pelletization. Choice of binders may differ from formulation to formulation and depends on the processing and physicochemical properties of the drug. The binders are commonly used in the range of 2-10% and should be optimized so that pellets are durable and not friable and yet to maintain the other desirable properties of pellets, such as releasing the drug at the intended rate.

Granulating fluid: Moisture content of the wet mass prepared is most crucial parameter for pellets growth as it imparts the required plasticity and cohesiveness to the wet mass to extrude it and spheronize it to give a perfect spherical shape. An optimum quantity of moisture content should be there to obtain a good quality pellets.

Different types of granulating fluid are used for the pelletization process. Besides the use of aqueous forms as a granulation liquid, use of alcoholic or hydroalcoholic systems, ethyl ether, dilute acetic acid, isopropyl alcohol has also been reported.

Spheronizing enhancer: Spheronization enhancers are formulation aids that improve the production of spherical pellets, mainly during spheronization and balling processes. They not only impart plasticity to the formulation but also impart binding properties that are essential for pellet strength and integrity.

Filler: These are the excipients used to form the bulk of the material, in the process of pelletization 70% to 80% of excipients is formed by fillers. Generally, microcrystalline cellulose is used for this purpose. Avicel PH 101 is considered to be the pelletization aiding excipient in this process. Other filler used in pelletization include glyceryl monostearate, starch RX1500, spray dried lactose etc.

Plasticizer: Plasticizers improve the flexibility of polymers by reducing the tensile strength and glass transition temperature of the material. Sometimes drugs and other excipients are employed as plasticizer. Plasticizer selection will depend upon its compatibility with the polymer and also solvent employed in casting of strip. These excipients used in hot melt extrusion can affect the release behaviour of the drug. The flow of polymer will be improved through the use of plasticizer that enhances the strength of the polymer. Glycerol, propylene glycol, low molecular weight polyethylene glycols, phthalate derivatives like dimethyl, diethyl and dibutyl phthalate, citrate derivatives such as tributyl, triethyl, acetyl citrate, triacetin and castor oil are some of the commonly used plasticizer excipients.

Lubricant: In the pelletization process, lubricants are rarely used as the high-speed rotary equipment are being used in the preparation of pellets. However, during compression and extrusion-spheronization, lubricants do play a crucial role in the successful manufacture of pellets. Their use reduces the friction between the die wall and material mix either during the compression process or in the ejection phase. They also play a significant role in the smooth discharge of the pellets from the Spheronizer.

Separating agents: These are materials which are adsorbed on the surface and promote the separation of pellets into individual units during a pelletization process separating agents are incorporated initially in the formulation or externally during processing to prevent pellets attracting one another due to surface charge development during the process. Binding the pellets together leads to the formation of aggregates due to subsequent addition of binding agents. Agglomeration of pellets due to the wetness of the surface of the pellets coupled with the local concentration of binding agents. The amount of separating agent used differs with the type of formulation and the manufacturing process. Separating agents are used in dry form during spheronization to prevent adhesion of the spheres to the friction plate and the cylindrical wall of the Spheronizer.

Surfactants: In most pelletization processes, the initial pellet formation and its subsequent growth depends to some extent, on the liquid bridges that hold the primary particles together. Therefore, effective wetting of particles is given more attention. Surfactants are added to the liquid to improve wettability by lowering the interfacial tension between the liquid and drug particles. Surfactants help to weaken the liquid bridges and results in more friable pellets. In extreme cases, excess fines might be produced which brings in the focus to addition of surfactants for pellet formulations. Care should be taken to avoid using surfactants unless it is absolutely essential for the production of pellets that possess specific properties.

pH adjusters: The pH adjusters are substances that are incorporated in pellet formulations which influence the microenvironment of drug molecules used for many reasons. Generally, acid-labile drugs are protected from the pH conditions of GIT by giving an enteric coating.

Buffer systems may also be added to the core formulation to maintain the stability of core in a favourable range. In addition, buffer systems may be included in pellet formulations to enhance the dissolution rate of drugs whose solubility's are influenced by changes in the pH this is particularly referred with pellets whose release rates are membrane-controlled as the solubility of drug plays a major role in determining rate of release. Therefore, specific buffer systems or dual buffer systems are incorporated in pellet formulations to adjust the solubility of drugs to fit a particular process.

Release modifiers: The main requirement of the pelletization process is to manufacture spherical drug cores that will be subsequently coated in a separate unit operation. It is also possible to prepare pellet cores that inherently possess specific release profiles in a single step which can be achieved by incorporation of release modifiers along with drug during the core formulation. Due to the diversity of chemical composition and physical properties of release modifiers, pellet formulations that provide a multitude of release profiles could be designed. Generally, water-soluble low molecular weight excipients, surfactants and disintegrates are incorporated in formulations to enhance drug release kinetics, while water-insoluble polymers, hydrophobic substances, inorganic salts and hydrophilic polymers that swell and/or form gels are incorporated in pellets that retard release kinetics.

Flavouring agents: The choice for the flavours changes from individual to individual depending upon the age, ethnicity and liking which plays a significant role in the taste fondness. Peppermint oil, cinnamon oil, spearmint oil, oil of nutmeg are examples of flavour oils while vanilla, cocoa, coffee, chocolate and citrus are fruity flavours. Apple, raspberry, cherry, pineapple are a few examples of fruit essence type. Cooling agents like monomethyl succinate, menthol can be added to improve the flavour strength and to enhance the mouth-feel effect of the product.

Sweetening agents: Natural sweeteners, as well as synthetic sweeteners, are used to improve the palatability of the formulations. The traditional source of sweetener is sucrose, dextrose, fructose, glucose, liquid glucose and maltose.

Colouring agents: Colouring agents are generally used in order to improve the appearance and make it more patient compliance. Pigments such as Titanium dioxide or FD&C approved colouring agents are used either in the dry form or mixed with the granulating fluid during the formulation.

Theory of Pellet Formation and Growth

It is important to understand the fundamental mechanisms of pellet formation and growth. Different theories have been postulated related to the mechanism of formation and growth of pellets. Some of these theories are derived from experimental results while others are derived from visual observations. The most convincing classification of the pelletization process involves three consecutive regions: nucleation, transition and ball growth. However, based on the experiments on the mechanism of pellet formation and growth, the following steps were proposed: nucleation, coalescence, layering and abrasion transfer.

Nucleation is a stage of the pelletization process that occurs whenever a powder is wetted with the solvent system. The primitive particles are drawn together to form a three-phase air-water-liquid nuclei system which is held together by liquid bridges that are pendular in nature. The reduction of particle size will improve the bonding strength between them. Further, size, rate and extent of nuclear formation depend upon the size of particles, moisture content, viscosity of binding particles, wettability of substrate and processing conditions, such as tumbling and drying rates.

Nucleation is followed by a transition phase where the growth mechanisms affecting are coalescence and layering. Coalescence is defined as formation of large-sized particles by random collision of well-formed nuclei, this mechanism requires slightly excess moisture on the surface of nuclei. Although number of nuclei is progressively reduced even though the total mass of the system remains unchanged during this operation. Layering is a slow growth mechanism and with successive addition of fragments and fines on already formed nuclei. In the layering step, number of particles remains constant while the total mass of the system increases due to increasing particle size as a function of time. The fragments or fine particles can be formed by particle size reduction.

The fines and the fragments produced through size reduction are taken up by larger pellets. Production of fines and subsequent coalescence and layering continues until the number of collisions declines rapidly, thereby leading to a reduction in rate of growth of pellets. At this point, the third phase, the ball growth region, is reached.

The main mechanism in the ball growth phase is the abrasion transfer which involves the transfer of materials from one granule formed to another without any preference in either direction. This phase does not result in any change in the total number or mass of the particles. However, the particles undergo a continuous change in their size as long as the conditions that lead to the transfer of material existence.

Pelletization Processes

Different techniques of pelletization processes:

1. *Agitation*

Balling is the process in which finely divided particles are converted upon the addition of appropriate quantities of liquid to spherical particles by a continuous rolling or tumbling motion. The liquid may be added prior to or during the agitation stage. Pans, discs, drums, or mixers may be used to produce pellets by the balling process.

2. *Compaction*

Compaction is a pelletization process in which mixtures or blends of active ingredients and excipients are compacted under pressure to generate pellets of defined shape and size. The pellets are small enough to be filled into capsules. The formulation and processing variables that govern the production of pellets during compression are similar to those that are routinely employed in tablet manufacturing. In fact, pellets produced by compression are nothing but small tablets that are approximately spheroidal in shape.

Extrusion/spheronization: Extrusion-spheronization is a multiple step process of making uniformly sized spherical particles. It is primarily used as a method to produce multi-particulates for controlled drug release applications. The major advantage over other methods of producing drug-loaded spheres or pellets is the ability to incorporate high levels of active ingredients without producing excessively large particles (*i.e.,* minimal excipients are necessary). The main steps of the process are:

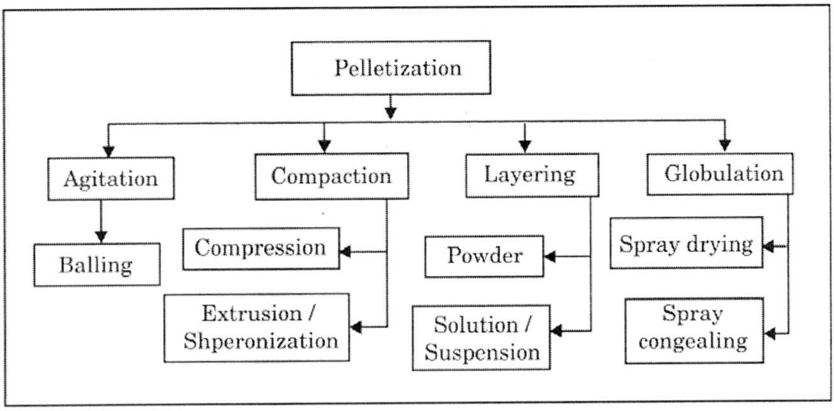

(i) Dry mixing of ingredients: Powders are dry mixed to achieve a homogeneous powder dispersion. It is generally carried out in same mixer used for the granulation; however, if a continuous granulator is used, a separate mixer is required for the dry mix. The uniformity of the dry mix has a significant effect on the quality of the granulation and, in turn, on the spherical particles produced.

(ii) Wet massing: A wet mass is prepared to produce a sufficiently plastic wet mass. With a few exceptions, this step is similar to conventional granulation techniques used to produce products for compression. It is typically carried out in a batch-type mixer-granulator; however, any equipment capable of producing a wet mass, including the continuous type can be used.

(iii) Extrusion: Extrusion consists of shaping the wet mass into rod-shaped particles of uniform diameter, which is more commonly termed 'extrudate'. The wet mass is forced through dies and shaped into small cylindrical particles having a uniform diameter. The extrudate particles break at similar lengths under their own weight.

There are many designs of the extruder but generally, they can be divided into three classes, based on their feed mechanism (Fig. 5.1):

- Screw-feed extruders (axial or endplate, dome and radial)
- Gravity-feed extruders (cylinder roll, gear roll, radial)
- Piston-feed extruders (ram).

(iv) Spheronization: The process of spheronization is carried out in relatively simple equipment to round off the extrudate (rods) into

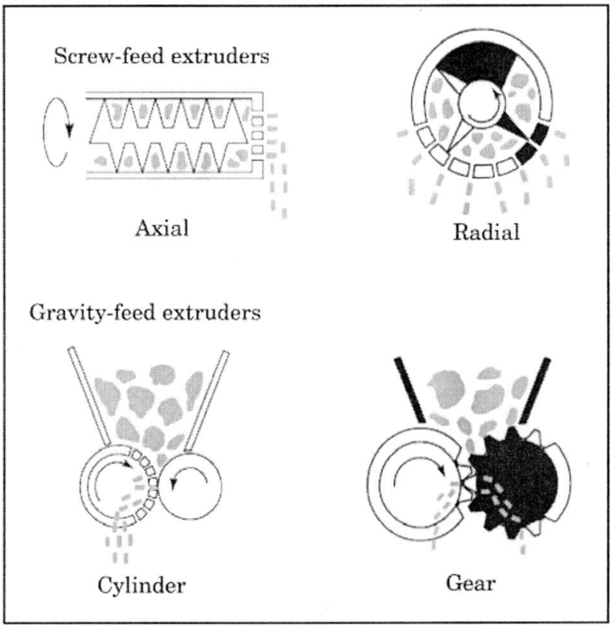

Fig. 5.1: Schematic representation of production extruders.

spherical particles. The rounding of the extrudate into spheres is dependent on frictional forces. The forces are generated by particle-to-particle and particle-to-equipment interaction.

(v) Drying: Drying of spherical particles to achieve the desired final moisture content. This can be accomplished in any dryer that can be used for conventional type granulations, including tray dryers, column-type fluid beds, and deck-type vibratory fluid beds. Fluidized bed dryers result in a much more rapid drying rate because of the higher air volumes and the potential use of higher inlet temperatures.

(vi) Screening: The process of screening is optional and is used to achieve the desired narrow size distribution.

Extrusion/ spheronization is a more labour intensive process than other forms of granulation and therefore should only be considered when other methods of granulation are either not satisfactory for that particular formulation or are inappropriate (*i.e.,* when spheres are required).

3. *Layering*

Layering processes are the most well-controlled and straightforward pelletization techniques that have been used over the years. They are classified into three categories: direct pelletizing, solution layering or suspension layering and powder layering.

Direct pelletizing: Direct pelletizing means manufacturing of pellets directly from powder.

It is an effective process; pellets are manufactured directly from powder with a binder or solvent with the very low usage of auxiliary materials.

In this process, the powder is mixed and moistened. A solvent or binder can also be added. The powder bed is set into a centrifugal motion. The impact and acceleration forces that occur in this process result in the formation of agglomerates, which become rounded out into uniform and dense pellets. The speed of rotation has a direct influence on the density and size of the pellets. The moist pellets are subsequently dried in the fluid bed. If required, the systems can be made inert for applications with organic solvents. Another alternative for direct pelletizing is spray granulation.

Powder layering: Powder layering involves the deposition of successive layers of dry powder of drug or excipients or both on performed nuclei or cores with the help of a binding liquid. Because powder layering involves simultaneous application of liquid and dry powder, it generally requires specialized equipment. Pieces of equipment revolutionized powder layering processing as pelletizing techniques are-tangential spray or centrifugal fluid bed granulators. In case of tangential spray, the rotating disk and fluidization air provides proper mixing.

Solution or suspension layering: Solution or suspension layering involves the deposition of successive layers of the solution and/or suspension of drug substances and binder on starter seeds, which may be inert materials or crystal/granules of the same drug. Suspension layering is usually used when the desired drug loading of the pellets is low because the production of pellets from low solids content formulation is not economically feasible.

An important factor that needs to be considered when suspensions are used as opposed to solutions is the particle size of the drug. If the size of the drug in suspension is large, the amount of binder required to immobilize the particles onto cores will be high, and consequently, pellets of low potency are produced.

Coating of Pellets

Fluid Bed Coating of Pellets

Advantages: i) Uniform, continuous product coating. ii) Aqueous or organic coatings can be applied. iii) Coating and drying take place in one machine. iv) Coating process, filling and emptying of the machine can be carried out in complete isolation and without product spreading into the environment.

The principle of operation of fluid bed coating;

With fluid bed coating, particles are fluidized and the coating fluid sprayed on and dried. Small droplets and a low viscosity of the spray medium ensure an even product coating. Different fluid bed systems are (Fig. 5.2):

Top spray coating
Bottom spray coating
Tangential spray coating

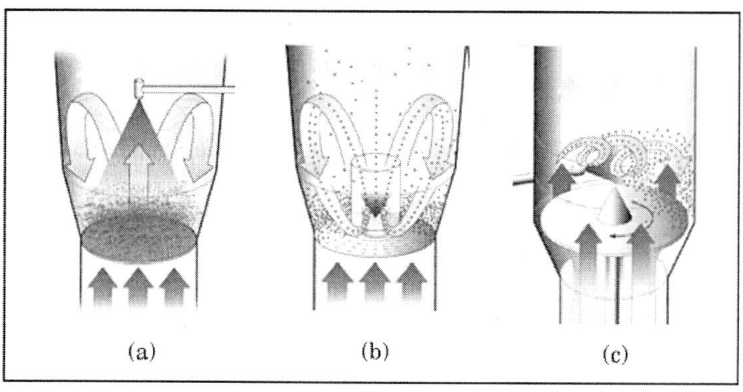

Fig. 5.2: (a) Principle of top spray fluid coating, (b) Principle of bottom spray fluid coating, (c) Principle of tangential spray fluid coating.

a) *Top spray coating*

This process is used for general coatings right up to enteric coating. With top spray coating in the fluid bed (batch and continuous), particles are fluidized in the flow of heated air, which is introduced into the product container *via* a base plate.

The coating liquid is sprayed into the fluid bed from above against the air flow (counter current) by means of a nozzle. Drying takes place as the particles continue to move upwards in the air flow. Small droplets and a low viscosity of the spray medium ensure that distribution is uniform. Coating in the continuous fluid bed is particularly suitable for protective coatings/colour coatings where the product throughput rates are high. The product is continuously fed into one side of the machine and is transported onwards *via* the sieve bottom by means of the air flow. Depending on the application, the system is sub-divided into pre-heating zones, spray zones and drying zones. The dry, coated particles are continuously extracted.

b) *Bottom spray coating (Wurster coating)*

This process is particularly suitable for a controlled release of active ingredients. In the Wurster process, a complete sealing of the surface can be achieved with a low usage of the coating substance. The spray nozzle is fitted in the base plate resulting in a spray pattern that is concurrent with the air feed. By using a Wurster cylinder and a base plate with different perforations, the particles to be coated are accelerated inside the Wurster tube and fed through the spray cone concurrently. As the particles continue travelling upwards, they dry and fall outside the Wurster tube back towards the base plate. They are guided from the outside back to the inside of the tube where they are once again accelerated by the spray. This produces an extremely even film. Particles of different sizes are evenly coated.

Bottom spray coating (continuous fluid bed); particularly suitable for protective coatings/ colour coatings where the product throughput rates are high. The product is continuously fed into one side of the machine and is transported onwards *via* the sieve bottom by means of the air flow. Depending on the application, the system is sub-divided into pre-heating zones, spray zones and drying zones whereby spraying can take place from below in the form of a bottom spray. The dry, coated particles are continuously extracted.

c) *Tangential spray coating*

Tangential spray coating is ideal for coatings with high solid content. The product is set into a spiral motion by means of a rotating base plate, which has air fed into the powder bed at its edge. The spray nozzle is arranged tangentially to the rotor disc and also sprays concurrently into the powder bed. Very thick film layers can be applied by means of the rotor method.

4. *Globulation*

Globulation or droplet formations describe the two related processes of spray drying and spray congealing.

Spray drying: During spray drying, drug entities in solution or in suspension form are sprayed, with or without excipients, into a hot air stream to generate dry and highly spherical particles. Though the technique is suitable for the development of controlled release pellets, it is generally employed to improve the dissolution rates and hence, the bioavailability of poorly soluble drugs.

Spray congealing: Spray congealing is a process in which a drug is allowed to melt, disperse, or dissolve in hot melts of gums, waxes, fatty acids, etc. and is sprayed into an air chamber where the temperature is below the melting points of the formulation components to provide, under appropriate processing conditions, spherical congealed pellets. Depending on the physicochemical properties of the ingredients and other formulation variables, pellets with immediate or controlled release behaviour can be produced.

Evaluation of Pellets

Size distribution: The sizing of pellets is necessary because it has a significant influence on the release kinetics. In most of the cases, particle size determination is carried out by a simple sieve analysis using a sieve shaker.

Pellets shape: Sphericity of the pellets is the most important characteristics and various methods have been used to determine the shape of pallets. Light microscope fitted to a camera Lucida, visual inspection of pellets by microscope and stereomicroscope etc.

Surface morphology: Scanning electron microscopy is used to examine the surface morphology and cross-section of pellets.

Specific surface area: Surface area of pellets is directly related with size and shape of the pellets. Knowledge of the surface area is desirable especially if film coating is considered. Knowledge about the surface area is important even in the case of uncoated pellets since drug release is influenced by the surface area. Specific surface area of pellets is determined by gas adsorption technique.

Hardness and friability: Pellets flake off during handling, shipping, storage coating process and other unit operations thereby resulting in the formation of dust. Variations in the formulation and/or process of pellets, as well as variability in the raw materials, can potentially result in significant variations with hardness and/or friability of pellets. The hardness of pellets can be determined using Kahl pellet-hardness tester but might not be accurate. Friability of pellets is determined by using Erkewa type tablet friabiliator or turbula mixer for a fixed period of time combined with glass beads of certain diameter in order to generate abrasion and to generate friability index. Friability can also be determined using the fluidized bed with Wurster insert by using a stream of air.

Tensile strength: The tensile strength of the pellets is determined by using tensile apparatus with a 5 kg load cell, the pellets are strained until failure occurs. The load is recorded and the tensile strength is calculated by applying the value for the failure load and the radius of the pellets.

Crushing strength: The crushing strength (the load needed to break the pellets) and elastic modulus of 15 pellets were determined using a material testing machine. The speed of the upper mobile plate fitted with a 1 kN load cell was set at 1 mm/min. Elastic modulus and force-displacement graphs were obtained by a computer system attached to the apparatus.

Density: Density of pellets (bulk and tapped) may affect other process or factors such as filling and packaging characteristic during capsule manufacture and tablet compression. Density of pellets is determined simply by density testing apparatus. The bulk density of pellets can be measured by using an automated tapper, while the true density of pellets can be determined by pycnometer or by solvent displacement method. Bulk density indicates the packing properties of pellets or spherical seeds which provide higher bulk densities due to small intraparticle porosities. True density indicates the extent of densification or compactness of pellets.

Porosity: The porosity of the pellets influences the release of drugs from the pellets by affecting the capillary action of the dissolved drug. The porosity of the pellets can be measured quantitatively by mercury porosimetry. The porosity of the pellets can also be determined qualitatively by SEM with image analysis and quantitatively by using optical microscopy rarely.

Disintegration time: Disintegration of pellets is one of the main characteristics for immediate release pellets. Disintegration test can be carried out by using the reciprocating cylinder method or in a tablet disintegration tester with certain modification.

In vitro dissolution studies: Release of the drug from pellet mainly depends on the composition, hardness and size of pellets and it is determined by using dissolution test apparatus. The drug release profiles from pellets also depend on the polymer and binder used, the aqueous solubility of the drug, physical state of the drug in the pellet, drug loaded into the pellet and the presence of additives such as surfactants. In the case of wax-based freeze-dried pellets, the drug release decreased as the hydrophobicity of wax increases and the drug release increased as the aqueous drug solubility increased.

Applications of Pellets

Pellets have varied applications in a number of industries and an innovative use of it's could achieve maximum profitability.

1. ***Taste masking:*** Pellets are ideal for products where perfect abatement of taste is required. Although various technologies have been utilized to mask the bitter taste of a drug such as the addition of sweeteners and flavours, filling in capsules, coating with water-insoluble polymers or pH dependent soluble polymers, complexing with ion-exchange resins, microencapsulation with various polymers, complexing with cyclodextrins and chemical modifications such as the use of insoluble prodrugs, few reports have described the masking of unpleasant taste without lowering of bioavailability especially for oral products. The pelletization technique solves difficult taste masking problem while maintaining a high degree of bioavailability due to their high surface area, especially for oral products.

2. ***Immediate release*:** Administering drugs in pellet form leads to an increased surface area as compared to traditional compressed tablets and capsules which would considerably reduce the disintegration time and have the potential for use in rapidly dispersible tablets.

3. ***Sustained release*:** The pellet form provides a smoother absorption profile from the gastrointestinal tract as the beads pass gradually through the stomach into the small intestine at a steady rate. Pellets are being increasingly used in the manufacture of sustained release dosage form of drugs.

4. ***Varying dosage without reformulation*:** Pellets have excellent flow properties, due to this, they can be conveniently used for filling capsules and the manufacturer can vary the dosage by varying the capsule size without reformulating the product tablets or capsules or packed simply as a single dose packet. They can be applied by both oral and buccal routes.

Glossary

Pellets	Pellets are small, free-flowing, spherical particulates manufactured by the agglomeration of fine powders or granules of drugs and excipients
Balling	It is pelletization process in which finely divided particles are converted, upon the addition of appropriate quantities of liquid, to spherical particles by a continuous rolling or tumbling motion
Compression	Compression is a pelletization process in which mixtures or blends of active ingredients and excipients are compacted under pressure to generate pellets of defined shape and size
Spray drying	During spray drying, drug entities in solution or in suspension f orm are sprayed with or without excipients into a hot air stream to generate dry and highly spherical particles
Spray congealing	The drug is allowed to melt, disperse, or dissolve in hot melts of gums, waxes, fatty acids and is sprayed into an air chamber where the temperature is below the melting points of the formulation components to forms spherical congealed pellets
Micronizing	Micronizing or finely milling the drug before layering improves the efficiency of the layering process
Extrudate	The wet mass is forced through dies and shaped into small cylindrical particles having a uniform diameter are extrudates

QUESTION BANK

Q. I: Multiple Choice Questions

1 Which method of pelletization does not involve the addition of water or other solvents?

a) Cryopelletization
b) Extrusion-spheronization
c) Hot melt extrusion
d) Balling

2 The particle size of pellets should be in the range of

a) 100 to 300 μ
b) 300 to 600 μ
c) 600 to 1000 μ
d) 1000 to 1400 μ

3 Which of the following dosage form limits localised build-up of the drug in GIT?

a) Pellets
b) Tablets
c) Capsules
d) Granules

4 Pelletization of powder leads to all of the followings EXCEPT

a) Dose uniformity
b) Improvement in flow property
c) Reduction in dust formation
d) Enhance solubility

5 ______ is considered as gold standard for the preparation of pellets by the extrusion-spheronization technique

a) Gelatin
b) Microcrystalline cellulose
c) Chitosan
d) Hydroxypropyl methylcellulose

Q. II: Very Short Answer Questions — 2 Marks

1. Add a short note on pellets
2. Enlist the application of pellets
3. Enlist the different techniques of pelletization
4. Give any four reasons for pelletization
5. Mention the requirements for good pellets

Q. III: Short Answer Questions — 5 Marks

1. Write the advantage and disadvantage of pellets
2. Explain extrusion-spheronization technique of pelletization
3. Discuss the various evaluation test for pellets

Q. IV: Long Answer Questions — 10 Marks

1. Define pellets and discuss pelletization techniques.
2. Discus the formulation aspects of pellets
3. Write a note on equipment used for the preparation of pellets.

UNIT-IV

CHAPTER 6

PARENTERAL PRODUCTS

INTRODUCTION

The term parenteral is derived from the Greek word para enteron its meaning “to avoid the intestines” includes any drug whose delivery does not utilize the alimentary canal for entry into body tissues.

Different routes of parenteral drug administration is depicted in Fig. 6.1.

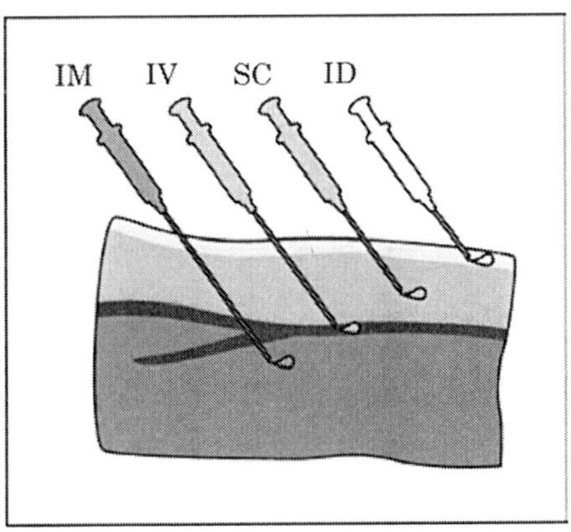

Fig. 6.1: Different routes of parenteral drug administration depicted are intramuscular (IM), intravenous (IV), subcutaneous (SC) and intradermal (ID) routes.

Parenteral preparations are sterile preparations containing one or more active ingredients intended for administration by injection, infusion or implantation into the body. They are packaged in either single-dose or multi-dose containers.

In other words, parenteral preparations bypass the gastrointestinal tract and liver. They directly enter into the systemic circulation hence, exhibit cent per cent bioavailability. These dosage forms used as implants, injections or infusions are meant to be administered directly into the blood vessels, tissues, tissue spaces or body compartments. In this chapter, we restrict our discussion to injectables (injections or infusions).

Classification of Parenteral Dosage Forms

1) *Small volume parenterals*: Volume of these parenteral varies from fractions of a millilitre to hundred millilitres (*i.e.,* up to 100 ml). Examples: Injections- furosemide, heparin, cimetidine, iron dextran etc.

2) *Large volume parenterals*: Volume of these parenteral varies from 100 ml and above. They are administered as single dose injections at a slow rate. Examples: Infusion fluids, total parenteral nutrition (TPN) solutions, patient-controlled analgesia, dialysis fluids etc.

Advantages

1. The parenterals are preferred when:
   - Rapid drug action is desired, as in emergencies;
   - The patient is uncooperative, unconscious, or unable to accept or tolerate oral medication
   - The drug itself is ineffective by other routes.
2. Drugs which cannot be delivered through the oral route can be administered through parenteral route.
3. As parenteral products bypass the gastrointestinal tract and liver, modification of the drug by enzymes of GIT and liver can be avoided.
4. Administration of the drug to the target area (site of action) is ensured.
5. Fluid and electrolyte balances can be rapidly corrected and maintained.

Limitations

1. Self-medication is not possible (except insulin injection in diabetic patients).
2. Proper care should be taken during its manufacturing, filling and packaging and strict sterility requirements are to be fulfilled.
3. Negligence during its administration can lead to infection. Hence, trained personnel are required for proper administration.
4. While injecting the drug, important structures such as nerve and arteries may be damaged this may lead to complete paralysis of the area to which it is supplied.
5. Parenteral products are quite expensive.

Essential Requirements for Parenteral Products

Following are the essential requirements for parenteral products

- All products must be sterile.
- All products must be free from pyrogenic (endotoxin) contamination.
- Injectable solutions must be free from visible particulate matter.
- Products should be isotonic, although strictness of isotonicity depends on the route of administration.
- All products must be stable chemically, physically and microbiologically (*i.e.,* sterility, free from pyrogenic and visible particulate contamination must be maintained throughout the shelf life of the product).
- Products must be compatible with other drug products co-administered.

Pre-formulation Factors Consideration

Pre-formulation consideration for parenteral products involves prior consideration of physicochemical properties of the drug substances, selection of the route of administration, selection of injection volume, pH and tonicity requirements, choice of excipients, sterility and packaging of the products.

1. *Active drug substance*

In order to produce a stable and safe parenteral dosage form, it is very essential to evaluate the properties of the active drug(s). These properties include physical state (crystal characteristics), polymorphism, solubility, pharmacokinetics, pH, stability and compatibility of the drug.

Physical state of the drug (crystal characteristics): Some drugs such as cephalosporins are available as dry solids which are prepared by sterile crystallization techniques. These techniques can be modified to enhance the rate of dissolution. Crystallization process should be designed in such a way that a uniform product free from particulate matter is obtained.

Some drugs associate with water to produce crystalline forms known as hydrates. Care should be taken while selecting the solvent for washing procedure of the crystals of hydrates. Absolute alcohol should not be used during washing procedure, as it may destroy the crystalline structure of the hydrates instead of which 95% ethanol should be used.

Polymorphism: It is defined as the phenomenon of the existence of several crystal forms of a given substance which exhibit different physico-chemical properties. When one polymorph gets converted to another, a considerable change in the physico-chemical properties of the drug may occur. Hence, chemical substances which exhibit polymorphism should be thoroughly evaluated prior to formulation. This is done in order to check whether the polymorphic form used in the formulation is stable in a particular solvent or solvent system.

Drug solubility: If the drug is insufficiently soluble in water at the required dosage, then the co-solvents must be included in the formulation. If relatively simple formulation additives do not result in a solution, then a dispersed system dosage form must be developed. Solubility also dictates the concentration of drug in the dosage form.

Pharmacokinetics of the drug: Rates of absorption (for routes of administration other than intravenous or intra-arterial), distribution, metabolism, and excretion for a drug have some effect on the selected route of administration and accordingly, the type of formulation. For example, if the pharmacokinetic profile of a drug is very rapid, modified release dosage formulations may need to be developed. The dose of drug and the dosage regimen are affected by pharmacokinetics, so the size (*i.e.,* concentration) of the dose will also influence the type of formulation and amounts of other ingredients in the formulation. If the dosage regimen requires frequent injections, then a multiple dose formulation must be developed, if feasible. If the drug is distributed quickly from the site injection, complexing agents or viscosity inducing agents may be added to the formulation to retard drug dissolution and transport.

pH: In the formulation of parenteral products (mainly solutions and suspensions). pH Vs solubility and pH Vs stability profiles are taken into consideration. This is done to ensure the physical and chemical stability of the formulation by either increasing or decreasing the solubility of the drug in vehicle.

Drug stability: If the drug has significant degradation problems in solution, then a freeze-dried or another sterile solid dosage form must be developed. Stability is sometimes affected by drug concentration that, in turn, might affect the size and type of packaging system used. Stability dictates the expiry date of the product that, in turn, determines the storage conditions. Storage conditions might dictate the choice of container size, formulation components, and type of container. If a product must be refrigerated, then the container cannot be too large, and formulation components must be soluble and stable at colder conditions.

Compatibility of drug: With potential formulation additives and packaging systems - It is well-known that drug-excipient incompatibilities frequently exist. Initial pre-formulation screening studies are essential to ensure that formulation additives, although possibly solving one problem, will not create another. Stabilizers, such as buffers and antioxidants, although chemically stabilizing the drug in one way, may also catalyze other chemical degradation reactions. Excipients and certain drugs can form insoluble complexes. Impurities in excipients can cause drug degradation reactions. Peroxide impurities in polymers may catalyze oxidative degradation reactions with drugs, including proteins, which are oxygen sensitive.

2. *Route of administration*

Injections may be administered by intravenous, subcutaneous, intradermal, intramuscular, intraarticular, intralesional and intrathecal. The type of dosage form (solution, suspension, etc.) determines the particular route of administration employed. Conversely, the desired route of administration places requirements on the formulation. For example, suspensions would not be administered directly into the bloodstream, due to the danger of insoluble particles blocking capillaries. Solutions administered subcutaneously require strict attention to tonicity adjustment, otherwise, irritation of the plentiful supply of nerve endings in this anatomical area would give rise to pronounced pain. Injections intended for intraocular, intraspinal, intracisternal and intrathecal administration require stricter standards of such properties as formulation tonicity, component purity, and limit of endotoxins, due to the sensitivity of tissues encountered to irritant and toxic substances.

3. *Selection of injection volume*

One of the first steps in the formulation of a parenteral products is to select the administration volume and concentration. This may be dictated primarily by physiological considerations, such as maximum injection volume or by pharmaceutical considerations. For example, if solubility is low, a larger volume/lower concentration formulation may be required, where as if stability were to improve at higher concentrations, then the converse would be true.

4. *pH and tonicity requirements*

pH considerations: A parenteral product should be formulated with a pH close to physiological unless stability or solubility considerations preclude this. Often, the pH selected for the product is a compromise between the pH of maximum stability, solubility and physiological acceptability.

The first step in selecting a suitable formulation pH will be the generation of pH/stability and pH/solubility profiles.

The target pH for maximum physiological acceptability is approximately pH 7.4. In practice, however, a reasonably wide pH range can be tolerated, particularly when dosing is *via* the IV route and dilution with blood is rapid. In these circumstances, pH ranging from 2 to 12 can be tolerated (although formulations at the extremes of this range are not recommended).

The dilution rate is slower when administration is *via* the intramuscular route and decreases further when the subcutaneous route is used. For this reason, pH ranges of 3 to 11 and 3 to 6, respectively, are recommended for these routes. Many products are formulated at a slightly acidic pH because of solubility or stability considerations and the vast majority of licensed products have a pH between 3 and 9. A pH outside this range should be avoided, if possible since a pH of greater than 9 can cause tissue necrosis, whereas a pH of less than 3 may cause pain and phlebitis.

Tonicity considerations: Wherever possible, parenteral products should be isotonic; typically, osmolarities between 280 and 290 mOsm/L are targeted during formulation. Isotonicity is essential for LVPs, but again, a wider range of osmolarities can be tolerated in SVPs, since either rapid dilution with blood will occur after injection, or the product itself will be diluted with an LVP prior to administration. Hypertonic solutions are preferable to hypotonic solutions because of the risk of haemolysis associated with the latter. Fortunately, hypotonic formulations can be easily avoided by the use of excipients, often sodium chloride to raise osmolarity. Mannitol, dextrose, or other inert excipients can also be used for this purpose and may be preferable if the addition of sodium chloride is likely to have an adverse effect on the formulation.

5. *Choice of excipients*

Wherever possible, formulations should be developed using excipients, which have an established use in parenteral products administered by the same route as the product under development. The excipient concentration, rate of administration and total daily dose should fall within the boundaries established by precedent in existing marketed products.

Another important consideration for excipients to be used in parenteral products is their quality, particularly in microbiological terms. Commonly used parenteral excipients can often be obtained in an injectable grade, which will meet strict bioburden and endotoxin limits. Pharmacopoeial grades of other excipients may be acceptable, but it is prudent to apply in-house microbiological specification limits, where none are present in the pharmacopoeias. For non-pharmacopoeial excipients, the best approach is always to purchase the highest grade available and apply internal microbiological specification limits.

6. *Sterility considerations*

The requirement for sterility in parenteral products is absolute and must be borne in mind at all stages of formulation and process development. The regulator now requires that parenteral products be terminally sterilized unless this is precluded, usually by reason of instability.

For a solution product, one of the earliest investigations carried out during formulation development will be a study of the stability to moist heat sterilization. The results of this study may impact the formulation selection; for example, the stability to autoclaving may be affected by solution pH. Where stability is marginal, attempts should be made through the formulation process to stabilize the product such that it can withstand the stresses of moist heat sterilization.

In many cases, however, the product will simply not withstand the stresses associated with autoclaving and in this case, the usual alternative is filtration through sterilizing grade filters followed by aseptic processing. This is likely to be the case for biologicals/ biopharmaceuticals, where heat may denature and deactivate them.

While the vast majority of parenteral products are rendered sterile either by moist heat sterilization or by filtration through sterilizing grade filters, other methods of sterilization should be considered, particularly in the development of non-aqueous formulations or novel drug delivery systems. For implants, for example, γ-irradiation is an option that should be explored early in development.

Preservatives: Preservatives should not usually be included in parenteral formulations except where a multi-dose product is being developed. The physical and chemical compatibility of the preservative (or antioxidant) with the other constituents of the formulation, the container and closure must be demonstrated during the development process. The key criteria for antimicrobial preservative selection are the preservative dose, antimicrobial functionality and effect on the active ingredient.

7. *Desired type of packaging*

Selection of packaging (*i.e.,* type, size, shape, colour of rubber closure, label and aluminium cap) is often based on marketing preferences and competition. Knowing the type of final package early in the development process aids the formulation scientist in being sure the product formulation will be compatible and elegant in that packaging system.

Formulation of Parenteral Products

Vehicles

Two types of vehicles are used in the preparation of parenteral based on the solubility and stability of drug substance.

1. *Aqueous vehicles*

'Water for injections' is the most common vehicle used for parenteral products. Water for injections is a highly purified grade of water which is subject to pharmacopoeial standards with respect to production methods and purity. Water is of course well tolerated by the body and it is a solvent for a wide range of drug substances.

For those drugs which are poorly soluble in water, water-miscible non-aqueous solvents such as ethanol, glycerol or propylene glycol may be added as co-solvents to improve the solubility of a drug substance.

Water for injection (WFI) – It is defined as pyrogen-free distilled water used as a vehicle in the preparation of parenteral products in a bulk. It is not required to be sterile but it should comply with the various tests for pyrogens. The residue on evaporation in water for injection should be $\leq$ 1 mg (0.001%).

Preparations of water for injection

The source water can be expected to be contaminated with natural suspended mineral and organic substances, dissolved mineral salts, colloidal material, viable bacteria, bacterial endotoxins, industrial or agricultural chemicals and other particulate matter. The degree of contamination varies with the source and will be markedly different, whether obtained from a well or from surface sources, such as a stream or lake. Hence, the source water must be pre-treated by one or a combination of the following treatments: chemical softening, filtration, deionization, carbon adsorption or reverse osmosis etc.

Water for injection can be prepared by distillation or by membrane technologies (*i.e.,* reverse osmosis or ultra-filtration).

Distillation: Distillation is a process of converting a liquid from of water to its gaseous form (steam) and that is subsequently condensed back to liquid form. Since steam is pure gaseous water, all other contaminants in the feed water are removed. There are two basic types of WFI distillation units — the vapour compression still and the multiple effects still are used for distillation of water.

Reverse osmosis (RO): As the name suggests, the natural process of selective permeation of molecules through a semipermeable membrane separating two aqueous solutions of different concentrations is reversed. Pressure, usually between 200 and 400 psi, is applied to overcome osmotic pressure and force pure water to permeate through the membrane. Membranes, usually composed of cellulose esters or polyamides are selected to provide an efficient rejection of contaminant molecules in raw water. The molecules most difficult to remove are small inorganic molecules, such as sodium chloride.

Storage and distribution: Water for injection is stored in a closed system with air exchange through a filter that removes micro-organisms. The water for injection is distributed to the plants by a pipe system continuously to avoid stagnation.

Sterile Water for Injection: Sterile water for injection (USP) is packaged in single-dose containers not larger than 1 L. As with water for injection, it must be pyrogen free but does have an allowable endotoxin level, not more than 0.25 USP endotoxin units per milliliter. Also, it may not contain any antimicrobial agent or other added substance. This water may contain slightly more total solids than water for injection because of the leaching of solids from the glass-lined tanks during sterilization. Hence, sterile water for injection has higher limits for residue on evaporation as compared to water for injection. The residue on evaporation should be $\leq$ 4 mg (0.004%) for containers of 10 ml or less and $\leq$ 3 mg (0.003%) for containers of more than 10 ml. Sterile Water for Injection is intended to be used as a solvent, vehicle, or diluent for already sterilized and packaged injectable medications. The 1-L bottles cannot be administered intravenously because they have no tonicity. Thus, they are used for reconstitution of multiple antibiotics. In use, the water is aseptically added to the vial of medication to prepare the desired injection. For instance, a suitable injection may be prepared from the dry powder Sterile Ampicillin Sodium, USP, by aseptic addition of sterile water for injection.

Bacteriostatic water for injection (USP): Is sterile water for injection containing one or more suitable antimicrobial agents. It is packaged in prefilled syringes or in vials containing not more than 30 ml of the water. The container label must state the names and proportions of the antimicrobial agent or agents. The water is employed as a sterile vehicle in the preparation of small volumes of injectable preparations. Theoretically, presence of the bacteriostatic agent gives the flexibility for multiple-dose vials. If the first person to withdraw medication inadvertently contaminates the vial contents, the preservative will destroy the microorganism, although there has been debate on how much protection the antimicrobial agent can provide in a multiple - dose vial. Because of the presence of antimicrobial agents, the water must be used only in parenterals that are administered in small volumes. Its use in parenterals administered in large volume is restricted by the excessive and perhaps toxic amounts of the antimicrobial agents that would be injected along with the medication. Generally, if more than 5 ml of solvent is required, sterile water for injection rather than bacteriostatic water for injection is preferred. In using bacteriostatic water for injection, due regard must also be given to the chemical compatibility of the bacteriostatic agent or agents with the particular medicinal agent being dissolved or suspended.

2. *Non-aqueous vehicles*

Even though an aqueous vehicle is generally preferred for an injection, it may be precluded by the limited water solubility of a medicinal substance or its susceptibility to hydrolysis. When such physical or chemical factors limit the use of a wholly aqueous vehicle, the pharmaceutical formulator must turn to onc or morc non-aqucous vehicles. The non-aqueous vehicles are used in case if:

i) The drug shows poor aqueous solubility.

ii) A prolonged action (sustained release effect) is desired through depot formation. Example: Steroids-hydroxy progesterone, testosterone, progesterone, estradiol etc.

iii) The drug is susceptible to hydrolysis (*e.g.,* barbiturates).

Among the non-aqueous solvents employed in parenteral products are fixed vegetable oils, glycerin, polyethylene glycols, propylene glycol, alcohol and a number of less often used agents, including ethyl oleate, isopropyl myristate, and dimethylacetamide.

- The selected vehicle must be non-irritating, nontoxic in the amounts administered and not sensitizing.

- Like water, it must not exert a pharmacologic activity of its own, nor may it adversely affect the activity of the medicinal agent.
- In addition, the physical and chemical properties of the solvent or vehicle must be considered, evaluated and determined to be suitable for the task at hand.
- Among the many considerations are the solvent's physical and chemical stability at various pH levels, viscosity which must be such as to allow ease of injection (suitable for use in syringes); fluidity, which must be maintained over a fairly wide temperature range; boiling point, which should be sufficiently high to permit heat sterilization; miscibility with body fluids; low vapour pressure to avoid problems during heat sterilization; and constant purity or ease of purification and standardization.

No single solvent is free of limitations; hence, cross consideration and assessment of each solvent's advantages and disadvantages help the formulator determine the most appropriate solvent for a given preparation.

Fixed vegetable oils: Fixed vegetable oils such as corn oil, cottonseed oil, peanut oil, sesame oil are used as parenteral vehicles. Of these sesame oil is the most preferred oil due to high stability (except in light). The fixed oil used as a vehicle for the preparation of parenteral should fulfil the following criteria.

i) It should be free from solid paraffin and mineral oils (If present may lead to tissue reactions and even tumour formation as they are not metabolized in the body).
ii) It should not be rancid.
iii) It must remain clear when cooled to 10°C
iv) It should meet the official requirement of iodine value and saponification value.

Note: Injections prepared from oily vehicles should not be administered intravenously as it may lead to occlusion of the pulmonary micro-circulation (*i.e.,* thromboembolism) which may be fatal.

Glycerin: Glycerin is a clear syrupy liquid with a sweet taste and is miscible with water and alcohol. In parenteral formulation glycerin is used mainly as a solvent, moreover, it is also used as co-solvent, wetting agent and tonicity adjusting agent.

Polyethylene glycols (PEG): It provides good cake structure and increases the viscosity of water. It is miscible with water and alcohol. The 2% solution of PEG has a critical temperature of - 22°C. Apart from lyophilization, it is also used as a co-solvent and viscosity modifier in parenteral including ophthalmics.

Propylene glycol: It is a viscous liquid which is miscible with water. It is non-toxic, as it gets rapidly metabolized and excreted. Drugs such as digoxin and phenobarbitone employ propylene glycol as a vehicle.

Note: Injections containing propylene glycol (vehicle) should not be given through intramuscular and subcutaneous route as it may cause severe irritation.

Alcohol: It is used as a solvent in some of the parenteral preparations where it is impractical to use aqueous vehicles. It is also used as a co-solvent with water, as it is miscible with it and can dissolve several water-insoluble drugs (*e.g.,* digoxin and ergotamine). It also imparts preservative action to the solution. Alcohol have the disadvantages such as: it causes pain and tissue damage and it exhibits pharmacological activity and may interfere with the activity of the main drug.

Excipients/added Substances

Excipients used in the parenteral preparation include antibacterial preservatives, buffers, solubilizers, antioxidants and other adjuncts. Agents employed solely for their colouring effect are strictly prohibited in parenteral products.

Antibacterial agents (preservatives): These are the substances which are added in order to prevent the growth of microbes. These agents either kill (bactericidal) or arrest the growth (bacteriostatic) of bacteria in the pharmaceutical preparations during their storage. Due to this the product does not deteriorate and remains stable for a longer period of time. Benzyl alcohol, phenol and the parabens are the most widely used antimicrobial preservative agents in injectable products.

Desirable features of antimicrobial agents

i) It should be able to arrest the growth or kill the micro-organisms which contaminate the product.

ii) It should be compatible with the therapeutic agent as well as other additives even on long storage.

iii) It should not be absorbed by rubber closure and should be compatible with the material with which they are made.

iv) It should not produce any toxic effects in the patients irrespective of the quantity used in the injections.

v) It should be stable throughout the shelf –life of the product.

It is better to avoid the use of antimicrobial agents wherever possible.

The formulator should be aware of the reactions which may take place between preservatives and other components of the formulation.

Basically, preservatives are included in multiple dose parenteral products. This is due to the reason that accidental contamination may take place while withdrawing individual doses.

Note: Antimicrobial agents or preservatives should not be included in parenteral preparations exceeding 15 ml (such as infusion fluid). Different preservatives with their % concentration ranges are given in Table 6.1.

Table 6.1: Preservatives with their concentration ranges

Examples	*Concentration range (%)*
Benzyl alcohol	0.5 – 10
Methylparaben (methyl p-hydroxybenzoate)	0.01 – 0.18
Propyl paraben (propyl p-hydroxybenzoate)	0.005 – 0.035
Thimerosal	
0.001 – 0.02	

Buffers: In order to maintain the physical and chemical stability of the parenteral preparation it is necessary to maintain the pH of the preparation at desired levels. The selected pH of the preparation should not destabilize or decrease the solubility of the drug in the vehicle. Alterations in the pH of a parenteral product occur due to the following reasons.

i) Degradation of the therapeutic agent.

ii) Incorporation of leached out alkali from the glass container into the product.

iii) The release of acid or alkaline impurities into the product from the rubber closure.

pH of the formulation is maintained at the desired level by incorporation of a suitable buffer.

The buffer should be selected such that it does not affect the pharmacological activity and solubility of drug. The most ideal pH of parenteral preparation is 7.4 (same buffer systems are composed of a combination as that of blood) of both a weak acid and its salts. Different buffers with their % concentration are given in Table 6.2.

Table 6.2: Buffers with their concentration ranges

Examples	***Concentration (%)***
Acetic acid	0.22
Benzoic acid and sodium benzoate	5
Potassium phosphate	0.1
Sodium bicarbonate	0.005
Sodium citrate	4

Antioxidants: These are the substances which are added to the formulation to prevent degradation of the therapeutic agent which may occur due to oxidation during accelerated conditions of heat sterilization and also during storage. Antioxidants act in four ways:

i) Undergoes oxidation in place of the therapeutic agent *i.e.,* they act as reducing agents and usually consumed as the shelf life of the product advances.

ii) Blocks an oxidative chain reaction without being consumed *i.e.,* they act as blocking agents.

iii) Some substance enhances the effect of antioxidants (especially of those antioxidants which blocks an oxidative chain reaction) which are termed as synergists.

iv) Some compounds prevent oxidation of the therapeutic agent by forming a complex with substances which catalyse the oxidative reaction (*i.e.,* chelating agents). Different antioxidants with their % concentration ranges are given in Table 6.3.

Chelating agents: These are the substances which form complexes with heavy metals such as copper, iron, lead, mercury, chromium etc.,

Table 6.3: Antioxidants with their concentration ranges

Category	*Examples*	*Concentration*	*Used in formulation*
Reducing agents	Ascorbic acid	0.01–0.1%	Aqueous
	Sodium bisulfate	0.1–0.15%	Neutral pH aqueous
	Sodium metabisulfite	0.01–0.1%	Acidic aqueous
Blocking agents	Ascorbic acid esters	0.01–0.015%	Non-aqueous
	Butyl hydroxyl toluene	0.005–0.02%	Non-aqueous
	Butyl hydroxyl anisole	0.005–0.01%	Non-aqueous
	Alpha-Tocopherols	0.001–0.05%	Non-aqueous
Synergists	Ascorbic acid	0.01–0.05%	Aqueous formulations
	Citric acid	0.3–2.0%	–
	Tartaric acid	0.01–0.02%	–
Chelating agents	Ethylenediamine tetra-acetic acid	0.0005–0.01%	–

thereby inactivating them. Due to this, the heavy metals cannot catalyse destructive changes (oxidative degradation) in the parenteral preparation. Raw materials, solvents (mainly water), containers, rubber closures and equipment employed act as sources of heavy metal contamination. The most commonly used chelating agents include ethylenediamine tetra-acetic acid, citric acid, tartaric acid etc.

Inert gases: Product stability and integrity of oxygen sensitive drugs can be maintained by the use of inert gases such as argon and nitrogen. During the manufacturing and filling of parenteral, the nitrogen-rich atmosphere should be maintained. Infilled vials, the air in the head-space is displaced by either nitrogen or argon before sealing. Examples of oxygen-sensitive drugs which are filled in this manner are ergotamine and tubocurarine injections.

Surfactants: These are the substances which are added to the formulation to disperse a water-insoluble drug to form a colloidal dispersion. In other words, they enhance the solubility of the drug. Surfactants are mainly used in parenteral suspensions and emulsions as wetting and solubilizing agents. While selecting the solubilizing agent the formulator should also see it is compatible with the therapeutic agent. Different surfactants and their % concentration ranges are given in Table 6.4.

Table 6.4: Surfactants and their concentration ranges

Examples	***Concentration range (%)***
Propylene glycol	0.2 – 50
Povidone	0.2 – 1
Polysorbate 80	0.04 – 4
Polyethylene glycol (PEG) 300	0.01 – 50
Lecithin	0.5 – 2.3
Glycerin	14.6 – 25
Dioctyl sodium sulfosuccinate (DOSS)	0.015

Tonicity contributing agents: Injections need to be isotonic with blood serum or any other body fluids. Tonicity of the solution depends upon the amount and nature of the solutes present. It is determined either by molecular concentration or estimation of the freezing point of the solution.

In some cases where tonicity is to be adjusted, it can be done by adding substances like NaCl, dextrose, borax etc., which should be compatible with other ingredients of the preparation.

When blood cells and other tissues come in contact with the isotonic solution they neither shrink nor swell. Due to this reason, isotonic solutions do not cause any discomfort. The solutions which are not isotonic are highly irritating. Hence, necessary tonicity adjustment is made by using 0.9% NaCl, 2% boric acid or 5% dextrose.

Protectants: These are the substances which are added to the parenteral preparation to prevent the loss of activity of the therapeutic agent. Different types of protectants includes:

1. *Lyoprotectants:* These are the substances which when incorporated into the parenteral preparations (mainly proteins) inhibits loss of integrity of the active substance caused due to freeze-drying. Examples: sucrose and trehalose.

2. *Cryoprotectants*: These are the substances which when incorporated into the parenteral preparation (mainly proteins) inhibits loss of integrity of the active substance caused due to freezing. Example: polyethylene glycol (PEG) - prevents the damage of enzymes such as lactate dehydrogenase and phosphofructokinase caused due to freezing.

The decrease in activity of the therapeutic agent may be caused due to the following reasons:

i) Stress caused by the manufacturing processes (freezing, drying as in lyophilization). Freeze-drying promotes loss of activity of the active substance. Hence, freeze-dried products (such as protein formulations, liposomal formulations and vaccines) should include protectants as one of the additives.
ii) Adsorption of the therapeutic agent by the equipment, container and closure.

During the manufacturing operations (such as filtration, supply, packaging etc.) active ingredient is adsorbed by the filters (especially if they are made of nylon), silicone tubings (used for transfer operations) as well as by polymeric packaging materials of plastic bags, infusion sets, inline filters, rubber closures etc. Example: Human serum albumin (HAS) acts as a protectant in the concentration range of 0.1-1% it prevents the adsorption of insulin hormone [which is present in very low concentration when compared to the protectant (HAS)] by itself being adsorbed.

Importance of Isotonicity in Parenteral

The term isotonic, meaning equal tone; the body fluids, including blood and tears, have an osmotic pressure corresponding to that of 0.9% solution of sodium chloride. Thus, 0.9% of sodium chloride solution is said to be iso-osmotic or isotonic means having an osmotic pressure equal to that of physiologic fluids. Solutions with a lower osmotic pressure than body fluids or a 0.9% sodium chloride solution are commonly called hypotonic, whereas solutions having a greater osmotic pressure are termed hypertonic.

Theoretically, a hypertonic solution added to the body fluid will have a tendency to draw water from the body tissues toward the solution in an effort to dilute and establish concentration equilibrium. In the bloodstream, a hypertonic injection can cause crenation (shrinking) of blood cells; in the eye, the solution can draw water toward the site of the topical application. Conversely, a hypotonic solution may induce haemolysis or passage of water from the site of an ophthalmic application through the tissues of the eye. In practice, the isotonicity limits of an ophthalmic solution in terms of sodium chloride or its osmotic equivalent may range from 0.6% to 2.0% without marked discomfort to the eye. Sodium chloride itself does not have to be used to establish a solution's osmotic pressure.

RBCs and other body cells may be damaged or destroyed if exposed to hypertonic or hypotonic solutions (Fig. 6.2). For this reason, most intravenous (IV) solutions, liquids infused into the vein are isotonic. Examples 0.9 % NaCl and dextrose 5% in water. Sometimes the infusion of a hypertonic solution such as mannitol is useful to treat patients who have cerebral oedema. Infusion of such a solution relieves fluid overload by causing osmosis of water from interstitial fluid into the blood. The kidneys then excrete the excess water from the blood into the urine. Hypotonic solutions, given either orally or through an IV, can be used to treat people who are dehydrated. The water in the hypotonic solution moves from the blood into interstitial fluid and then into body cells to rehydrate.

Tonicity agents are used in many parenteral and ophthalmic products to adjust the tonicity of the solution. Although it is the goal for every injectable product to be isotonic with physiologic fluids, this

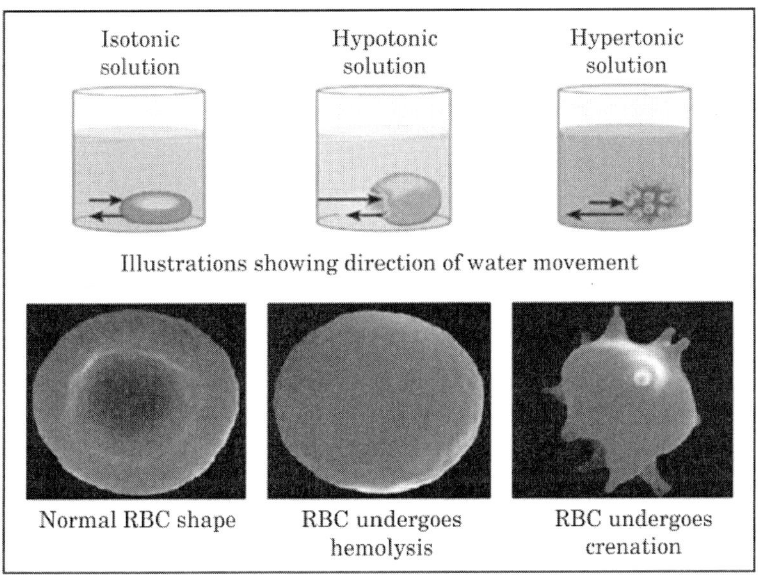

Fig. 6.2: Effect of hypertonic or hypotonic solutions on body cells (RBC).

is not an essential requirement for small volume injectables administered intravenously. However, products administered by all other routes, especially into the eye or spinal fluid, must be isotonic. Injections into the subcutaneous tissue and muscles should also be isotonic to minimize pain and tissue irritation. The agents most commonly used are electrolytes and mono or disaccharides.

Pharmacists are often called upon to calculate the quantity of solute that must be added to adjust a hypotonic solution of a drug to isotonic. Since, all the solutes incorporated in the parenteral and ophthalmic preparations, including the active and inactive ingredients, contribute to the osmotic pressure of a solution.

Hypotonic injection solutions are made isotonic by the addition of tonicity adjusting agents such as sodium chloride, dextrose or mannitol. Hypertonic injection solutions must be made isotonic by dilution prior to administration.

There are a number of methods available for calculating the amount of additional substance to be added to a hypotonic drug solution to render it isotonic, including freezing point depression, the use of sodium chloride equivalents, molar concentrations and calculations based on serum osmolarity. Isotonicity calculation based on freezing point depression and sodium chloride equivalent method are demonstrated below:

Isotonicity Calculation

a) Based on freezing point depression

Colligative properties of solutions like osmotic pressure, vapour pressure, boiling point and freezing point depend on the number of particles in solution. The presence of solutes in water will increase osmolarity and depress the freezing point of water. Consequently, the freezing point of a solution can be used as a measure of its osmolarity. The freezing point of blood serum/plasma and tears is -0.52°C. Therefore, an aqueous solution that freezes at -0.52°C is isotonic.

The amount of adjusting substance required to make a hypotonic solution to isotonic. It is given by the equation:

$$W = \frac{0.52 - a}{b}$$

where W is the % w/v of adjusting substance in the final solution, a is the freezing point depression of unadjusted solution (*i.e.*, freezing point depression of 1% solution × strength in %w/v) and b is the freezing point depression of water due to 1% w/v of adjusting substance, usually sodium chloride or glucose.

Example 1: Make a solution containing 0.28% w/v potassium chloride isotonic by the addition of anhydrous glucose using the given data.

Data: The freezing point depression of 1% solution of potassium chloride is 0.439 and for anhydrous glucose, it is 0.101.

Solution:

- 1% solution of potassium chloride depresses the freezing point of water by 0.439°C. Thus, the freezing point depression of unadjusted solution = 0.28 × 0.439 = 0.123°C.
- 1% solution of anhydrous glucose depresses the freezing point of water by 0.101°C.

$$W = \frac{0.52 - 0.123}{0.101} = \frac{0.397}{0.101} = 3.93$$

Thus, it requires the addition of 3.93% w/v (*i.e.*, 3.93 g per 100 ml) anhydrous glucose to make the potassium chloride solution isotonic with plasma.

Example 2: What is the concentration of NaCl required to make 1% solution of cocaine HCl isotonic with blood plasma? The freezing point of 1% w/v solution of NaCl is -0.576°C and freezing point of 1% w/v of cocaine HCl is -0.09°C.

Solution:

- 1% solution of cocaine HCl depresses the freezing point of water by 0.09°C.
- 1% solution of NaCl depresses the freezing point of water by 0.576°C.

$$W = \frac{0.52 - 0.09}{0.576} = \frac{0.43}{0.576} = 0.7465$$

Thus, it requires the addition of 0.7465% w/v (*i.e.,* 0.7465 g per 100 ml) NaCl to make the 1% w/v solution of cocaine HCl solution isotonic with plasma.

b) Based on sodium chloride equivalent method

Another method frequently used for calculating the quantity of sodium chloride necessary to prepare an isotonic solution is the *sodium chloride equivalent method.* A sodium chloride equivalent is the amount of sodium chloride that is osmotically equivalent to 1 g of the drug. For example, the sodium chloride equivalent of ephedrine sulfate is 0.23; that is, 1 g of ephedrine sulfate is equivalent to 0.23 g of sodium chloride.

How much sodium chloride is required to make the following prescription isotonic?

Rx

Ephedrine sulfate 2%

Sterile water, q.s. 30 ml

Molar isotonic with sodium chloride

- Amount of ephedrine sulfate required to prepare 30 ml of 2% solution $= \frac{30 \times 2}{100} = 0.6$ g
- To prepare 30 ml of 0.9% w/v sodium chloride requires $= \frac{30 \times 0.9}{100}$ = 0.270 g sodium chloride
- 1 g of ephedrine sulfate is equivalent to 0.23 g of sodium chloride
- Hence, 0.6 g of ephedrine sulfate is equivalent to $= \frac{0.6 \times 0.23}{1} =$ 0.138 g of sodium chloride
- Since 0.270 g sodium chloride is required if only sodium chloride is used and the quantity of sodium chloride that is equivalent to 0.6 g of ephedrine sulfate is 0.138 g, then 0.270 g - 0.138 g = 0.132 g of sodium chloride required to render the solution isotonic.
- Therefore, the solution requires ephedrine sulfate 0.6 g, sodium chloride 0.132 g, and sufficient sterile water to make 30 ml.

Production Procedure and Aseptic Processing for Parenteral

An inherent requirement for parenteral preparations is that they must be of the very best quality and provide maximum safety for the patient.

Constant adherence to high moral and professional ethics on the part of the responsible persons is most vital to achieving the desired quality in the products prepared. Once the formulation for a particular parenteral product is determined, including selection of the proper vehicles and additives, the production pharmacist must follow rigid aseptic procedures in preparing the products. The general production procedure for parenteral products is given in Fig. 6.3.

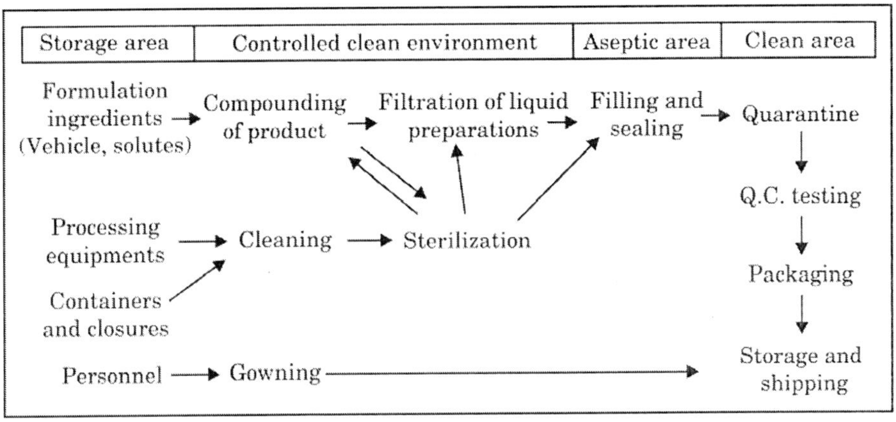

Fig. 6.3: Flow diagram of production parenteral products.

Production procedure for parenteral products includes:

a) Maintenance of production environment (or facilities)

b) Cleaning and sterilization of equipment, containers and closures

c) Compounding (filtration, filling and terminal sterilization) of parenterals

a) *Maintenance of production environment and facilities*: As parenterals are sterile preparations hence, maintenance of production environment and cleanliness is of utmost importance. These can be achieved by the strict control on:

***i) Personnel requirements*:** Personnel employed in the manufacturing of parenterals should be physically fit. They should not be suffering from any infectious disease which might increase microbial contamination. Periodically, the physical and medical examination should be done. If any worker is suffering from a cold, sore throat or allergy, he must report it to the higher authority and should be restricted from entering into the aseptic area. Proper training is to be given to the operators of the aseptic area as per good manufacturing practice (GMP) rules. The uniform of employees should be sterile and made of Dacron (effective barriers to discharged particles). They should also wear head-covers, shoe covers, face masks, gloves while working in aseptic rooms. The air shower is necessary as it removes any loose particles (dust, lint etc.) present on the uniforms of the employees. The employees entering the aseptic room should wash their hands with antiseptic soap. Frequent inward and outward movement in the aseptic room should be avoided during processing and filling operations.

ii) Environmental control and its evaluation: The environmental control maintained is different for different areas (*i.e.,* clean-up area, compounding area, filling and packaging areas). Stringent environmental control is required before and during processing of parenterals. This is to assure an area free from contamination and where, there is no accumulation of dust particles, lint, viable micro-organisms etc.

The production environment is monitored and evaluated to check whether the required sterility conditions are maintained or not. If any discrepancy is noted in the action levels then possible corrective measures should be taken. Various evaluation tests are available to evaluate the environmental control. These tests are as follows:

Particle count: The number of particles in a volume of sample air is measured. This is done by particle measuring systems which not only count the particles but also provide size distribution details based on light scattered from the particles. This test is used to detect the presence of dust particles but viable forms such as bacteria and fungi cannot be detected.

Slit to agar (STA) sampler: This device consists of a rotating agar plate comprising of a slit through which air is drawn out by applying vacuum. This air comes in contact with the surface of the agar plate. Viable microorganisms such as bacteria, fungi etc. stick to the surface of the agar plate and start growing in the form of colonies (colony forming units-CFU).

Rodac plates: These plates consist of nutrient agar with a convex surface. The plate is rolled on the surface to be tested wherein micro-organisms sticks to the surface of the agar plate. These plates are incubated during which, the micro-organisms start growing. The tested surface should be thoroughly cleaned after the completion of the test.

iii) Traffic control: Traffic includes the supply of materials and entry and exit of the workers in the production area. Traffic should be strictly controlled in aseptic rooms. A prescribed procedure should be followed which is applicable to every person who enters the aseptic areas. They should change their clothes, cover their faces with masks, wear hand gloves, head covers or caps and shoes. Once the person enters the aseptic area, he or she cannot leave until the completion of the manufacturing cycle. Entry of unauthorized persons in this area should be restricted.

iv) *General cleaning:* A cleaning schedule should be developed and followed on a daily or periodic basis, based on sterility requirements. Separate workers should be appointed for maintenance to clean all the equipment, walls, ceilings and floors before and after production at the end of the day.

General cleaning and surface disinfection: Sanitization is carried out using disinfectants or UV radiation before starting the production. Cleaning and sanitization are carried out in two ways. 1) By spraying a suitable liquid disinfectant over all the surfaces in aseptic areas. 2) An effective surface disinfection is achieved by the use of germicidal UV lamps. Irradiation of UV light rays is done to decrease the population of bacteria in aseptic areas.

Cleaning of air: Air entering in the aseptic area is the greatest source of contamination, as it contains most of the bacteria. It is important to clean the air before it enters the aseptic area to avoid contamination. The cleaning of air is mainly carried out by conventional systems or laminar flow systems.

Conventional systems/class 10000: Conventional clean room system consists of two air conditioners fixed at the ceiling and at the bench level respectively. This area is responsible for the control of dust particles, humidity and temperature. Before entering, the air is dehumidified, cooled and filtered. This filtered air is allowed to enter at a velocity of 800 ft/min. This room is also known as 10000 class because it contains not more than 10000 particles (of size $> 0.5\ \mu$) per cubic feet. As there is a high degree of air fluctuation, it is highly difficult to maintain and control temperature, humidity and dust particles. Hence, a high proportion of cleanliness cannot be maintained. As a result, conventional systems are used for the purpose of cleanliness in general areas or surrounding areas but not in aseptic rooms.

Laminar flow systems: Laminar flow systems are used for cleaning air in the aseptic rooms. Cleaning of air is done in order to remove bacteria or dust particles which may cause contamination during production of sterile preparations. In laminar air flow systems, clean air is obtained through high-efficiency particulate air (HEPA) filters. This clean air flows at a uniform velocity of 100 ± 20 ft/min in parallel lines. The air sweeps the dust particles and makes the entire area of the aseptic room free from dust particles.

In conventional systems, the sterile area attained is of low degree, whereas in laminar systems it is of high degree. Hence, conventional systems are not used for maintaining sterility of air in aseptic areas, but laminar systems are used. * Laminar airflow system used in parenterals is discussed at the end of this chapter.

b) Cleaning and sterilization of equipment, containers and closures: Equipment, containers and closures are in intimate contact with the parenteral preparations. Hence, they are thoroughly cleaned and sterilized before use.

Cleaning of equipment: The equipment used for the manufacturing of parenteral preparations should be opened and all detachable parts are separated from the main body. This is done to facilitate easy and thorough cleaning of internal structures such as joints, crevices, screw threads etc. an effective detergent and a stiff brush should be used for cleaning purpose. The walls of stationary tanks, spigots (taps) and pipes and the areas which are not easily accessible may contain debris which can be removed by exposing them to a stream of clean steam.

Presently automated systems are available which help to accomplish cleaning through high pressure rinsing treatments with hot detergent, hot water and final rinse with distilled water. Such equipment does not require manual cleaning and can be cleaned and sterilized while they are in place. Hence, they are also known as clean-in-place (CIP) equipment and sterilization-in-place (SIP) equipment respectively.

Sterilization of equipment: The equipment which is intended for use in the aseptic area should be rendered sterile. The sterilizations temperature and time duration vary with the material of construction of the equipment.

For equipment which is sensitive to temperature, gas sterilization by ethylene oxide is the method of choice for sterilizing such equipment. The equipment which is exclusively employed in the sterile area such as bottles, filling machinery, sterilizing membranes, stoppering equipment, tanks, utensils, vent filters, must be sterilized just before the commencement of the sterile operation.

Cleaning of containers: Parenteral preparation should always be packed in new containers. Use of detergents for cleaning the containers should be avoided because improper rinsing may leave detergent residues which may enter into the parenteral preparation. Instead, thermal shock treatment should be carried out. In this treatment, the containers are heated and subsequently cooled. Due to this, expansion followed by contraction of the containers may take place which results in loosening of debris from the container walls. Sometimes an air rinse is sufficient to get rid of loose debris from the container walls. All the containers should be finally rinsed with water for injection (WFI). Cleaning of containers is carried out in specially designed machines. These machines include:

i) Manual loading type rinse: This machine comprises jet tubes and a central post which is meant for the introduction of treatments (hot or cold treatment). The jet tubes are arranged as spokes of a wheel onto the arms. The unclean containers are manually loaded onto the arms. The stream of hot or cold treatment from jet tubes cleans the containers.

ii) Conveyor type rinsers: This machine uses a row of jet tubes across a conveyor belt. These are a programmed series of treatments at various points. Inverted containers are placed on the conveyor belt. When the machine starts working, these containers are moved past the series of treatments (hot, cold, WFI treatments). Cleaned containers are conveyed to a sterilizing oven where they are sterilized and then finally delivered into a clean room where the aseptic filling is carried out.

Sterilization of containers: Dry heat sterilization is the method of choice for sterilizing glass containers. In this method, sterilization is carried out at 250°C for 4 h in a typical hot air sterilizer. The sterile containers free from pyrogens are then stored in stainless steel trays and delivered to a clean room with a facility of laminar air flow.

Owing to the low melting point, plastic containers cannot be sterilized by moist heat and dry heat sterilization. Instead, they are sterilized by gas sterilization method using ethylene oxide. During the gas sterilization process, spore strips and colour change strips are included in the sterilization chamber along with the plastic containers. After completion of the process, these strips are examined to ensure that sufficient exposure to ethylene oxide gas has taken place. Once the sterilization process has been completed the plastic containers are removed. Deaeration is carried out in a forced draft hot air oven at 60-100°C or in a laminar airflow hood for several hours. Apart from gas sterilization, plastic containers can also be sterilized by radiation. This method employs cobalt 60 γ rays or high energy electron beam source.

Cleaning of closures: Rubber closures and plastic caps are most commonly used for sealing the parenteral products. Closures are washed with or without the use of detergents. When detergent is used for washing, copious amounts of water should be used for rinsing. The method involves washing the closures with 0.5% sodium pyrophosphate (hot detergent solution) in a larger tank which is under mechanical agitation or tumbling action. Final rinses should be done with pyrogen-free water for injection (WFI).

An ideal washing machine should be used for washing rubber closures and caps. The primary goal of this machine is to remove debris which was accumulated onto the closures during the moulding process, minimizes abrasion of closures and removal of loose debris.

After washing, closures are packed either in glass polypropylene synthetic bags which are non-shedding or stainless steel containers provided with intact seals. They are then transferred to the sterilization chamber.

Sterilization of closures: Rubber closures can neither be sterilized through dry heat sterilization nor through gas sterilization. Since rapid head penetration upon dry heat sterilization may lead to the development of cracks in rubber closures. Upon gas sterilization with ethylene oxide, the gas may get associated with rubber matrix and is difficult to escape during deaeration.

Hence, moist heat sterilization is considered to be the ideal method to sterilize rubber closures. After sterilization, the closures are allowed to dry and stored in clean rooms preferentially provided with laminar air flow hood.

c) Compounding (filtration, filling and terminal sterilization): In the preparation of parenteral solutions, the required ingredients are dissolved in solvent, or in a combination of solvents. The solutions are usually filtered through a membrane until sparkling clear. After filtration, the solution is transferred as rapidly as possible and with the least possible exposure into the final containers. The product is then sterilized, preferably by autoclaving and samples of the finished product are tested for sterility and pyrogens. If sterilization by autoclaving is impractical because of the nature of the ingredients, the individual components of the preparation that are heat or moisture labile may be sterilized by other appropriate means and added aseptically to the sterilized solvent or solution of components that can be autoclaved.

Suspensions of drugs for parenteral use may be prepared by reducing the drug to a very fine powder with a ball mill, micronizer, colloid mill, or other appropriate equipment and then suspending the material in a liquid in which it is insoluble. It is frequently necessary to sterilize separately the individual components of a suspension before combining them, as frequently the integrity of a suspension is destroyed by autoclaving. Autoclaving of a parenteral suspension may alter the viscosity of the product, affecting the suspending ability of the vehicle, or change the particle size of the suspended particles, altering both pharmaceutical and therapeutic characteristics. If a suspension remains unaltered by autoclaving, this method is generally employed to sterilize the final product. Because parenteral emulsions, which are dispersions of a liquid throughout into another liquid, are generally destroyed by autoclaving, an alternative method of sterilization must be employed for this type of injectable.

Some injections are packaged as dry solids rather than in conjunction with a solvent or vehicle because the therapeutic agent is unstable in the presence of the liquid component. These dry powders are packaged in the final container to be reconstituted, generally to a solution or less frequently a suspension. The method of sterilization of the powder may be dry heat or another appropriate method.

Area for Production of Sterile Preparations

During sterile preparation, two types of rooms are to be maintained.

i) Class 100: This class can be achieved by laminar air flow. This area contains not more than 100 particles of 0.5 μ and larger size per cubic feet (ft^3) of air.

ii) Class 10000: This class can be achieved by a conventional air flow system (air conditioning). This area contains not more than 10000 particles of 0.5 μ and even large per cubic feet (ft^3) of air.

Different sectional areas for sterile preparations:

a) Clean-up section: In this area, cleaning of the bottles, vials or ampoules is carried out. Proper care should be taken while cleaning procedure is carried out. The cleaning area has walls and ceiling which are made up of film coating materials.

This area should be free from holes, corners or projections which may otherwise lead to accumulation of dust. The air inside the clean area should be free from dust and micro-organisms. This is ensured through high efficiency (95%) filters. Existing air in the clean area should be frequently replaced (10-15 air changes per hour).

b) Compounding section: In this area, the actual compounding is carried out. Unlike the aseptic area, maintenance of sterile conditions is not needed. But necessary measures should be adopted to control the dust generated from "raw material at the time of weighing and compounding. Generally, stainless steel cabinets and counters are seen in this section.

c) Aseptic section: In this area, strict control measures should be adopted to avoid contamination of the preparations. There should not be any provision for the dust to enter this area, hence, for this reason, the ceiling floor and walls are sealed properly and should be washed frequently with disinfectant. The stainless steel counters and cabinets should be such that they do not allow dirt particles to accumulate. The mixing and storage of the compounded preparations should be done outside the aseptic area. The compounded preparations are then transferred to the aseptic area through pipelines where the filling operation is carried out.

d) Quarantine section: This area consists of the store where the in-process batches, as well as the approved batches, are stored separately. This allows easy location of a particular batch during re-sampling. This area has limited access. A responsible person is in charge of this area.

Without the consent of the in-charge other personnel cannot enter into this particular area.

e) Packing and labelling section: In this area, the batches are packed and labelled. Labels are obtained by overprinting devices and packing is carried out by packaging machines. At a time, only one product labels are printed.

Examples of Parenteral Formulations

The preparation of parenterals should be accomplished in clean, aseptic rooms. Stringent sterility conditions as per standards should be maintained to prevent particle and microbial contamination.

1) *Formulation of injections*

Injections are sterile solutions, emulsions or suspensions. They are prepared by dissolving, emulsifying or suspending the active ingredient(s) and any added substances in water for injection or in a suitable non-aqueous vehicle, or in a mixture of the two if they are miscible. Injections that are emulsions should not show any evidence of separation and show a uniform appearance after shaking. The diameter of the globules of the dispersed phase of emulsions intended for intravenous injection must be decided with regard to the use of the preparation. Injections that are suspensions may show sediment which is readily dispersible on shaking. The suspension remains sufficiently stable to enable a homogenous dose to be withdrawn from the container. Examples for injections are shown in Table 6.5, Table 6.6, Table 6.7 and Table 6.8.

1. *Diazepam injection I.P. (I.P. 2007)*

Table 6.5: Diazepam injection I.P.

Ingredients	*Role*	*Quantity (%)*	*Overages*
Diazepam	Active ingredients	0.5	
Propylene glycol	Co-solvent	40	
Ethanol, absolute	Co-solvent	10	
Benzyl alcohol	Preservative	1.5	10 %
Sodium benzoate	Preservative	4.9	
Benzoic acid	Preservative	0.1	
Water for injection (q.s)	Solvent	100	

Route of administration: Intravenous or intramuscular use only

Method

1. Take a measured volume of propylene glycol and heat it to about 70°C. Start passing nitrogen gas.
2. Dissolve diazepam in previously heated benzyl alcohol (30 to 35°C) and add to propylene glycol.
3. Dissolve sodium benzoate in some quantity of water and add to propylene glycol solution.
4. Adjust the pH to 6.2 to 6.9. Make up the volume to the final level and check the pH.
5. Filter through a sterile 0.45 μ membrane filter.
6. Fill the required quantity under nitrogen, sterilize by dry heat before filling at 160° for 1 h.

2. *Ascorbic acid injection I.P. (I.P. 2007)*

Table 6.6: Ascorbic acid injection I.P.

Ingredients	***Quantity (%)***	***Overages***
Ascorbic acid	25	
Disodium edetate	0.025	15%
Sodium bicarbonate	1	
Water for injection (q.s)	100 %	

Route of administration: Intravenous or intramuscular or subcutaneous use only

Method

1. In 2/3rd of volume of water for injection, suspend ascorbic acid under dark slowly with continuous stirring; this should be done in an open vessel.
2. Add slowly sodium bicarbonate with vigorous stirring.
3. The level of the liquid will rise considerably because of profuse effervescence.
4. As this subsides add further sodium bicarbonate. Continue this process until ascorbic acid is completely dissolved.
5. Adjust the pH between 5.5 to 7.0 using sodium hydroxide or hydrochloric acid
6. Filter through G-3 and G-4 sintered filters or through a pre-sterilized assembly using 0.22 μ final filter and 0.45 μ pre-filter
7. Make up the volume with Water for injection. Fill the required volume into amber coloured ampoules and seal it.

8. Sterilize by steaming at 121° C for 30 min. Label the containers and evaluate as per monograph.

3. *Paracetamol injection*

Table 6.7: Paracetamol injection 75 mg/ml

Ingredients	***Role***	***Quantity***
Paracetamol	Active ingredient	7.5 g
Propylene glycol	Co-solvent	80.0 ml
Benzyl alcohol	Preservative	1.5 ml
Tween 80	Surfactant	1.0 g
Lignocaine HCL	Local anaesthetics	0.5 g
EDTA sodium	Chelating agent	0.1 g
Water for injection	Solvent	100.0 ml

Method

1. Take 80 ml of propylene glycol in a suitable vessel
2. Add to it benzyl alcohol and Tween 80
3. Stir to mix well
4. Heat the above mixture to 60°C
5. Add paracetamol slowly with continuous stirring until it dissolves completely
6. Cool to room temperature, check the volume and calculate water required to adjust up to 100 ml
7. Take calculated volume of water and dissolve it in EDTA and lignocaine HCL
8. Add the resultant solution to bulk and stir well to mix.
9. Check the pH and adjust the pH to 6.2 by using citric acid.
10. Filter through 0.22-μ membrane and fill into pre-sterilized vials aseptically

4. *Triamicinole diacetate suspension for injection*

Method

1. Prepare a saturated solution of sodium chloride (85 g) and triamicinole diacetate (40 g)
2. Put a required quantity of water for injection into a suitable vessel, add PEG 4000 (3 g) and agitate slowly until a clear solution is formed.

Table 6.8: Triamicinole diacetate 40 mg/ml suspension for injection.

Ingredients	*Role*	*Quantity*
Triamcinolone diacetate	Active ingredient	40 g
Polysorbate 80	Dispersing agent	2.0 g
Polyethylene glycol 4000	Co-solvent	3.0 g
Sodium chloride	Tonicity agent	85 g
Benzyl alcohol	Preservative	9.0 g
Sodium hydroxide or hydrochloric acid qs	Buffering	pH 6.0
Water for injection qs	Solvent	1000 ml

3. Preparation of polysorbate 80 solution: Place 2 g of polysorbate 80 into a suitable container and add sufficient quantity of water for injection
4. Take sterile water for injection for final volume adjustment for the suspension
5. Preparation of preservative solution: Dissolve benzyl alcohol in a small quantity of water for injection in a suitable container, mix well and transfer into a suitable vessel.
6. Place the following containers in a steam autoclave
   - Insoluble drug slurry in saturated sodium chloride
   - PEG 4000 solution
   - Polysorbate 80 solution
   - Preservative solution
   - Water for injection
7. Close the autoclave. The autoclave is then charged with steam at a sufficient pressure to yield 121°C maintain the conditions for 30 min.
8. After 30 min remove the containers from the autoclave when sufficiently cool to handle after the completion of the cycle.
9. Place the following preparation in a sterile room and allowed to cool to room temperature
10. Aseptically pour all the containers into the final volume container
11. Aseptically homogenise the sterile suspension with suitable homogenizer and transfer into the final container

Table 6.9: Common examples of large-volume parenterals

Large volume parenterals	***Ingredients***	***Category***
Amino acid	3.5, 5, 5.5, 7, 8.5 and 10% crystalline amino acid with or without varying concentrations of electrolytes or glycerin	Fluid and nutrient replenisher
Dextrose Injection, USP	2.5, 5 and 10% dextrose, other strengths	Fluid and nutrient replenisher
Dextrose and sodium chloride injection, USP	Dextrose 2.5% – 10%; NaCl 0.11% – 0.9% (19–154 mEq sodium)	Fluid, nutrient, electrolyte replenisher
Mannitol injection, USP	5, 10, 15, 20 and 25% mannitol	Diagnostic aid in renal function;diuretic; fluid and nutrient replenisher
Ringer's injection, USP	147 mEq sodium, 4 mEq potassium, 4.5 mEq calcium, and 156 mEq chloride per liter	Fluid and electrolyte replenisher
Lactated Ringer's injection, USP	2.7 mEq calcium, 4 mEq potassium, 130 mEq sodium, and 28 mEq lactate per liter	Systemic alkalinizer; fluid and electrolyte replenisher
Sodium chloride injection, USP	0.9% NaCl	Fluid and electrolyte replenisher; isotonic vehicle

Formulation of large volume parenterals are shown in Table 6.10 and Table 6.11.

1. *Sodium chloride injection I.P. (I.P. 2007)*

Table 6.10: Sodium chloride injection I.P.

Ingredients	***Quantity***	***Overages***
Sodium chloride	0.9 %	
Activated charcoal	q.s	4%
Water for injection (q.s)	100 %	

Route of administration: Intravenous use only

2. *Large volume parenterals*

Large volume parenterals are terminally sterilized aqueous injectable drug products packaged in a single dose container with a capacity of 100 ml or more and administered as intravenous injections, irrigating solutions, peritoneal dialysates etc.

Common examples of large-volume parenterals in use today are presented in Table 6.9 and are administered by IV infusion to replenish body fluids or electrolytes or to provide nutrition. They are usually administered in volumes of 100 ml to 1 L or more per day by slow IV infusion with or without a controlled-rate infusion system. Because of the large volumes administered, these solutions must not contain bacteriostatic agents (preservatives) or other pharmaceutical additives. They are packaged in large single-dose containers.

Method

1. Add sodium chloride to water for injection at 60°C & mix for 5 min
2. Add activated charcoal and mix for 15 min
3. Filter the solution through filter pads to get a clear charcoal free solution
4. Again filter through 0.45 μ membrane filter before filling into infusion bottles
5. Fill into the bottles calculated volume at 45° to 50°C immediately

2. *Dextrose injection I.P. (I.P. 2007)*

Table 6.11: Dextrose injection I.P.

Name of ingredients	*Quantity*	*Overages*
Dextrose	5 %	
Activated charcoal	q.s	4%
Water for injection (q.s)	100 %	

Route of administration: Intravenous use only

Method

1. Add dextrose to water for injection at 60°C and mix for 5 min
2. Add activated charcoal and mix for 15 min
3. Filter the solution through filter pads to get a clear charcoal free solution
4. Again filter through 0.45 μ membrane filter before filling into infusion bottles
5. Calculated volume is filled into the bottles at 45° to 50°C immediately

As indicated previously, energy source, electrolytes and vitamins are frequently incorporated into large-volume parenterals for co-administration to the patient in the form of parenteral nutrition.

Parenteral nutrition

Parenteral nutrition (PN) involves intravenous administration of nutrients to patients that require nutritional support and are anorectic despite correction of dehydration and other metabolic derangements. PN solutions are usually mixtures of dextrose solutions, lipid emulsions and amino acid solutions that variably contain electrolytes, vitamins and mineral supplements. When dextrose, lipids and amino acids are used together in a PN formulation; the resulting mixture is called a three-in-one solution or total parenteral nutrients (TPN).

TPN are easy to administer; provide a patient's short-term amino acid, glucose and energy needs in one solution; and are well tolerated by patients. Dextrose and amino acid solutions—without lipids - are given to patients as well. The use of these solutions can help to avoid negative side effects of lipid administration. Dextrose and amino acid solutions do not need to be replaced on a daily basis as with lipid-containing admixtures but, because they contain fewer kilocalories per millilitre, require substantially greater volumes of delivery to meet caloric needs.

The principal indication for TPN is a seriously ill patient where enteral feeding is not possible. It may also be used to supplement inadequate oral intake. The successful use of TPN requires proper selection of patients, adequate experience with the technique, and awareness of its complications. Some of the more important indications of TPN are listed below.

Indications for TPN

General indications for TPN

TPN may be indicated in the short term for patients who are malnourished or who are at risk of malnutrition and who have reversible loss of gastrointestinal function, *i.e.,* the gastrointestinal tract cannot be accessed, is not functional because it is either obstructed, inflamed, fistulated or leaking and the patient cannot achieve adequate nutrition by oral or enteral means. Less commonly, where there is irreversible loss of alimentary function (*e.g.,* short gut syndrome), TPN can be life-saving and may be considered long term.

Specific clinical situations

In pre-operative nutritional support: Patients who are identified as being severely malnourished pre-operatively and who cannot be adequately fed *via* oral or enteral routes may benefit from 7-10 days of parenteral nutrition prior to surgery to improve postoperative outcomes.

Patients with high-risk of prolonged postoperative ileus: Post-operative TPN is recommended in patients who cannot meet their caloric requirements within 7-10 days *via* oral or enteral routes.

Pancreatitis and pancreatic fistulae: Patients with severe pancreatitis, its complications there of or the need for surgery, benefit from early nutritional support. Jejunal feeding, *via* a naso-jejunal feeding tube or jejunostomy, is the preferred route for nutrition with improved outcomes compared to TPN.

Palliative surgical and non-surgical oncology: This is controversial and requires broad and extensive consultation. In patients with intestinal failure where enteral nutrition is insufficient and expected survival due to disease progression is longer than 3 months, long-term TPN may be considered in motivated patients.

There are several special formulations available for specific clinical situations; an outline of basic TPN solution is given below.

Fluid requirements: 100 ml/kg body weight for the first 10 kg, 50 ml/kg for next 10 kg and 20 ml/kg for each additional kg of body weight. Compensations should be made for additional losses *e.g.,* from a fistula.

Calories: Glucose is the major carbohydrate which supplies calories, and this is administered in the form of 25% or 50% solution. Total energy requirement may vary considerably between 2000 to 4500 or more calories daily.

Fats: In order to avoid essential fatty acid deficiency at least 4% of calories should be supplied as fats.

Proteins: Protein requirement varies from 1.5 to 2.5 g/kg of body weight per day. The ratio of nitrogen to calories should be 1: 100–150. Branched-chain amino acids have been recommended as an integral part of TPN. However, their benefits have so far not been conclusively proved.

Electrolytes: Daily maintenance requirements of sodium are 1–1.5 mEq/kg; potassium 1 mEq/kg; chloride 1.5–2 mEq/kg; calcium 0.2 mEq/kg and magnesium 0.35 – 0.45 mEq/kg.

Micronutrients: Trace elements are an important component of TPN. Zinc 5 mg, copper 1 mg, chromium 10 μg, manganese 0.5 mg and iron 1–2 mg are required daily.

Vitamins: Vit K-1 10 mg and folic acid 5 mg should be administered intramuscularly once a week. Vit B 12 1 mg is given once a month. Water-soluble vitamins should be given daily.

Nutritional monitoring: It is recommended that the following parameters be measured daily during TPN: Body weight estimation; 12-hourly intake-output chart; 8-hourly urine-sugar estimation; serum sodium, potassium, bicarbonate, calcium and chloride; blood urea and serum creatinine. Liver function tests and serum proteins should be measured twice daily.

3. *Sterile powders*

Sterile powders or powders for injection are sterile, solid substances which are distributed in their final containers and which, when shaken with the prescribed volume of the appropriate sterile liquid, rapidly form clear and particle-free solutions or uniform suspensions.

Injections of medicaments that are unstable in aqueous solution must be made immediately prior to use. The ingredients are presented as sterile powders in ampoules or vials. Sufficient diluent, *e.g.,* sterile water for injections, is added from a second container to produce the required drug concentration and the injection is used immediately. The powder may contain suitable excipients in addition to the drug, *e.g.,* sufficient additive to produce an isotonic solution when the injection is reconstituted. The technologies available to produce sterile dry powder drug, a product includes freeze-drying, sterile crystallization or spray-drying and powder filling.

Sterile powders must be prepared using materials and methods designed to ensure sterility and to avoid the introduction of contaminants and the growth of micro-organisms.

The label for powders for injection should state i) the amount of active ingredient contained in the sealed container, ii) the directions for preparing the injection or intravenous infusion from the powder and iii) that when dissolved or suspend the preparation is intended for parenteral use.

Following are most important sterile dry powders without any adjutants:

Ampicillin sodium injection

Streptomycin sulphate injection

Penicillin-G sodium injection

Kanamycin sulphate injection

Hydrocortisone sodium succinate injection

For example ampicillin sodium injections are generally prepared as sterile dry powders without any adjuvants in sterile clear glass vials. Water for injection required for reconstitution of sterile powders.

The general method of preparation of sterile powders

1. Sterilize vial, rubber closure, aluminium seals and disinfect the dry powders filling machine.
2. Aseptically transfer sterile drug powders in the pre-sterilized hopper of the filling machine.
3. Fill the powder aseptically into sterile vials using a suitable sterile powder filling machine.
4. Some products need sterile nitrogen gas is used for purging.
5. Sterilize the filled vial containing dry powder.

4. *Lyophilized products*

Lyophilisation or freeze-drying is the most common unit process for manufacturing drug products which are unstable to be marketed as solutions. Many parenteral drugs, particularly biopharmaceuticals, are too unstable in solution to be available as ready-to-use liquid dosage forms. Such drugs can still be filled as solutions, placed in a chamber, where the combined effects of freezing and drying under low pressure will remove the solvent and residual moisture from the solute components, resulting in a dry powder that has sufficient long-term stability. Example for preparation (or formulation) a lyophilized sterile injectable is given in Table 6.12.

Table 6.12: Formula for preparation of a lyophilized sterile injectable.

Ingredients	***Quantity***
Soluble drug (active drug substance)	1000 mg
Mannitol (bulking agent or tonicity adjusting agent)	q. s.
Sodium hydroxide (pH adjusting agent) or	q. s.
hydrochloric acid	pH 6.8 – 7
Water for injection (solvent or vehicle)	up to 100 ml

***The general method of lyophilisation*:** Initially q. s. solution is frozen by subjecting it to a process of mechanical freezing in the presence of circulating fluid such as silicone oil at -35 to -45°C. Freezing facilitates the formation of large ice-crystals with large holes. Preferably such crystals are of great importance in freeze drying because they form a porous product on drying. While freezing low temperature (-50°C) is maintained in the freezing chamber (Fig. 6.4). After solidification of the product, the pressure in the freeze-drying chamber is decreased to a pressure less than that of the vapour pressure of the ice (*i.e.,* below its eutectic point) at the same working temperature of the *i.e.,* -50°C the product is then subjected to heating by increasing the temperature of the circulating fluid (silicone oil). At this temperature, (*i.e.,* the temperature below the triple point of water) the frozen product sublimes to vapour. This is referred to as primary drying which leads to the removal of about 98-99% of moisture from the material, forming a cake. Remaining 1-2% of moisture is removed by increasing the temperature to about 30°C, this is called secondary drying which takes more than 10 hours. To avoid re-absorption of moisture, the freeze-dried product should be removed and sealed as early as possible under vacuum and controlled low humidity conditions.

The formulation should take into consideration the critical quality attributes such as maintenance of chemical or biological activity of the product even after reconstitution, rapid and complete dissolution upon

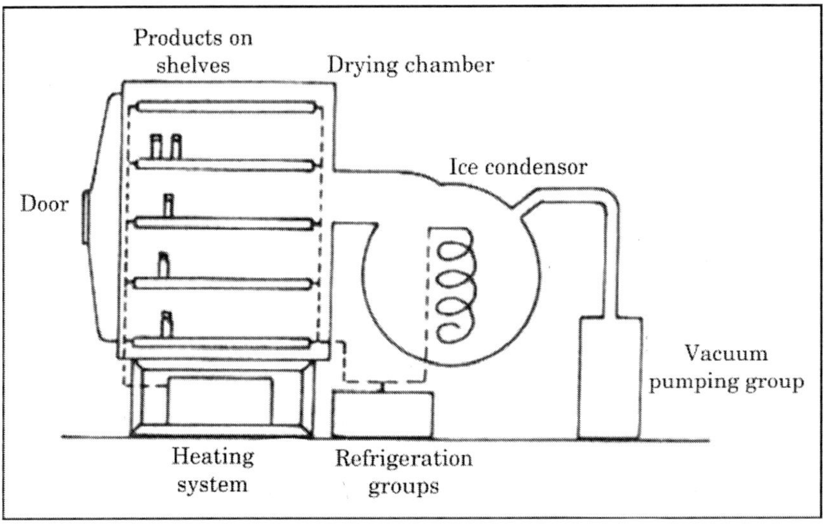

Fig. 6.4: Freeze dryer

reconstitution, minimum moisture level etc. process conditions such as temperature, pressure, humidity etc. should be chosen such that the efficiency of the process is maximized which in turn maintains the quality attributes of the product.

Before the commencement of freeze-drying process, the formulator should characterize physical state of the solutes and should accordingly select the product temperature for primary drying which does not affect the quality of the product.

Advantage

1. Thermolabile drugs, biological preparations, tissue secretion and viable microorganisms which are unstable in aqueous solution can be manufactured as dry powders which remain stable for prolonged storage period due to least moisture content.
2. Freeze-drying enhances the specific surface are of the drug which enable rapid and complete reconstitution of the solid drug.
3. Fill dose for vials can be maintained as the drug is filled as a solution and then it is freeze dried. This is not possible when the drug is filled into vials as a powder. No loss of material due to

drying and ease of recovery. Also applicable for volatile materials. Uniform and porous product is obtained.

In case of vials and ampoules, the material is dried directly inside the containers, hence useful to maintain sterility of products.

Disadvantages

1. Biologicals such as hormones, vaccines, liposomal systems etc. are susceptible to damage by freeze-drying. This problem is of great concern and can be minimized by adding protective agents in the formulation.
2. This method is not applicable for non-aqueous preparations.
3. Product is prone to oxidation, if not packed under vacuum or with inert gas.
4. If a drug is available in the solid state it is very essential to consider the physical state of the drug (crystalline or amorphous). If the resultant free-dried product is amorphous in nature which is undesired due to its instability, then for such a product, freeze-drying cannot be applied.
5. Time-consuming process (requires more than 10 h). Operation cost is high.

Containers and Closures

Containers and closures and their components used for packing of parenteral preparations should be extensively studied as they can affect the stability, potency, toxicity and safety of these products. The packaging components of containers and closures should be given primary consideration and should be evaluated before selection.

The containers used for packing of parenterals should have the following properties.

1. It should not absorb the medicament or release any substance into the product.
2. It should not alter the stability or therapeutic activity of the preparation.
3. It should withstand sterilization procedure.
4. It should facilitate easy handling and withdrawal of the contents.

Containers

For parenteral preparations, most commonly employed container are made up of glass, plastic rubber and stainless steel. But glass and plastic are more preferable.

Glass containers: Glass containers are the most preferred containers for parenteral preparations. Prior to selection, glass containers are evaluated for its chemical resistance and physical characteristics.

Physical characteristics

a) The glass containers should provide protection against degradative effect of UV rays. This is ensured by using amber coloured glass containers incorporated with iron oxide. But the parenteral preparations which are prone to degradation in the presence of heavy metal catalysts such as iron, amber glass cannot be used. This is because traces of iron may be leached into the parenteral preparation and may degrade the product. In such case, the product must be packaged in a transparent glass container which is inturn packed in an opaque container or carton.

b) Glass container used for packaging of parenteral preparations should be sufficiently strong to tolerate high pressure and temperature differentials during autoclaving, risks of handling during processing, storage and transport. In order to withstand temperature fluctuations during sterilization, the glass should have a low coefficient of thermal expansion.

c) Glass containers should be transparent to facilitate inspection of the contents to ensure the quality of the product.

d) Containers should have uniform dimensions to facilitate handling by the mechanical machinery used for automatic production operation.

e) The containers which require thin, uniform wall thickness (ampoules, small vials and cartridges) should be manufactured through glass tubing method large vials and bottles require greater wall thickness as well as strength. Hence, they are made only by blow moulding method.

f) Possible variations in the physical dimensions of glass containers can be done to meet the design needs especially for those containers which are made by blow moulding method. Examples: Freeze-dried products (lyophilized drug) and vehicle for reconstitution can be packed in a single as well as double-chambered container. In dried product where upper chamber vehicle meant for reconstitution of the lyophilized drug.

g) Adherence of costly suspensions and emulsions to the inner walls of the glass containers (especially syringes) is prevented by coating the inner walls. As a result, a hydrophobic surface is formed which prevents adherence of the formulation onto the inner walls and also increase the slippage of a plunger in a syringe barrel.

Evaluation of chemical resistance

The evaluation of chemical resistance of glass containers is done under controlled conditions of accelerated temperature and time. The detail principle and procedure for evaluation of chemical resistance of glass containers are discussed in Chapter 10. On the basis of powdered glass test and whole container test, glass is classified into 4 types, which are given in Table 6.13.

Small volume parenterals (SVPs) such as injections and infusion solutions are packed in single-dose containers which are made of type I glass. The volume ranges from 1 ml to 1000 ml multiple dose vials are also made up of type I glass.

Table 6.13: Classification of glass based on hydrolytic resistance test.

Types of glass	***Hydrolytic resistance***	***Uses***
Type-I or borosilicate glass or Neutral glass.	Highly resistant	Used for ampoules and vials for buffered and un-buffered aqueous solutions.
Type-II or soda-lime glass (surface treated)	Highly resistant	Used for buffered aqueous preparations (with pH below 7 and dry powders and non-aqueous solutions).
Type-III or soda-lime glass	Moderately resistant	Used for non-aqueous solutions and dry powders.
Type-IV or NP (*i.e.,* not for parenterals)	Low resistant	It is not meant for packing parenterals. instead used for packing tablets, oral solutions, suspensions, emulsions, ointments etc.

Large volume parenterals (LVPs) such as infusion fluids, parenteral nutrition solutions etc., are a packaged in glass bottles of 500 ml capacity but they have been largely replaced by plastic bags.

Sterilization of glass containers is done through dry heat sterilization method. The mouths of the containers are plugged with non-absorbent cotton and placed inside the dry heat sterilization equipment. The equipment used for this purpose is hot air oven. The temperature is maintained at 150-160°C for 60 min.

Plastic containers: Plastic containers meant for packing of sterile products (infusion and dialysis fluids, ophthalmic preparation and few injections) are made from thermoplastic polymers of high molecular weight. Plastic containers are preferred over glass containers due to the following characteristics.

a) They are light in weight.
b) They are non-breakable.
c) Show low toxicity and low reactivity towards the products when they have a low amount of added ingredients (plasticizers, fillers, antistatic agents, antioxidants etc.)

Like glass, plastic is also selected on the basis of physical and chemical properties for the manufacture of containers.

Polyvinyl chloride (PVC) collapsible bag: They are used for packaging large volume parenterals such as infusion fluids, parenteral nutrition solutions etc.

Advantages

a) Highly resistant to impact.
b) More flexibility and collapsibility and hence, do not require an air-inlet system.

Disadvantages

a) Moisture permeation is high
b) Shows high reactivity with the product
c) They must be sterilized for an extended sterilization time as PVC exhibits high thermal resistance.

Different types of thermoplastics and their nature is given in Table 6.14.

Table 6.14: Thermoplastics and their nature

Types of thermoplastic	*Autoclavable*	*Nature*
1. Polyethylene		
a) Low density	No	Translucent and semi-rigid
b) High density	Yes	Translucent and semi-rigid
2. Polypropylene	Yes	Translucent and semi-rigid
3. Polyvinyl chloride (PVC)		
a) Flexible	Yes, but used with caution	Transparent and flexible
b) Rigid	Yes, but used with caution	Transparent and rigid
4. Polyamide	Yes	Transparent and rigid
5. Polystyrene	No	Translucent in appearance, tough, rigid, resistant to temperature.

Semi-rigid polythene containers: They are used for packing lectrolyte solution, total parenteral nutrition solutions and dialysis solutions to a range 100 ml, 3 L and 5 L respectively.

Advantages

a) More compatible with the drug content when compared to PVC containers.

b) They are rigid and hence difficult to break.

Disadvantages

a) They must be sterilized for an extended sterilization time.

b) Require an air inlet system.

Closures

Closures are made up of natural or synthetic rubber. They are in intimate contact with the contents and hence, there is a need to carefully study and evaluate them before selection. Openings of cartridges, vials and bottles are sealed with rubber closures which must possess the following characteristics.

a) They should have good ageing qualities.

b) They should have satisfactory hardness and elasticity so as to permit the entry and withdrawal of the needle.

c) They should be resistant to sterilization conditions.

d) They should be impermeable to moisture and air.

e) The amount of undesirable substance released should be negligible.

f) They should extract negligible amount of substances from injection solutions.

Different natural and synthetic rubber components used for closure are given in Table 6.15.

Closures are available in various shapes based on their intended use. They include flanged closure, slotted closures for vials, punctured closure (with a provision for the attachment of adapters for infusion sets), plunger type closures for disposable syringe and cartridges.

Metal closures are sterilized through dry heat sterilization whereas plastic screw caps lined with rubber as well as rubber closures are sterilized by moist heat sterilization (autoclaving at 115-116°C for 30 min).

Table 6.15: Different natural and synthetic rubber components used for closure.

Types of rubber	*Autoclavable*	*Nature*
1. Natural	Yes	Opaque and flexible
2. Synthetic		
a) Butyl	Yes	Opaque and flexible
b) Neoprene	Yes	Opaque and flexible
c) Polyisoprene	Yes	Opaque and flexible
d) Silicone	Yes	Translucent and flexible

Filling and Sealing of Ampoules, Vials and Infusion Fluids

Filling

During the filling of containers with a product, the most stringent requirements must be exercised to prevent contamination, particularly if the product has been sterilized by filtration and will not be sterilized in the final container. Under the latter conditions, the process is called an 'aseptic fill' and is validated with media fills.

Filling of sterile liquids into containers

For smaller volumes of liquids, delivery usually is obtained from the stroke of the plunger of a syringe, forcing the liquid through a two-way valve, providing for alternate filling of the syringe and delivery of mobile liquids. For heavy, viscous liquids, a sliding piston valve, the turn of an auger in the neck of a funnel, or the oscillation of a rubber diaphragm may be used.

For large volumes, the quantity delivered is measured in the container by the level of fill in the container, the force required to transfer the liquid being provided by gravity, a pressure pump, or a vacuum pump.

There are three main methods for filling liquids into containers with high accuracy: i) volumetric filling, ii) time/pressure dosing and iii) net weight filling.

i) Volumetric filling machines: Employing pistons or peristaltic pumps, are most commonly used. When high-speed filling rates are desired but accuracy and precision must be maintained, multiple filling units are often joined in an electronically coordinated machine. When the product is sensitive to metals, a peristaltic- pump filler may be used, because the product comes in contact only with silicone rubber tubing. However, this sacrifices filling accuracy.

ii) Time-pressure (or time-gravity) filling machines: Are gaining popularity in filling sterile liquids. A product tank is connected to the filling system equipped with a pressure sensor. The sensor continuously measures pressure and transmits values to the PLC system controlling the flow of product from tank to filling manifold. Product flow occurs when tubing is mechanically unpinched and stops when tubing is mechanically pinched. The main advantage of time/pressure filling operations is that these filling apparatus do not contain mechanical moving parts in the product stream. The product is driven by pressure (usually nitrogen) with no pumping mechanism involved. Thus, especially for proteins that are quite sensitive to shear forces, time/ pressure filling is preferable.

The filling of a small number of containers may be accomplished with a hypodermic syringe and needle, the liquid drawn into the syringe and forced through the needle into the container. An example of such a device that provides greater speed of filling is the Cornwall Pipet (Becton Dickinson). The device has a two-way valve between the syringe and the needle and a means for setting the stroke of the syringe, so the same volume is delivered each time. Clean, sterile, disposable assemblies operating on the same principle have particular usefulness in hospital pharmacy or experimental operations.

Filling of sterile dry powders in containers

1. ***Conventional method*:** Fine powders do not have sufficient flow property. They show a slow and irregular flow. Hence, they are subdivided into containers by individual weighing. A scoop is used as a measure to approximate the amount of dry powder required to fill each container. Then the powder s weighed on an electronic balance.

2. ***Advanced method or machine filling methods*:** Granular dry powders possess good flow property. So, machine filling methods can be employed for sterile subdivision of granular dry powders. The machines are calibrated to adjust the fill weight for each individual unit (vials, bottles or plastic minibags). Basically, two types of machines are available for sterile subdivision of granular powders. They are:

   a) Auger filler.
   b) Vacuum – pressure displacement filler.

Auger filler: Powder filling machine working on auger mechanism employs an auger which is present in the stem of the hopper. According to the required fill weight of dry powder for an individual unit, the size and rotation of the auger can be manipulated.

Sterile dry powder is placed in a funnel-shaped hopper. The powder flows down the funnel and reaches the funnel stem which bears an adjustable auger. The auger turns and picks up a specified amount of powder and delivers it to the empty vial or bottle.

Vacuum pressure displacement filler: This machine comprises of a hopper, a filling wheel with an adjustable cavity in the rim. The dry powder is placed in the hopper. As the machine is turned on, the filling wheel which bears an adjustable cavity starts rotating. When it moves beyond the stem of the hopper the cavity gets filled with vacuum.

Difficulties in subdivision of sterile dry powders

1. Equal distribution of powder in individual units is difficult.
2. Differences in flow properties of powders hinders effective and accurate filling. For instance, fine powder shows slow and

irregular flow and is difficult to subdivide in individual containers while granular powder flows evenly and is easy to subdivide.

3. Spillage of powder during filling operation may alter the amount of sterile drug powder in individual container. Thus, accuracy of the quantity delivered cannot be assured.

Sealing of containers

Filled containers should be sealed as soon as possible, to prevent the contents from being contaminated by the environment.

Sealing of ampoules

Ampoules are sealed by melting a portion of the glass neck. Two types of seals are employed normally: tip-seals (bead-seals) or pull-seals.

Tip-seals: Tip-seals are made by melting enough glass at the tip of the neck of an ampoule to form a bead and close the opening. These can be made rapidly in a high-temperature gas-oxygen flame. To produce a uniform bead, the ampoule neck must be heated evenly on all sides, such as by burners on opposite sides of stationary ampoules or by rotating the ampoule in a single flame. Care must be taken to properly adjust the flame temperature and the interval of heating to completely close the opening with a bead of glass. Excessive heating results in the expansion of the gases within the ampoule against the soft bead seal, which causes a bubble to form. If the bubble bursts, the ampoule is no longer sealed; if it does not, the wall of the bubble will be thin and fragile. Insufficient heating will leave an open capillary through the centre of the bead. An incompletely sealed ampoule is called a 'leaker'.

Pull-seals: Pull-seals are made by heating the neck of the ampoule below the tip, leaving enough of the tip for grasping with forceps or other mechanical devices. The ampoule is rotated in the flame from a single burner. When the glass has softened, the tip is grasped firmly and pulled quickly away from the body of the ampoule, which continues to rotate. The small capillary tube, thus, formed is twisted closed. Pull-sealing is slower, but the seals are more secure than tip-sealing. Ampoules having a wide opening must be sealed by pull-sealing. Fracture of the neck of ampoules during sealing may occur if wetting of the necks occurs at the time of filling. Also, wet necks increase the frequency of bubble formation and unsightly carbon deposits, if the product is organic.

Sealing of vials and bottles

Glass or plastic vials and bottles are sealed by closing the opening with a rubber closure (stopper). This must be accomplished as rapidly as possible after filling and with reasoned care, to prevent contamination of the contents. The large opening makes the introduction of contamination much easier than with ampoules. Therefore, during the critical exposure, the open containers should be protected from the ingress of contamination, preferably with a blanket of HEPA-filtered laminar airflow. The closure must fit the mouth of the container snugly enough, so its elasticity seals rigid to slight irregularities in the lip and neck of the container. However, it must not fit so snugly that it is difficult to introduce into the neck of the container. Preferably, closures are inserted mechanically, using an automated process, especially with high-speed processing. To reduce friction, so the closure may slide more easily through a chute and into the container opening, the closure surfaces are halogenated or treated with silicone. When the closure is positioned at the insertion site, it is pushed mechanically into the container opening. When small lots are encountered, manual stoppering with forceps may be used, but such a process poses greater risk of introducing contamination than automated processes. This is a good test for evaluation of operator aseptic techniques, but not recommended for any product filling and stoppering. Container-closure integrity testing has become a major focus for the industry, due to emphasis by regulatory agencies. Container- closure integrity measures the ability of the seal between the glass or plastic container opening and the rubber closure to remain tight and fit and to resist any ingress of microbial contamination during product shelf life. Rubber closures are held in place by means of aluminium caps. The caps cover the closure, crimped under the lip of the vial or bottle to hold them in place. The closure cannot be removed without destroying the aluminium cap; it is tamperproof. Therefore, an intact aluminium cap is proof that the closure has not been removed intentionally or unintentionally. Such confirmation is necessary to ensure the integrity of the contents, as to sterility and other aspects of quality. The aluminium caps are designed so the outer layer of double- layered caps, or the centre of single-layered caps, can be removed to expose the centre of the rubber closure, without disturbing the band that holds the closure in the container. Rubber closures for use with intravenous administration sets often have a permanent hole through the closure. In such cases, a thin rubber disk, overlayed with a solid aluminium disk, is placed between an inner and outer aluminium cap, thereby providing a seal of the hole through the closure. Single-layered aluminium caps may be applied using a hand crimper. Double- or triple-layered caps require greater force for crimping; therefore, heavy-duty mechanical crimpers are required.

Quality Control Tests of Parenteral Products

The importance of undertaking every possible means to ensure the quality of the finished product cannot be overemphasized. Every component and step of the manufacturing process must be subjected to intense scrutiny to be confident quality is attained in the finished product. The following tests are performed on the finished parenteral products to maintain quality control:

1. Clarity test
2. Leakage test
3. Sterility test
4. Pyrogen test

1. *Clarity test (or test to detect particulate matter):* The parenteral products must be free from particulate matter such as glass, fibre, floaters etc. if the particle size is more than RBC, then it can cause obstruction of blood vessels leading to severe consequences like emboli in the vital organs of the body.

Particulate matter: Is defined as presence of unintentional and undesirable extraneous, mobile and un-dissolved substances (other than gas bubbles) within the parenteral preparations. Permissible limits (maximum limits) for particulate matter according to IP is given in Table 6.16.

Table 6.16: Permissible limits for particulate matter as per IP

Particle size $\geq$ ***(μ)***	***Maximum number of particles/ml***
10	50
25	5
50	Nil

Injectable solutions in containers with 100 ml or more of a single dose large volume injection intended for administration by intravenous infusion comply with the above limits of particulate matter.

Methods: The following methods are used to detect the presence of particulate matter:

a) Visual method: The filled containers are examined by holding the neck of the container against strong illuminated screen. The containers are slowly inverted and rotated and the contents are examined for the presence of any foreign particles. The black surface is used for the detection of light coloured particles and white surface for dark coloured particles. If any foreign particle is visible, then that container is discarded.

b) Microscopic count method (or membrane filtration method): A measured sample solution is filtered through a membrane filter. The collected particles on the surface of the filter are then counted with the help of a microscope at 100X magnification the whole method is carried out under aseptic conditions. However, it is a time-consuming process.

c) Light obscuration (obstruction) method: This method uses an electronic instrument that produces a light beam of high intensity. The solution is allowed to pass under this bright light. If the particle present in the solution passes through, a shadow cast is produced due to the obstruction of light by the particle. The particles are measured and counted automatically by the device by means of the shadow castings. Limits for sub-visible particulate matter in injectable preparations as prescribed in USP is given in Table 6.17.

Table 6.17: Limits for sub-visible particulate matter in injectable preparations by light obscuration method.

Particle size	*Small volume injectables*	*Large volume injectables*
≥ 10 μ	6000 particles/container	25 particles/ml
≥ 25 μ	600 particles/container	3 particles/ml

d) Coulter counter method: This electronic method is used to detect the particles and also to determine the particle size. The sample solution is added to an electrolyte solution (*e.g.,* NaCl). This solution is drawn through a small orifice of the device. Positive and negative electrodes are present one on either side of an orifice. As the particle passes through the orifice, it displaces its own volume of electrolyzed and at the same moment, an increase in electrical resistance is observed between the two electrodes. The resulting voltage pulses which are proportional to the particle size, are amplified and are measured and counted. Particles below 0.2 μ can also be detected by this method. Limits for sub-visible particulate matter in injectable preparations as prescribed in USP is given in Table 6.18.

Table 6.18: Limits for sub-visible particulate matter in injectable preparations by Coulter counter method.

Particle size	***Small volume injectables***	***Large volume injectables***
≥ 10 μ	3000 particles/container	12 particles/ml
≥ 25 μ	300 particles/container	2 particles/ml

2. *Leakage test:* Ampoules are subjected to leakage test because ampoules are sealed by fusion. Therefore, there is a chance for incomplete sealing or presence of micropores, allowing the contents to leak or micro-organisms and other contaminants to enter the ampoules.

Methods:

a) This test is performed by immersing the ampoules in a vacuum chamber consisting of a dye such as 1% methylene blue solution.

b) A vacuum (negative pressure) of about 27 inch Hg or more is created for about 15 to 30 minutes.

c) This negative pressure causes the methylene blue solution to enter the ampoules with defective sealing.

d) The vacuum is released, ampoules are washed externally and observed for the presence of dye in the ampoules.

e) The coloured (blue) solution because of the dye in the ampoules confirms the leakage and hence those ampoules are discarded.

Detection of leakage is more effective when the ampoules are subjected to autoclaving in the presence of a dye. This method has the advantage that both detections of leakage and sterilization can be done in a single operation. Bottles and vials are not subjected to vacuum test because of the flexibility of the rubber closures.

High-frequency spark test which detects pin holes in the ampoules is another means of detecting leakage. This has been developed by the Nikka Densok company of Japan.

The advantages of this test are:

a) High accuracy of inspection and
b) High speed of processing.

3. *Sterility test*

The sterility test is based on the principle that when micro-organisms are supplied with nutrient medium and water and incubated at a favourable temperature, then the micro-organisms will multiply. The presence of micro-organisms can be identified by the turbidity in the clear medium.

Steps involved in sterility test

a) Preparation of culture media
b) Sampling
c) Sample quantities to be used in each culture medium
d) Test methods
e) Interpretation of results

a) *Preparation of culture media*

The culture media used for sterility test must be capable of promoting the growth of a wide range of micro-organisms such as aerobic bacteria, anaerobic bacteria and fungi. Two types of media are available:

i. Fluid thioglycollate medium, and
ii. Soybean-casein digest medium

Fluid thioglycollate medium: This medium is used primarily to support the growth of anaerobic bacteria. It also supports the growth of aerobic bacteria to some extent. The composition of fluid thioglycollate medium is given in Table 6.19.

Agar is added to increase the viscosity of the medium, thereby reducing the diffusion of oxygen into the medium. Resazurin is added as an oxidation-reduction indicator.

Soybean-casein digest medium: It is used to support the growth of aerobic bacteria and fungi. The composition of soybean-casein digest medium is given in Table 6.20.

Table 6.19: Composition of fluid thioglycollate medium.

Ingredients	*Quantity (for 1000 ml)*
L-cystine	0.5 g
Sodium chloride (Nacl)	2.5 g
Dextrose	5.5 g
Agar	0.75 g
Yeast extract	5.0 g
Pancreatic digest of casein	15.0 g
Sodium thioglycollate	0.5 g
Resazurin (0.1% fresh solution)	1.0 ml
Distilled water	Up to 1000 ml

Table 6.20: Composition of soybean-casein digest medium.

Ingredients	*Quantity (for 1000 ml)*
Pancreatic digest of casein	17.0 g
Peptic digest of soybean meal	3.0 g
Sodium chloride	5.0 g
Di-basic potassium phosphate	2.5 g
Dextrose	2.5 g
Distilled water	up to 1000 ml

b) *Sampling (selection of the size of samples)*

The selection of samples and the number of samples to be taken from any given batch of sterile product is important. The material must be thoroughly mixed if the sample is to be taken from the bulk. The sample is taken at random from the batch of final containers. Minimum sample size related to batch size is given in Table 6.21.

A batch refers to a homogeneous collection of sealed containers the possibility of microbial contamination is uniform in all the units of that batch.

c) *Sample quantities to be used in each culture medium*

I.P. has recommended the following guidelines for determining the minimum number of items to be tested in relation to the number of items in the batch. Determination of samples quantities to be used in each culture medium: IP has recommended the minimum quantities of samples to be used in each culture medium for injectable preparations is mentioned in the Table 6.22.

Table 6.21: Selection of the size of samples

No. of items in the batch	*Min. No. of item recommended to be tested*
1. ***Injectable preparations***	
Up to 100 containers	10% or 4 containers whichever is greater.
> 100 but ≤ 500 containers	10 containers.
> 500 containers	2% or 20 containers whichever is less.
2. ***Ophthalmic and other non-injectables***	
Up to 200 containers	5% or 2 containers whichever is greater.
> 200 containers	10 containers.
3. ***Bulk solids***	
< 4 containers	All containers.
4-50 containers	20% or 4 containers whichever is the greater
> 50 containers	2% or 20 containers whichever is greater.
4. ***Surgical dressings***	
> 100 packages	10% or 4 package whichever is greater.
> 100 but ≤ 500 packages	10 packages
> 500 packages	2% or 20 package whichever is less.

Table 6.22: Minimum quantities of samples for injectable preparations (IP).

Quantity of each container	*Minimum quantity to be used for each culture medium*
1. *For liquids*	
<1 ml	Total contents of a container
≥1 ml and but < 4 ml	Half of the contents of a container.
≥4 ml but < 20 ml	2 ml
≥20 ml but < 100 ml	10% of the contents of a container.
≥100 ml	Not less than half of the contents.
2. *For solids*	
< 50 mg	Total contents of a container.
≥50 mg but <200 mg	Half of the contents of a container.
≥200 mg	100 mg

d) Test methods

The sterility test can be carried out by

i. Membrane filtration method

ii. Direct inoculation method

Membrane filtration method: The method is employed if the test substance is:

a) An oily preparation
b) An ointment that can be placed into solution.
c) A soluble powder or a liquid with antimicrobial properties.
d) A solid without antimicrobial properties and is not readily soluble in the culture medium.

Procedure: Membrane filters of pore size not greater than 0.45 μ and diameter of about 47 mm that are effective in retaining microorganisms are employed for sterility test. The filtration system and the membrane are sterilized.

The test substances are filtered through the membrane under aseptic conditions.

If the test substance has antimicrobial properties, the membrane is washed with 3 successive 100 ml quantities of sterile diluents.

The membrane is then aseptically cut into two equal halves. One half of the membrane is immersed in 100 ml of soybean-casein digest medium and incubated at 20-25°C. the other half of the membrane is immersed in 100 ml of fluid thioglycollate medium and incubated at 30-35°C both the media are incubated for not less than 7 days.

Direct inoculation method: The quantity of the test substance to be used in each culture medium is directly transferred or inoculated into culture media under aseptic conditions. Mix the inoculated liquid with the medium. If the test substance contains antimicrobial properties then it is neutralized by adding suitable inactivating substances (example: penicillinase in case of penicillins) to the medium. Incubate the inoculated media at 20 – 25°C in case of soybean-casein digest medium and at 30 – 35°C in case of fluid thioglycollate medium for not less than 14 days. Positive and negative controls are performed along with the main tests.

e) *Interpretation of results:* Examine the culture media during and after the incubation period to detect the possible microbial growth.

i. The sample passes the test for sterility if microbial growth is not found.
ii. If there is an evidence of microbial growth, the test containers are kept aside. A retest is performed by repeating the original

test. If microbial growth is not found then the sample passes the test for sterility.

iii. If microbial growth is found in the retest, isolate and identify the organisms. If same organisms are found as in the first test, the sample fails the test for sterility.

If the micro-organisms found in the retest are different from that of the first test, a second retest is performed using twice the number of samples. If microbial growth is not found in the second retest, the sample passes the test.

4. *Pyrogen test*

Pyrogens are fever producing metabolic products of micro-organisms. The most potent pyrogens are the high molecular weight endotoxins found in the outer membrane of Gram-negative bacteria. Pyrogens are lipopolysaccharides that may be soluble, insoluble or colloidal in nature. Pyrogens can pass through bacteria-proof filters and are thermostable. Even minute amount of pyrogens can cause fever, platelet aggregation, alterations in blood coagulation etc. in large amounts, pyrogens can also produce shock and eventually death. So, the detection of pyrogens and their elimination from parenteral preparations is very essential.

Test for pyrogens can be carried out by two methods:

a) Rabbit test (*in-vivo*)
b) LAL (Limulus amoebocyte lysate) test (*in-vivo*)

a) *Rabbit test* (*in-vivo*): The test involves measurement of rise in body temperature of the rabbits following the intravenous injection of a sterile solution of the substance to be tested. The body temperature of the rabbit's increases if pyrogens are present in the injected test solution.

Selection of test animals: Healthy, adult rabbits of either sex, each weighing not less than 1.5 kg, fed on a balanced diet are used for the test. Do not use any rabbit for main test if:

i. It shows a temperature variation greater than 0.2°C between two successive readings noted during the determination of initial temperature and /or.

ii. Their body temperatures are higher than 39.8°C or lower than 38°C.

Equipment required for the test

i. All glassware, syringes, needles and thermometer must be thoroughly washed with water for injection and heated in a hot air oven at 250°C for 30 min or at 200°C for 1 h.
ii. Retaining boxes for rabbits.

Test

i) *Preliminary test*: This test is performed to identify and exclude any rabbit with an unusual response to the trauma of the injection.

The test is performed by taking pyrogen-free saline solution (10 ml/kg of body weight) warmed to about 38.5°C and injected intravenously to the rabbits. The temperatures of the rabbits are recorded 90 min before the injection and continued for 3 hours after the injection. Any animal showing a temperature variation of 0.6°C or more must not be used for the main test.

ii) Main test: The test is carried out on a group of 3 rabbits.

Procedure

1. *Preparation of the sample:* Dissolve the test substance in, or dilute with a pyrogen-free saline solution. Warm the solution to about 38.5°C before the injection.

2. *Determination of initial temperature of rabbits:* Insert a clinical thermometer into the rectum of each rabbit and normal readings of body temperature (rectal temperature) are taken prior to the injection of test solution. Two such readings are taken at an interval of 30 min and the mean is calculated. This mean reading is taken as the initial temperature of the rabbits.

3. *Determination of the response of the rabbits:* The test solution is injected into the ear vein of each rabbit. The volume of injection is not less than 0.5 ml /kg and not more than 10 ml/kg of the body weight. This volume varies according to the test substance and is prescribed in the individual monograph.

Record the temperature of each rabbit at an interval of 30 min for 3 h after the injection. This is the maximum temperature recorded for the rabbit. The difference between maximum temperature and initial temperature is taken as its response. If this difference is negative, it is taken as a zero response.

Interpretation of results: If the response of any individual rabbit is less than 0.6°C and if the sum of the responses of the 3 rabbits is more than 1.4°C, the preparation being examined passes the test.

If the response of any rabbit is 0.6°C or more or if the sum of the responses of the 3 rabbits is more than 1.4°C, then the same test is repeated on another 5 rabbits. If not more than 3 of the 8 rabbits show individual responses of 0.6°C or more and if the sum of the responses of the 8 rabbits is not more than 3.7°C, the preparation being examined passes the test.

Advantage: It is used to identify the presence of a wide range of pyrogens.

Disadvantage: It is a time-consuming method.

b) *LAL (Limulus amoebocyte lysate) test (in-vivo):* This is a sensitive test used to detect endotoxins from gram-negative bacteria. Therefore, it is also called as bacterial endotoxin test.

The endotoxins upon reaction with lysate form an insoluble gel clot. The lysate is obtained by the lysis of amoebocytes (blood cells) of the horseshoe crab, *Limulus polyphemus.*

The sensitivity of lysate is expressed in terms of endotoxin units (EU).

The test is based on the principle of formation of a gel (Fig. 6.5) in the presence of bacterial endotoxins and the lysate solution. The lystate consists of a proclotting enzyme and coagulogen (clottable protein) which are required for the reaction to occur.

There are 3 types of LAL tests:

1. Gel clot test.
2. Turbidimetric test
3. Kinetic chromogenic test

1. *The gel-clot test:* It is based on the formation of a solid gel clot.

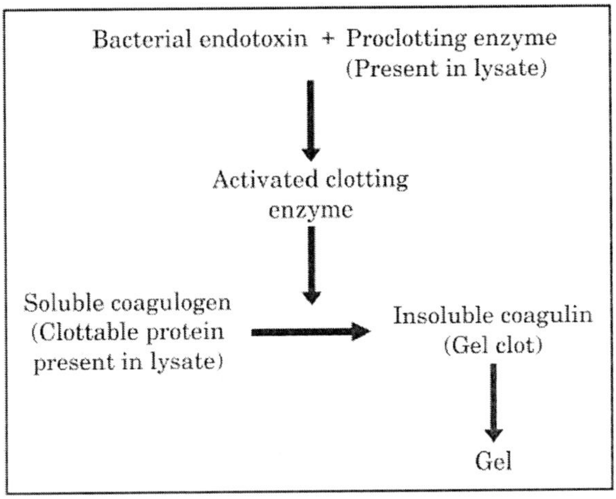

Fig. 6.5: Mechanism of lysate clotting

Procedure: The lysate solution is mixed with an equal volume of the test solution in a pyrogen-free test tube. The test tube is allowed to stand for about 60 min. Now, the tube is inverted and observed for the formation of gel clot. The formation of solid gel confirms the presence of endotoxins. If the solid gel is not formed, it indicates the absence of endotoxins and the test solution passes the test.

The test requires positive and negative controls

Positive control: A known concentration of endotoxin added to the lysate solution is used as a positive control.

Negative control: water (free from endotoxins) added to the lysate solution can be used as a negative control.

2. *Turbidimetric test:* This test is based on the measurement of opacity change in the LAL test due to the formation of a gel clot (insoluble coagulin). Opacity is directly proportional to the endotoxin concentration.

The test is used for water systems and simple pharmaceutical product

3. *Kinetic chromogenic test:* The test is based on the measurement of colour change which is caused by the release of chromogenic chemical, para-nitroanilide. This p-nitro-anilide is a byproduct of the clotting reaction during the LAL test. The quantity of para-nitroanilide produced is directly proportional to the endotoxin concentration.

Advantages of LAL test over rabbit test:

1. It is easy to perform
2. It is a rapid method
3. It is an economical method
4. It is more sensitive test than rabbit test. Even the minute amounts of endotoxin can be detected by LAL test.

LAL test is used to identify the presence or absence of viable forms of micro-organisms in sterile preparation (injectables and ophthalmic products) and the other materials (*e.g.*, absorbent cotton) that are required to be sterile. The test is carried out under aseptic conditions to avoid contamination of the product during the test.

Laminar air flow systems

Laminar air flow systems are generally of three types: i) Downward flow system, ii) Horizontal flow system, iii) Wall to floor flow system.

i. Downward flow system:

This system consists of false floor and ceiling. The air is filtered through pre-filters, electrostatic filters and HEPA filters in sequence. These three filters are placed in the false ceiling. The filtered air is devoid of particles ranging from 0.1-0.3 µ or even larger. This phenomenon of obtaining the filtered air is known as false ceiling washing. This filtered air enters into the false floor through second set of HEPA filters. From the false floor, small proportion of filtered air is re-circulated into the false ceiling through a re-circulation duct. In this system, vertical flow of air is seen.

Advantages

- During the handling of chronic and hazardous materials, the vertical airflow pattern provides protection to the operator against these substances.
- The operating area is provided with exhaust filters which removes the remaining portion of the air. This provides protection to the operator.

Disadvantages

- It is a costly and expensive system as it requires the double installation of HEPA filters.

- Vertical air flow is focused on the working area. Due to this air flow pattern, the dust particles may contaminate the undergoing process.

ii. Horizontal flow system:

The air is filtered through pre-filters and HEPA filters. In this system, the flow of air is horizontal. The filters are placed in the lateral walls and are re-circulated through a recirculation duct.

Disadvantages

- As the flow of the air is horizontal which is not directly focused on working area, the undergoing process is not carried out under completely sterile conditions.
- During the handling of materials like anti-neoplastic drugs, this system provided no protection to the operator against such drugs.

iii. Wall to floor flow system:

The filtered air enters from the lateral wall with an inclined flow towards the floor. In this system, the working area is offered with high aseptic conditions.

Advantages

a) The wall to floor flow system is portable.

b) This system offers aseptic and non-sterile conditions.

Working: The laminar air flow system is placed at such an area where the flow of air is minimum. The system is started 15 min before the actual operation is carried out to make the area free of particulate matter. Cleaning of HEPA filters is carried out and the working area is cleaned before the operation.

HEPA filters or absolute filters are protected with grills. Before using the filters these grills are vacuumed. The workspace should be cleaned with disinfectant before carrying out the actual operation (Fig. 6.6).

Maintenance of HEPA filters: The filters should be properly installed for its proper functioning. It should be changed on monthly basis. Filters should be immediately replaced if the velocity of air across the working

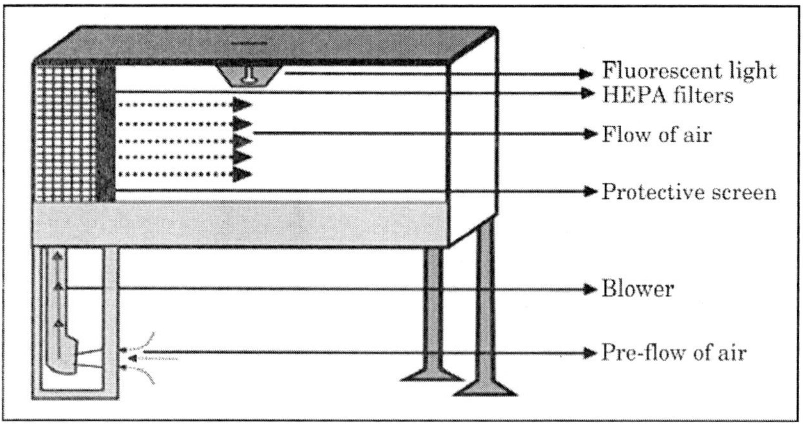

Fig. 6.6: Laminar air flow

surface area falls below 22 m/min. any leakage in the filters can be detected through smoke photometer. For this purpose, dioctly phthalate (DOP) smoke is used. DOP smoke consists of very minute particle of size 0.34 μ which cannot pass through the filters. This particular substance forms an invisible smoke. If the filter shows presence of leakage, then the smoke passes through the filter and can be detected by smoke photometer.

The velocity of air should be maintained at 230 ± 90 cm/min. if any change occurs in the velocity of air then it can be detected through an anemometer (measure velocity or pressure of the air). Every six months, laminar hood installation should be properly checked for leaks and its functioning. If the laminar air flow hood is properly maintained then it provides the aseptic environment. Because of this the pharmacist can prepare and handle the sterile preparation with ease.

Glossary

Parenteral	Drug delivery does not utilize the alimentary canal for entry into body tissues
Small volume parenterals	Volume of these parenterals less than 100 ml
Large volume parenterals	Volume of these parenterals 100 ml and above
Polymorphism	Phenomenon of existence of several crystal forms of a given substance which exhibit different physical properties

Water for injection	It is defined as pyrogen-free distilled water used as a vehicle in the preparation of parenteral products
Antioxidants	These are the substances which are added to the formulation to prevent degradation of the therapeutic agent due to oxidation
Antimicrobials	These are the substances which are added in order to prevent the growth of microbes
Buffers	Buffers maintain the pH of preparation after addition of small quantity of acids or bases
Chelating agents	These are the substances which form complexes with heavy metals such as copper, iron, lead, mercury, chromium etc., thereby inactivating them
Inert gases	Product stability and integrity of oxygen sensitive drugs can be maintained by the use of inert gases such as argon and nitrogen
Tonicity contributing agents	Injections need to be isotonic with blood serum or any other body fluids and tonicity can be adjusted by adding substances like NaCl, dextrose, borax etc.
Protectants	These are the substances which are added to the parenteral preparation to prevent the loss of activity of the therapeutic agent
Isosmotic	0.9% sodium chloride solution is said to be isosmotic or Solutions having an osmotic pressure equal to that of physiologic fluids
Hypotonic	Solutions with a lower osmotic pressure than body fluids or a 0.9% sodium chloride solution are commonly called hypotonic
Hypertonic	Solutions having a greater osmotic pressure than body fluids or a 0.9% sodium chloride solution are termed hypertonic
Colligative property	A property which depends on number of molecules irrespective of their size, shape and nature
Class 100	This area contains not more than 100 particles of 0.5 μm and larger size per cubic feet of air
Class 10000	This area contains not more than 10000 particles of 0.5 μm and even large per cubic feet of air
HEPA	High-Efficiency Particulate Air Filters
Quarantine section	This area consists of store where the in-process batches as well as the approved batches are stored separately. Without the consent of the in-charge other personnel cannot enter into this particular area
Bacteriostatic agent	These prevent the microbial growth in the solutions
Auger filler	Powder filling machine working on auger mechanism employs an auger which is present in the stem of the hopper
Pyrogens	Pyrogens are fever producing metabolic products of micro-organisms and most potent pyrogens are the high molecular weight endotoxins found in the outer membrane of gram-negative bacteria
LAL	Limulus amoebocyte lysate

QUESTION BANK

Q.I. Multiple Choice Questions

1 What is the concentration of NaCl required to make 1% solution of cocaine HCL isotonic with blood plasma? Freezing point of 1% w/v solution of NaCl is -0.576°C and freezing point of 1% w/v cocaine HCL is -0.09°C

a) 0.746 % w/v
c) 0.5 % w/v
b) 0.9 % w/v
d) 0.373 % w/v

2 What is the proportion of NaCl required to render a 1.5 5 solution of drug isotonic with blood plasma? The freezing point of 1% w/v solution of drug is -0.122°C and that of NaCl is -0.576°C

a) 0.65 %
c) 0.9 %
b) 0.585 %
d) 0.5 %

3 How many grams of drug is required to prepare 500 ml of a 1: 2500 solution?

a) 0.2
c) 0.4
b) 0.02
d) 1.25

4 One thousand nanogram equals to

a) Centigram
c) Kilogram
b) Gram
d) Microgram

5 The colligative property of a solution is related to the:

a) Total number of solute particles
c) Number of ions
b) pH
d) Number of ingredients

6 An antioxidant commonly used in the formulation of a non aqueous parenteral preparation is

a) Thioglycolic acid
c) Sodium metabisulphite
b) Ascorbic acid
d) Butylated hydroxytoluene

7 Which of the following is used as a local anaesthetic in the formulation of parenteral products?

a) Acetic acid
c) Ethyl alcohol
b) Benzyl alcohol
d) Sorbitol

8 A co-solvent used in the preparation of parenteral product is

a) Benzyl alcohol
c) Dimethyl acetamide
b) Methyl alcohol
d) Phenol

9 Bulking agent used for parenteral preparation is

a) Sodium metabisulphite
c) Carbolic acid
b) Benzyl alcohol
d) Sorbitol

10 Which of the commonly available large volume dextrose solution for intravenous use is isotonic

a) 2.5 %w/v
c) 10 %w/v
b) 5 %w/v
d) 20 % w/v

11 As per GMP permitted limit of solid contents in water for injection is

a) 100 ppm
c) 0.1 ppm
b) 1.0 ppm
d) 10.0 ppm

12 Water attack test is used to identify alkalinity in

a) Type I glass
c) Type III glass
b) Type II glass
d) All the 3 types

13 The formula for the preparation of ascorbic acid injection I.P. include

a) Glacial acetic acid
c) Propylene glycol
b) Dilute hydrochloric acid sodium
d) Sodium carbonate or bicarbonate or sodium hydroxide in water

14 For drying blood plasma the following technique is used

a) Spray drying
c) Vacuum drying
b) Freeze drying
d) Fluid bed drying

15 Limulus test is rapid *in vitro* test for parenterals to detect the presence of

a) Particulate matter
c) Pyrogens
b) Fungus
d) Bacteria

16 Water for injection differs from sterile distilled water as it is free from

a) Carbon dioxide
c) Preservatives
b) Pyrogens
d) Antioxidant

17 Sterilization temperature for aqueous solution in autoclave (Moist heat) is:

a) 72°C
c) 147°C
b) 121°C
d) 160°C

18 LAL test is used as an in-process control in parenteral preparation to examine the presence of

a) Pyrogens
c) Endotoxins
b) Exotoxins
d) proteinaceous matter

19 To remove bacteria, virus and pyrogens from water with efficiency of about 90-99 % which method can be employed?

a) Sterilization
c) Reverse osmosis
b) Ultrafiltration
d) Nano filtration

20 Addition of which the following to a large volume parenteral product is not advised?

a) Active pharmaceutical ingredient
b) Preservatives
c) Buffering agents
d) Tonicity adjusters

21 For determining the efficacy of sterilization in an autoclave, the spores of the following organisms are used as test organisms.

a) *Bacillus cereus*
b) *Clostridium perfringens*
c) *Bacillus stearothermophilus*
d) *Clostridium histolytium*

22 A co-solvent used for parenteral preparation is

a) Benzyl alcohol
b) Dimethylacetamide
c) Methyl alcohol
d) Phenol

23 Listed below are some of the common vehicles, which one is most appropriate for the intravenous admixture of ampicillin 500 mg/50 ml?

a) 5% dextrose injection
b) 5% dextrose and 0.9 % sodium chloride solution
c) 2.5% dextrose & 0.45% sodium chloride injection
d) 0.9% sodium chloride injection

24 Before washing the ampoules the mouth of each ampoule is rotated in Bunsen flame to melt down the rough edges. This process is called as

a) Flaming
b) Charging
c) Annealing
d) Crounding

25 A drug which is unstable to light, susceptible to oxygen and gets degraded in presence of metallic ions, has to be formulated in the form of a solution for injection. Choose a suitable additive to improve the stability of the injection

a) Preservative
b) Chelating agent
c) Buffer
d) Tonicity contributor

26 10 ml ampoule of KCl injection is available with a labeled strength of 22.5 mg/ml but about requirement is 175 ml of 1 mg/ml. How will you reconstitute?

a) 10 ml of ampoule solution diluted to 175 ml of water
b) 22.5 ml of ampoule solution diluted to 175 ml of water
c) 7.78 ml of ampoule solution diluted to 175 ml of water
d) 2.25 ml of ampoule solution is diluted upto 175 ml of water

27 What concentration of dextrose will be used for preparation of 100 ml of dextrose isotonic with blood serum?

a) 0.95 g
b) 10 g
c) 2.5 g
d) 5 g

28 A hypertonic injection can cause

a) Shrinking of blood cells c) Fever

b) Haemolysis d) All of the above

29 a hypotonic solution may induce

a) Shrinking of blood cells c) Fever

b) Haemolysis d) All of the above

30 Hypotonic injection solutions are made isotonic by the addition of

a) Tonicity adjusting agents c) Chelating agents

b) Buffers d) None of the above

Q. II. Very Short Answer Questions 2 Marks

1. In what way small volume parenterals are different from large volume parenterals?
2. Classify vehicles used in parenterals.
3. Classify non-aqueous vehicles used in parenterals.
4. What are the requirements of oily vehicles used in parenterals?
5. Classify antioxidants used in parenterals.
6. List the preservatives used in parenterals.
7. Why is preservative in general not suitable for large multidose vials?
8. What is the use of buffers in parenteral formulation?
9. Name the methods of adjustment of isotonicity.
10. How are isotonic solutions different from paratonic solutions?
11. Name the methods to prepare sterile powders for injection.
12. Enumerate the glass containers used to supply parenterals. Suggest corresponding tests to determine their chemical resistance.
13. What is the rationality in conducting water attack test only on type II glass containers?
14. What is the maximum quantity of injection can be stored in ampoule, vial, and infusion bottle?
15. What is the composition of rubber?
16. Write the examples of polymers used in the manufacture of rubber closures.
17. What should be the properties of rubber closures?
18. What are the disadvantages of rubber closures?
19. Define pyrogens.
20. List two sources of pyrogens. Suggest two methods of eliminating the pyrogens.

21. What for LAL test is performed? How can the results be interpreted?
22. What is the full form of LAL in LAL test? What is the use of this test?
23. What are the different methods of sealing of ampoules?
24. Name the materials used to coat the walls and floor of aseptic area.
25. How is surface disinfection done in parenterals manufacturing area?
26. What is the full form of HEPA? Write its efficiency.
27. What do you mean by 'class 100' clean area?
28. How is class 100 clean room is different from class 10,000 clean room.

Q. III. Short Answer Questions **5 Marks**

1. Explain how clarity test is performed?
2. Write *in vitro* method for testing of pyrogens.
3. Write the significance of isotonicity in parenteral products.
4. How is leakage test performed for parenterals?
5. Compare pull sealing technique and tip sealing technique
6. What are the materials used to manufacture the uniforms of personnel working in parenterals?
7. How is rubber evaluated for its quality?
8. Isotonicity contributors in parenterals.
9. LAL test.
10. Enumerate the methods of adjustment of isotonicity for parenterals solution.
11. Add a note on manufacture of water for injections.
12. Add a note preparation of sterile dry powder injections
13. Write a note on environment control during manufacturing of parenterals.
14. Add a note on pyrogen test.
15. Explain filling of parenterals liquids

Q. IV. Long Answer Questions **10 Marks**

1. Explain lyophilisation and preparation of sterile powders.
2. Discuss quality control test for parenterals
3. Explain the excipients used in the manufacture of parenterals giving their functions and examples.
4. Describe the formulation requirements for the manufacture of parenterals.
5. Describe in detail the production facilities required to be maintained for parenterals.

6. With a layout, explain the facilities required in production of parenterals.
7. Describe environmental control and maintenance of environment in parenteral production in detail along with cleaning and sterilization techniques.
8. Explain preformulation factors considered for parenteral preparations.
9. Explain the importance of air control and the methods to control. Explain the sources of contamination in parenteral production giving the methods to overcome.
10. Define pyrogens. What are the sources of pyrogens and methods to eliminate the same? Explain the method to determine the presence of pyrogens in parenteral products using animals.
11. Describe LAL test and rabbit method to determine the presence of pyrogens in parenteral products.
12. Explain the methods of sterilization of parenteral products. How is test for sterility performed for injections?
13. Describe briefly the production of parenterals.

CHAPTER 7

OPHTHALMIC PREPARATIONS

INTRODUCTION

Ophthalmic preparations are sterile, liquid, semi-solid, or solid (powders for reconstitution) preparations that may contain one or more active pharmaceutical ingredient intended for application to the conjunctiva or conjunctival sac of the eyelids.

Ophthalmic preparations are applied topically to the eye to treat surface or intraocular conditions. These are used in bacterial, fungal, and viral infections of the eye or eyelids. These are also used in allergic or infectious conjunctivitis or inflammation; elevated intraocular pressure and glaucoma; and dry eye due to inadequate production of fluids bathing the eye.

The major categories of drugs applied topically to the eye:

- Local anaesthetics
- Antibiotic and antimicrobial agents
- Antifungal agents
- Anti-inflammatory agents
- Antiviral agents
- Astringents
- Beta-adrenergic blocking agents
- Miotics and other glaucoma agents
- Mydriatics and cycloplegics

- Protectants and artificial tears
- Vasoconstrictors and ocular decongestants

The most commonly used ophthalmic dosage forms are solutions, lotions, suspensions and ointments. The other dosage forms for ophthalmic drug delivery are gels, gel-forming solutions, ocular inserts, intravitreal injections and implants.

Formulation Considerations

Ophthalmic preparations should require special consideration with regard to the sterility, ocular toxicity and irritation, clarity, isotonicity, hydrogen ion concentration (pH), purity, stability, viscosity and surface activity.

Sterility: Every ophthalmic product must be manufactured under the condition validated to render it sterile in its final container for the shelf life of the product. Sterility testing is conducted on each batch of ophthalmic product. To maintain sterility during use, preservatives are included in all ophthalmics except those meant for traumatized eyes and those used during surgery. Preservatives can destroy the vegetative bacteria in small numbers, within one hour to few hours that enter the solution when the container is opened.

Ophthalmic preparations contaminated with microorganisms may cause corneal damage and finally leads to blindness, especially if the micro-organisms are *Pseudomonas aeruginosa*. This organism occurs as a common contaminant of distilled water. It can also survive better under conditions of less nutrient supply. Moreover, it shows resistance to many preservatives in safer concentrations.

Ocular Toxicity and Irritation: Assessment for potential ocular irritation and toxicity of active pharmaceutical ingredients and additives used in the preparation represent an extremely important step in the development of ophthalmic preparations.

Advances in design and use of ophthalmic drugs and devices have brought ocular toxicity into sharp focus. More interior structure of eye adjacent to target tissues or which are the targets of newer therapies themselves can suffer irritable damage so safety evaluation must be compressive.

Clarity: All ophthalmic solutions should be clear and free from any particulate matter. The inflamed eye is very sensitive to particulate matter which not only causes discomfort but also abrades the corneal epithelium and facilitates invasion by pathogens. Filtering the solutions with a 0.4 μ filter should remove all harmful particulate matter. Clear solutions can be obtained by the use of clean manufacturing area, laminar-flow hoods and clean equipment, also, the containers and closures must be thoroughly clean and contribute no particulate matter to the solution during storage. The use of HPMC over other viscosity agents can improve the clarity of ophthalmic solutions.

Adding Polysorbate 20 and Polysorbate 80, in a maximum concentration of 1%, can also improve the clarity of ophthalmic solutions. Polysorbates, also known as polyoxyethylene sorbitan fatty acid esters, are solubilizing agents that help dissolve poorly soluble ingredients.

Isotonicity: Two solutions are said to be isotonic when the magnitudes of the colligative properties of both the solutions are equal. An isotonic ophthalmic solution exerts the same osmotic pressure as that of 0.9% sodium chloride solutions.

Solutions which are hypotonic result in painful swelling of ocular tissues (adjacent to the site of administration of the solution) due to the entry of solvent into them. Hypertonic solutions cause shrinkage of tissues at the site of administration. The damage caused by a hypotonic solution is quite severe. So the ophthalmic solution should be isotonic. The tonicity adjusting agents like sodium chloride, boric acid etc. are used to adjust the isotonicity, solutions equivalent to 0.5 – 1.8% sodium chloride solutions do not cause marked discomfort to the eye, isotonicity is a must for intraocular preparations.

Hydrogen Ion Concentration (pH): The pH of the ophthalmic solutions should be adjusted in order to prevent irritation or pain to the eye. Ideally, an ophthalmic solution should have a pH equivalent to the tear fluid. But this is not attainable due to decreased stability, decreased solubility or decreased bioavailability of the drug at that pH. Tears have buffering action and they neutralize the ophthalmic solutions to some extent and decrease the discomfort caused by them.

A solution of low pH (acidic pH) will not cause discomfort to the eye. Discomfort result when the buffer used resists the pH adjustment by tear fluid. So the buffer selected should not disturb the pH of tear fluid for more than few moments and should maintain the pH within the selected range throughout the shelf-life of the preparation. Ophthalmics with a pH ranging from 6.5-8.5 does not cause any corneal damage.

The pH of an ophthalmic preparation may be adjusted and buffered for one or more of the following purposes: (a) for greater comfort to the eye, (b) to render the formulation more stable, (c) to enhance the aqueous solubility of the drug, (d) to enhance the drug's bioavailability (*i.e.,* by favouring unionized molecular species) and (e) to maximize preservative efficacy.

Purity and Stability: A stable and therapeutically active ophthalmic preparation contains pure ingredients. It has no chemical, physical and microbial contaminants. To maintain stability, additives like antioxidants, buffers and preservatives should be used. Examples for antimicrobial preservative is given in Table 7.1.

Table 7.1: Antimicrobial preservative and their concentration.

Antimicrobial preservative	***Concentration range (%)***
Benzethonium chloride	0.01 – 0.02
Benzalkonium chloride	0.01 – 0.02
Chlorobutanol	Up to 0.5
Chlorhexidine	0.002 – 0.01
Phenylmercuric borate	0.002 –0.004
Thiomersal	0.001 – 0.15
Methylparaben	0.015 – 0.05
Phenyl ethyl alcohol	Up to 0.5
Propylparaben	0.005 – 0.01
Phenylmercuric acetate	0.001 – 0.002

Viscosity: The optimum range of viscosity of ophthalmic preparations is 15-25 cps. The viscous preparations remain in contact with the tissues for more time and facilitate better drug bioavailability. Viscosity imparting polymers are used which thicken the tear film and decrease the rate of clearing of the preparation by the tear fluid. The viscous suspensions do not allow the drug particles to settle down for few months. The particles remain suspended for a longer period of time and hence, facilitate uniform dosing. Examples of viscosifiers are mentioned in Table 7.2.

Table 7.2: Viscosity enhancers

Viscosity enhancer	*Concentration range (%)*
Methylcellulose	0.2 – 2.5
Hydroxypropyl cellulose	0.2 – 2.5
Hydroxypropyl methylcellulose	0.2 – 2.5
Hydroxyethyl cellulose	0.2 – 2.5
Carboxymethylcellulose sodium	0.2 – 2.5
Polyvinyl alcohol	0.1 – 5.0
Povidone	0.1 – 2.0
Polyethylene glycol 400	0.2 – 1.0
Carbomer 940/934P	0.05 – 2.5

Surface Activity: The ophthalmic preparations' should have the property of wetting the ocular tissues whereby the drug penetrates into the cornea and other tissues and exerts its effects. The wetting property or surface activity can be increased by the use of surfactants in the smallest concentration. Non-ionic surfactants which are less irritating to the ocular tissues like polysorbate 20, Polysorbate 80 etc. are used. The surfactant selected should be compatible with the drug and other additives.

EYE DROPS

Eye drops are sterile aqueous or oily solutions or suspensions or powders for reconstitution intended for instillation into the conjunctival sac. The use of eye drops remains the major method of administration for the topical ocular route. The usual method of self-administration is to place the eye drop from a dropper or dropper bottle into the lower cul-de-sac by pulling down the eyelid, tilting the head backward and looking at the ceiling after the tip is pointed close to the sac and applying a slight pressure to the rubber bulb or plastic bottle to allow a single drop to form and fall into the eye. Most people become quite adept at this method with some practice and may develop their own modifications. However, elderly, arthritic, low-vision and glaucoma patients often have difficulty in self-administration and may require another person to instil the drops.

The pharmacist should instruct patients to keep in mind the following considerations in administering drops to help improve the accuracy and consistency of dosage and to prevent contamination:

- Make sure that the hands are clean;
- Do not touch the dropper tip to the eye, surrounding tissue, or any surface;
- Prevent squeezing or fluttering of lids which causes blinking;
- Place the drop in the conjunctival sac, not on the globe;
- Close the lids for several moments after instillation.

Eye drops are one of the few dosage forms not administered by exact volume or weight dosage, yet this seemingly imprecise method of dosing is quite well established and accepted by ophthalmologists. The volume of a drop is dependent on the physiochemical properties of the formulation, particularly surface tension; the design and geometry of the dispensing orifice; and the angle at which the dispenser is held in relation to the receiving surface. The manufacturer of ophthalmic products controls the tolerances necessary for the dosage form and dispensing container to provide a uniform drop size.

The normal tear volume is about 7 µl and with blinking about 10 µl can be retained in the eye. Approximately 1.2 µl of tears is produced per minute for about a 16% volume replacement per minute. Commercial ophthalmic droppers deliver drops of about 30-50 µl. Therefore, the volumes delivered normally are more than three-fold larger than the eye can hold and the fluid that does remain in the eye is continuously being removed until the normal tear volume is attained. It can be seen, that the use of more than 1 drop/dose must take into account the fluid volume and dynamics of the lacrimal system of the eye. If the effect of multiple drops is desired, they should be administered 1 drop at a time with a 3- to 5-min interval in between dosing. Some doctors may prescribe more than 1 drop/dose to ensure that the patients retain at least 1 drop in the eye.

Eye Drop Dosage Forms

Solutions

The two major physical forms of eye-drops are aqueous solutions and suspensions. Nearly all the major ophthalmic therapeutic agents are water-soluble or can be formulated as water-soluble salts. The homogeneous solution offers the assurance of greater uniformity of dosage and bioavailability and simplifies large-scale manufacture. The selection of the appropriate salt form depends on its solubility, therapeutic concentrations required, ocular toxicity, the effect of pH, tonicity and buffer capacity, its compatibility with the total formulation and the intensity of any possible stinging or burning sensations (*i.e.,* discomfort reactions). The most common salt forms used are the hydrochloride, sulfate, nitrate, phosphate, salicylate, hydrobromide and bitartrate salts are also used. For drugs that are acidic, such as the sulfonamides, sodium and diethanolamine salts are used.

One disadvantage of solutions is their relatively *short residence time in the eye*. This has been overcome to some degree by the development of solutions that are liquid in the container and thus can be instilled as eye drops but gel on contact with the tear fluid. This provides increased contact time with the possibility of improved drug absorption and increased duration of therapeutic effect.

Suspension

If the drug is not sufficiently soluble, it can be formulated as a suspension. A suspension may also be desired to improve stability, bioavailability, or efficacy. The major topical ophthalmic suspensions are the steroid, anti-inflammatory agents, prednisolone acetate, dexamethasone, fluorometholone and rimexolone. Water-soluble salts of prednisolone phosphate and dexamethasone phosphate are available; however, they have a lower steroid potency and are poorly absorbed.

In some cases, it may be advantageous to convert a water-soluble active ingredient to an insoluble form for development as an ophthalmic suspension dosage form. This could be the case when it is beneficial to extend the practical shelf life of the water-soluble form, to improve the compatibility with other necessary compositional ingredients, or to improve its ocular tolerability. Such an example is the β-blocker betaxolol HCL, which is an effective intra ocular pressure-lowering agent with clinically significant safety advantages for many asthmatic patients. With the ophthalmic solution dosage form, some patients experienced discomfort characterized as a transient stinging or burning upon instillation. Although this did not interfere with the safety or efficacy of the product, it was desirable to improve the patient tolerability.

An ophthalmic suspension should use the drug in a micro-fine form; usually, 95% or more of the particles have a diameter of 10 μ or less. This is to ensure that the particles do not cause irritation of the sensitive ocular tissues and that a uniform dosage is delivered to the eye. Since a suspension is made up of solid particles, it is at least theoretically possible that they may provide a reservoir in the cul-de-sac for slightly prolonged activity. However, it appears that this is not so, since the drug particles are extremely small, and with the rapid tear turnover rate they are washed out of the eye quickly.

Pharmaceutical scientists have developed improved suspension dosage forms to overcome problems of poor physical stability and patient-perceived discomfort attributed to some active ingredients. An important development aspect of any suspension is the ability to resuspend easily any settled particles prior to instillation in the eye and ensure that a uniform dose is delivered. It would be ideal to formulate a suspension that does not settle since the patient may not always follow the labelled instructions to shake well before use. However, this is usually not feasible or desirable since the viscosity required to retard settling of the insoluble particles completely would likely be excessive for a liquid eye drop. The opposite extreme of allowing complete settling between doses, usually leads to a dense layer of agglomerated particles that are difficult to resuspend.

Powders for reconstitution

Drugs that have only limited stability in liquid form are prepared as sterile powders for reconstitution by the pharmacist prior to dispensing to the patient. In ophthalmology, these drugs include Q-chymotrypsin, echothiophate iodide, dapiprazole HCl and acetylcholine. The sterile powder is usually manufactured by lyophilization in individual glass vials. In powder form, these drugs have a much longer shelf life than in solution. Mannitol is usually used as a bulking agent and lyophilization aid and is dissolved in the solution with the drug prior to drying. In the case of echothiophate iodide, it was found that potassium acetate used in place of mannitol as a drying aid produced a more stable product. Apparently, the presence of potassium acetate with the drug allows freeze-drying to lower residual moisture content.

A separately packaged sterile diluent and sterile dropper assembly is provided with the sterile powder and requires aseptic technique to reconstitute. The pharmacist should only use the diluents supplied by the manufacturer since it has been developed to maintain the optimum potency and preservation of the reconstituted solution. The storage conditions and expiration dating for the final solution should be emphasized to the patient.

Formulation of eye drops

The therapeutically inactive ingredients in ophthalmic solution and suspension dosage forms are necessary to perform one or more of the following functions, adjust tonicity, buffer and adjust pH, stabilize the active ingredients against decomposition, increase solubility, impart viscosity and act as a solvent. The use of unnecessary ingredients is avoided and the use of ingredients solely to impart a colour, odour, or flavour is prohibited.

The choice of a particular inactive ingredient and its concentration is based not only on physical and chemical compatibility but also on biocompatibility with the sensitive and delicate ocular tissues. The possibility of systemic effects due to nasolacrimal drainage should also be kept in mind.

a) *Vehicle:* Special vehicles available for use in ophthalmic include boric acid vehicle, isotonic phosphate vehicle, special boric acid vehicle etc. purified water is used in the preparation of these vehicles.

Boric acid vehicle

1. It consists of 1.9% boric acid and phenylmercuric nitrate or acetate or any other bactericide.
2. The pH is 4.7.
3. It should be stable during heat sterilisation and storage.
4. It should be isotonic with lacrimal fluid.
5. It should not alter the activity of medicaments.
6. The additional buffer is not required, as it is acidic and readily neutralized by tears.
7. This is used as a vehicle in case of drugs like cocaine, phenylephrine etc.

Isotonic phosphate vehicle

1. This is a buffered solution.
2. It is a mixture of anhydrous sodium acid phosphate and anhydrous sodium phosphate in different concentrations.
3. Sodium chloride is added to the mixture in sufficient quantity in order to make it isotonic with lacrimal secretions.

Special boric acid vehicle

1. It is boric acid vehicle which consists of an antioxidant.
2. This antioxidant is sodium sulphite (0.1%), which prevents oxidative degradation of drugs like adrenaline, physostigmine etc.

b) *Tonicity agents:* These agents adjust the tonicity of the solution to that of lacrimal fluid. The quantity of tonicity agent to be used depends on the concentration of drug and additives. This can be determined by i) Freezing point depression method and ii) sodium chloride equivalent method discussed in detail in chapter 6.

In compounding an eye solution, it is more important to consider the sterility, stability, and preservative aspects and not jeopardize these aspects to obtain a precisely isotonic solution. A range of 0.5–2.0% NaCl equivalency does not cause a marked pain response and a range of about 0.7–1.5% should be acceptable to most persons. The eye seems to tolerate hypertonic solutions better than hypotonic ones. Common tonicity-adjusting ingredients include NaCl, HCl, buffer salts, dextrose, glycerin, propylene glycol, boric acid and mannitol.

c) *pH adjustments and buffers:* The pH and buffering of an ophthalmic solutions are probably of equal importance to proper preservation, since the stability of most commonly used ophthalmic drugs is largely controlled by the pH of their environment. In addition to stability effects, pH adjustment can influence comfort, safety and activity of the product. Comfort can be described as the subjective response of the patient after instillation of the product in the cul-de-sac. Eye irritation is normally accompanied by an increase in tear fluid secretion to aid in the restoration of normal physiological conditions. Accordingly, in addition to the discomfort encountered, products that produce irritation will tend to be flushed from the eye and hence a more rapid loss of medication may occur with a probable reduction in the therapeutic response.

Ideally, every product would be buffered to a pH of 7.4, considered the normal physiological pH of tear fluid. The argument for this concept is that the product would be comfortable and have optimum therapeutic activity.

d) *Viscosity imparting agents (or viscosifiers):* Polyvinyl alcohol, methylcellulose, hydroxypropyl methylcellulose, hydroxyethyl cellulose and one of the several high molecular weight cross-linked polymers of acrylic acid known as carbomers, are commonly used to increase the viscosity of ophthalmic solutions and suspensions. Although they reduce surface tension significantly, their primary benefit is to increase the ocular contact time, thereby decreasing the drainage rate and increasing drug bioavailability. A secondary benefit of the polymer solutions is a lubricating effect that is largely subjective, but noticeable to many patients. One disadvantage to the use of the polymers is their tendency to dry to a film on the eyelids and eyelashes; however, this can be easily removed by wiping with a damp tissue. Requirements of viscosifier are:

- It should not alter the activity of drugs and other additives.
- It should not pose any problem of sterilisation.
- The solution of the viscosifier should be easy to filter.
- It should give a clear solution.

e) *Stabilizers:* Stabilizers are ingredients added to a formula to decrease the rate of decomposition of the active ingredients. Antioxidants are the principal stabilizers added to some ophthalmic solutions, primarily those containing epinephrine and other oxidizable drugs. They reduce the degradation of the solution by preventing oxidation during storage. Examples: sodium metabisulphite (0.05-0.5%), sodium thiosulphate (0.1 – 0.2%). Several patented antioxidant systems consist of ascorbic acid and acetylcysteine, and sodium bisulfite and 8-hydroxyquinoline.

f) *Antibacterial agents (preservatives):* These are the substances which are added in order to prevent the growth of microbes. These agents either kill (bactericidal) or arrest the growth (bacteriostatic) of bacteria in the pharmaceutical preparations during their storage. Due to this the product does not deteriorate and remains stable for a longer period of time. For example benzalkonium chloride (0.01% w/v), chlorhexidine acetate (0.01% w/v). Other preservatives used in eye drops are chlorbutol, thiomersal and phenylethyl alcohol.

g) *Surfactants:* The use of surfactants is greatly restricted in the formulation of ophthalmic solutions. The order of surfactant toxicity is anionic > cationic >> nonionic. Several nonionic surfactants are used in relatively low concentrations to aid in dispersing steroids in suspensions and to achieve or to improve solution clarity. The lowest concentration possible is used to perform the desired function. Their effect on preservative efficacy and their possible binding by macromolecules must be taken into account, as well as their effect on ocular irritation.

Methods of preparation of eye drops

Apart from drug safety, stability, efficacy and shelf-life considerations associated with tonicity, pH and buffer capacity, the major design criteria of an ophthalmic pharmaceutical product are the additional safety criteria of sterility, preservative efficacy and freedom from extraneous foreign particulate matter. Good Manufacturing Practices (GMP) provide for the use of specially designed environmentally controlled areas for the manufacture of sterile large- and small-volume preparations for terminal sterilization. These environmentally controlled areas must meet the requirements of class 100,000 space in all areas where open containers and closures are not exposed, or where product filling-and-capping operations are not taking place. The latter areas must meet the requirements of class 100 space. As defined in Federal Standard 209E, class 100,000 and 100 spaces contain not more than 100,000 or 100 particles, respectively, per cubic foot of air of a diameter of 0.5 μ or larger.

In general, aqueous ophthalmic solutions are manufactured by methods that call for the dissolution of the active ingredient and all or a portion of the excipients into all or a portion of the water and the sterilization of this solution by heat or by sterilizing filtration through sterile depth or membrane filter media into a sterile receptacle. If incomplete at this point, this sterile solution is then mixed with the additional required sterile components, such as previously sterilized solutions of viscosity-imparting agents, preservatives, and so on, and the batch is brought to final volume with additional sterile water.

Example: Preparation of atropine eye drops (B.P.C.). Ingredients and their quantities are given in Table 7.3.

Method

1. Dissolve phenylmercuric nitrate in purified water and prepare 0.002 % solution.
2. Dissolve atropine sulphate in 50 ml phenylmercuric nitrate solution.
3. Add purified water to make 100 ml. Filter the solution through a membrane filter.
4. Transfer the solution to the final container and sterilize it by autoclaving at 115°C for 30 min.

Table 7.3: Atropine eye drops B.P.C.

Ingredients	*Quantity*
Atropine sulphate	1 g
Phenylmercuric nitrate solution 0.002%	50 ml
Purified water	up to 100 ml
Make an eye-drops	

Aqueous suspensions: The method of preparation is similar to that of eye drops except that before bringing the batch to final volume with additional sterile water, the solid that is to be suspended is previously rendered sterile by heat, by exposure to ethylene oxide or ionizing radiation (gamma or electrons), or by dissolution in an appropriate solvent, sterile filtration and aseptic crystallization. The sterile solid is then added to the batch, either directly or by first dispersing the solid in a small portion of the batch. After adequate dispersion, the batch is brought to final volume with sterile water. Because the eye is sensitive to particles larger than 25 μ in diameter, proper raw material specifications for the particle size of any dispersed solids must be established and verified on each lot of raw material and final product. The control of particle size of the final suspended material is very important, not only for the comfort of the product but also for improving physical stability and resuspendability of the suspension throughout the shelf life. Manufacturing of some suspension products may require modified processes in order to control particle size and obtain a sterile product.

The *sterile powder* is usually manufactured by lyophilization in individual glass vials. Sterile powders are sterile, solid substances which are distributed in their final containers and which, when shaken with the prescribed volume of the appropriate sterile liquid, rapidly form clear and practically particle-free solutions or uniform suspensions.

Container: Ophthalmic liquid products were traditionally packaged in glass containers fitted with an eye dropper. Today glass containers have limited use except where product stability or compatibility issues exclude the use of flexible plastic containers made of polyethylene or polypropylene. Most commercial liquid ophthalmic products are packaged in plastic containers fitted with nozzles from which, by gentle squeezing, the contents may be delivered as drops. Many ophthalmic liquids can be packaged in sterile plastic bottles with self-contained dropper tips or in glass bottles with separate droppers. Whichever container type is selected, all containers must be adequately sealed to prevent contamination.

Labelling: The label of eye drop should state (1) concentration of active ingredients and (2) name and concentration of antimicrobial agent used in the eye drops.

Eye drops should be labelled "For External Use Only" along with storage conditions to maintain full activity.

EYE LOTIONS

Eye lotions are sterile aqueous solutions intended for use in rinsing the eye or for impregnating eye dressings. It may allow a large volume of fluid to flow quickly over the eye. Eye lotions are iso-osmotic to tears, because compared to eye drops, lotions cause much greater dilution of the lachrymal fluid, hence cause discomfort if not adjusted. Thus their preparations should be very simple as well as the most common eye lotion consists of sterile normal saline.

Eye lotions may contain excipients, for adjusting tonicity, viscosity and pH of the preparation. These substances do not adversely affect the intended action at the concentrations used and cause undue local irritation.

Eye lotions supplied in multi-dose containers contain a suitable antimicrobial preservative in appropriate concentration except when the preparation itself has adequate antimicrobial properties. The antimicrobial preservative chosen is compatible with the other ingredients of the preparation and remains effective throughout the period of time during which the eye lotions are in use.

If eye lotions do not contain antimicrobial preservatives, they are supplied in single-dose containers. Eye lotions intended for use in surgical procedures or in first-aid treatment do not contain an antimicrobial preservative and are supplied in single-dose containers.

Eye lotions, examined under suitable conditions of visibility, are practically clear and practically free from particles. The containers for multi-dose preparations do not contain more than 200 ml of eye lotion unless otherwise justified and authorised.

B.P.C. describes two types of eye lotions

1. Sterile aqueous solutions:
   - Contains no bactericidal agent
   - Intended for first aid or other purposes over a maximum period of 24 h
   - These are supplied in a single dose container

Example: Sodium chloride eye lotion B.P.C. used to remove a foreign substance from the eye.

2. Aqueous solutions:
   - It contains a bactericidal agent
   - Used for intermittent domiciliary administration for up to seven days
   - These are supplied in the multi-dose container.

Example: Soothing lotions for tired eyes

Sodium bicarbonate eye lotion is used for emergency treatment of acid burns of the eye and is known as 'Factory Eye Drops No. 2'. Sodium chloride eye lotion is an isotonic solution which is occasionally used for irrigating the eye. These preparations are prepared by conventional sterilization methods. Example for preparation eye lotion is given in Table 7.4.

Table 7.4: Formulation of eye lotion

Ingredients	*Quantity (%)*
Boric acid	2
Zinc sulphate	0.4
Purified water	Up to 100 ml
Use with an equal volume of warm water in an eye bath	

Procedure: The zinc sulphate and boric acid are dissolved in purified water, the solution is clarified by filtration and transferred to a fluted bottle, closed with a screw- cap and sterilized by heating in an autoclave. It is instructed to avoid contamination of the solution during use as far as possible.

Containers: Eye lotions are dispensed in colour fluted bottles closed with a screw cap. It is important to ensure that the liner of the screw-cap not made of cork since it may be a source of microbial contamination. Rubber or plastic liners are suitable and screw cap may be either metallic or plastic.

Labelling: In addition to the word 'For external use only', if the eye lotion is used for first aid purpose *i.e.,* Sodium bicarbonate eye lotion, should be labelled as 'Discard any lotion remaining after use when the seal is first broken'.

Eye lotions which are used for domiciliary purposes should be labelled to indicate that they are not to be used more than 24 h (or seven days if bactericide is added) after first opening the container *e.g.*, with words 'Discard any lotion remaining 24 h after the container has been first opened.

Comparison between eye drops and eye lotions is given in Table 7.5.

OPHTHALMIC OINTMENTS

Drugs are frequently applied topically to the eye as ophthalmic ointments. Ophthalmic ointments must be sterile and free of grit. In addition, ophthalmic ointments must meet the USP sterility tests and the test for metal particles in ophthalmic ointments.

Compared with ophthalmic solutions, ophthalmic ointments provide extended residence time on the surface of the eye, increasing the

Table 7.5: Comparison between eye drops and eye lotions

Eye drops	*Eye lotions*
1. Less amount used	1. Used in a large volume to mechanically remove foreign materials.
2. Medicament is necessary	2. The medicament is not necessary
3. Adjustment of isotonicity is not strictly essential	3. Must be isotonic to tears due to larger amount use
4. It is used as treatment purpose	4. It is used for the first aid or irrigation or washing purpose
5. Dilution is not strictly considered	5. It must be undiluted
6. This is domiciliary use, should be discarded in 4 weeks after first opening. But in hospital wards should be discarded 1 week after opening.	6. Should be discarded in 24 h (or seven days if bactericide is added) after first opening.

duration of their surface effects and bioavailability for absorption into the ocular tissues. Ophthalmic ointments are cleared from the eye as slowly as 0.5% per minute, compared with solutions, which can lose up to 16% of their volume per minute.

The chief disadvantages of the use of ophthalmic ointments are their greasy nature and the blurring of vision. They are most often used as adjunctive night time therapy, with eye drops administered during the day. The nighttime use obviates the difficulties produced by blurring of vision and is stated to prolong ocular retention when compared with drops. Ointments are used almost exclusively as vehicles for antibiotics, sulfonamides, antifungal and anti-inflammatories. The petrolatum vehicle is also used as an ocular lubricant following surgery or to treat various dry eye syndromes. Anesthesiologists may prescribe the ointment vehicle for the non-ophthalmic surgical patients to prevent severe and painful dry eye conditions that could develop during prolonged surgeries.

Formulation of eye ointments

Medicinal agents are added to an ointment base either as a solution or as a finely micronized powder. The ointment is made uniform and smooth by fine milling process.

Ointment bases:

a) It should be non-irritant to the eye.

b) It should allow the drug to diffuse into the lacrimal secretions.

c) The temperature at which the base softens should be close to body temperature.

d) Bleached bases like white soft paraffin should not be used, as the residues of the bleaching process may damage the ocular tissue.

e) The composition of the most commonly used base is: yellow soft paraffin 80 parts, liquid paraffin 10 parts and wool fat 10 parts

f) Mainly anhydrous types of bases are used in ophthalmic ointments.

The principle semisolid dosage form used in ophthalmology is an anhydrous ointment with a petrolatum base. The ointment vehicle is usually a mixture of mineral oil and white petrolatum. The mineral oil is added to reduce the melting point and modify the consistency. The principal advantages of the petrolatum-based ointments are their blandness and their anhydrous and inert nature, which make them suitable vehicles for moisture sensitive drugs. Excipients used in eye ointments are shown in Table 7.6.

Table 7.6: Excipients used in eye ointments

Excipients	***Role***	***Examples***
Antioxidants	They prevent the oxidation of the bases and keep it stable.	Butylated hydroxyl toluene, tocopherol etc.
Buffers	They maintain the pH of the preparation within the selected range.	Sodium acetate, sodium citrate, potassium meta phosphate etc.
Surfactants	These are rarely used to solubilise the drug in the base.	Polyoxyl 40 stearate, polyethylene glycol etc.
Preservatives	To prevent the growth of microorganisms.	Methylparaben (0.1 – 0.2%), propylparaben ($\cong$ 0.04%), phenylmercuric acetate (0.0008%), chlorobutanol (0.5%), and benzal konium chloride (0.008%).

Preparation of ophthalmic ointments

Ophthalmic ointments are sterile preparations involves aseptic handling using previously sterilized medicaments they are seldom dispensed extemporaneously. Hence, when an ophthalmic ointment is manufactured, all raw material components must be rendered sterile before compounding unless the ointment contains an aqueous fraction that can be sterilized by heat, filtration, or ionizing radiation.

The ointment base is sterilized by heat and appropriately filtered while molten to remove extraneous foreign particulate matter. It is then placed into a sterile steam-jacketed kettle to maintain the ointment in a molten state under aseptic conditions and the previously sterilized active ingredient(s) and excipients are added aseptically. While still molten, the entire ointment may be passed through a previously sterilized colloid mill for adequate dispersion of the insoluble components. Two commonly employed methods for the preparation of ophthalmic ointments are:

1. *Fusion method*

   a) The drug and the additives are milled to get particles of a fine size, under aseptic conditions.
   b) The base which is previously sterilized is melted under aseptic conditions.
   c) The drug and the additives are slowly added to the base present in the rotation mixer and mixing is carried out until the preparation attains uniformly.
   d) The finished product is processed through a roller mill to get a uniform dispersion and break the aggregates if any.
   e) The ointment is immediately packed under aseptic conditions into sterile containers.

2. *Levigation method*

   a) This method is suitable for drug substances which are insoluble in the base.
   b) The drug and the additives are milled to get particles of a fine size, under aseptic conditions.
   c) The drug is mixed thoroughly with a small quantity of the sterile base or with any miscible liquid like propylene glycol, light mineral oil etc.
   d) The drug mixture is mixed with the additives homogenously.
   e) The above mixtures diluted geometrically with the base.

f) The finished product is passed through a roller mill to get a uniform dispersion which is smooth.

g) The ointment is immediately packed under aseptic conditions into sterile containers.

Example: Preparation of atropine eye ointment and ointment base B.P. is given in Table 7.7 and 7.8 respectively.

Table 7.7: Atropine eye ointment B.P.

Ingredients	***Quantity***
Atropine sulphate	1 g
Sterile base	100 g

The sterile base is prepared by using following ointment bases:

Table 7.8: Preparation eye ointment base B.P.

Ingredients	***Quantity***
Liquid paraffin	10 g
Wool fat	10 g
Yellow soft paraffin	80 g

Method

1. Heat the liquid paraffin, yellow soft paraffin and wool fat in a suitable vessel.
2. Filter while still hot through a coarse filter paper in a heated funnel into a container which can withstand a temperature of 160° C for 2 h.
3. Sterilized atropine sulphate is dissolved in minimum quantity of water for injection and incorporated gradually in the melted sterilized base with continuous stirring.
4. Transfer the eye ointment to the final sterile container under aseptic condition label and dispense.

Dry heat sterilization may decrease the stability of the drug and may result in separation of the ointment base from other ingredients. Ethylene oxide and steam cannot penetrate the ointment base hence; they are not suitable for sterilization purpose. Also, sterilization of the preparation after manufacturing is not possible. Strictly, aseptic techniques are followed during preparation to get a sterile product.

Container: Ophthalmic ointments should be supplied in metal or plastic collapsible tubes.

Ophthalmic ointments are filled into previously sterilized containers. Commonly employed methods of sterilization of packaging components include exposure to heat, ethylene oxide gas, and ^{60}Co (gamma) irradiation.

Labelling: The label on the tube or outer sealed envelope should state that the contents are sterile provided that the container has not been opened.

Storage: Eye ointment should be stored in a cool place

Ophthalmic marketed preparations are shown in Fig. 7.1.

Evaluation of Ophthalmic Preparations

Ophthalmic preparations can be evaluated by performing the following general tests:

a) Test for sterility.
b) Test for ocular toxicity and irritation.
c) Test for preservative efficacy.

a) Test for sterility

All the ophthalmic preparations should be sterile. A sterile preparation should be free from any viable living organism and its spores.

The following criteria should be followed while carrying out sterility testing. Two sterile culture media are prepared for the detection of aerobic and anaerobic bacteria and fungi. These media are as shown in Table 7.9.

Table 7.9: Medium type and organism detection.

Medium	*Micro-organism*
Fluid thioglycollate medium	Detects the presence of aerobic and anaerobic bacteria
Soya bean casein digest medium	Detects the presence of fungi and aerobic bacteria.

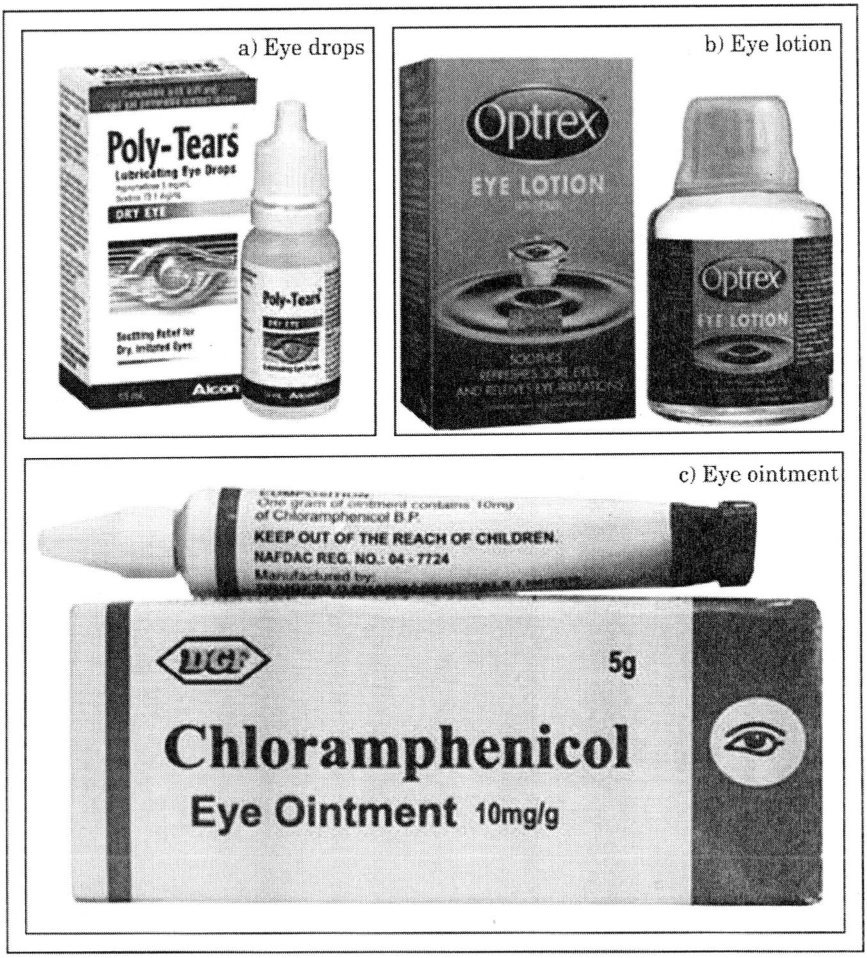

Fig. 7.1: Ophthalmic marketed preparations A) Eye drops B) Eye lotion and C) Eye ointment

Samples which are to be tested are transferred into test tubes containing a clear medium. Detection of microorganisms can be done on the basis of turbidity of the media. If the sample contains microorganisms, then the medium becomes turbid. If the sample is free from microorganisms, then the medium remains clear. The tests should be carried out it aseptic conditions.

Various controls are to be considered before carrying out the actual sterility testing. These are as follows:

First control: Incubation of the medium is done for 7 days for the detection of viable forms of bacteria and fungi. For bacteria 30-35°C and for fungi, 20-25°C temperature is maintained. If there is no growth of micro-organism, then it indicates that the media is sterile.

Second control: In each medium, suspensions of microorganisms (aerobic and anaerobic) are added separately and then they are incubated at a specified temperature for 7 days. The quick and ample growth of micro-organism indicates that the media is not sterile and can support the growth of micro-organism at existing conditions.

Third control: In this test, two media are prepared separately. Each medium is divided into two portions. To one portion, either aerobic or non-aerobic microbe suspension is added, and to another portion, a suspension of a fungus is added to one of the portions of the medium. These media are then incubated for about 7 days at a temperature of about 35°C if growth occurs, then it indicates that the preparation under test is not sterile.

The test for sterility is carried out by two methods:

1. *Membrane filtration method:* It is also known as method A. This method is generally followed for the products which can be easily filtered. This method is carried out under aseptic conditions.

The method consists of sterilized filter unit with a sterile membrane filter of 0.45 μ pore size. A specified quantity of parenteral preparation (sample) is filtered through the membrane filter. In this method, two sterile membrane filter can be used or a single membrane filter which is divided into two equal halves. Incubation is carried out by keeping one half of the membrane in fluid thioglycollate medium at 30-35°C and another half of the membrane in soybean casein digest medium at 20-25°C for 7 days.

Result: if the medium shows no growth, then the sample solution passes the test. If the medium shows growth, then the test is repeated. If the growth is observed again, then the sample solution fails the test.

2. *Direct inoculation method*: This method is also known as method B. In this method also, direct inoculation is carried out on both aqueous solutions and oily solutions.

The specified quantity of the solution to be tested is drawn through a sterile syringe or pipette. This is mixed with the medium and incubated; a portion of the medium is transferred to fresh medium. This is done if the medium shows turbidity, then both the media old and fresh are incubated for 14 days.

Result: If the medium shows no growth, then the sample solution passes the test. If the medium shows growth, then the test is repeated. If growth is observed again, then the sample fails the test.

Ophthalmic ointments are diluted with a specified volume of non-aqueous fluid and are tested in the above manner.

b) Test for ocular toxicity and irritation

1. This test is to assess whether the preparation is isotonic, the pH is within tolerable limits and the drug and the additives are safe for use.
2. Five albino rabbits are selected, the iridal vessels of which can be easily observed for toxicity and irritation.
3. Based on the type of dosage form the medicament is extracted using cottonseed oil (or) saline.
4. Small quantities of the extract are instilled into one eye of all the rabbits.
5. The sterile saline solution is instilled into the second eye of all the rabbits.
6. After one hour all the rabbits are observed for irritation, swelling or shrinkage of the eye.
7. No change in the eye into which the preparation is instilled indicated that the preparation under test is safe for use.

c) Test for preservative efficacy

1. Cultures of micro-organisms like *Aspergillus niger*, *Candida albicans*, *Escherichia coli* and *Pseudomonas aeruginosa*, each containing about 10000-1000000 organisms per ml are selected.
2. Three to four samples of each preparation are taken in sterile test tubes and inoculated with few ml of each culture separately.
3. They are incubated at 20-25°C for a period of 28 days and weekly observations are carried out for the appearance of turbidity.

4. No growth of micro-organisms occurs if the preservative is totally effective.

Glossary

Sterile	Preparation contains no living microorganisms
Eye drops	Sterile aqueous or oily solutions or suspensions intended for instillation into the conjunctival sac
Eye-lotions	Sterile aqueous solutions having no bactericide for first aid purposes for the period of 24 h
Para-tonic	Solutions which are not isosmotic with body fluids

QUESTION BANK

Q. I: Multiple Choice Questions

1 Cryoscopic method is familiar in the calculation of isotonic solution. This method is based on

a) Freezing point depression of the drug c) Solubility of the drug

b) pH of the drug d) None of the above

2 Which of the following is used as a preservative in ophthalmic preparations

a) Benzalkonium chloride c) Benzoic acid

b) Phenol d) Chlorocresol

3 Eye lotions are supplied in ______ form

a) Concentrated c) Powder

b) Diluted d) All of the above

4 Ophthalmic preparations should be _______ with lachrymal secretions

a) Paratonic c) Compatible

b) Isotonic d) None of these

5 pH of the ophthalmic preparations may be adjusted and buffered for

a) For greater comfort to the eye c) To maximise preservative efficacy

b) To render the formulation more stable d) All of the above

6 Sterility test for ophthalmic is carried out by

a) Membrane filtration method c) Both (a) and (b)

b) Direct inoculation method d) None of these

7 Ophthalmic injections and sterile powders are packed in

a) Type I glass
c) Type III glass
b) Type II glass
d) Type IV glass

8 Plastic containers used in the packing of ophthalmic products generally made up of

a) Low-density polyethylene
c) Both (a) and (b)
b) Polypropylene
d) None of these

9 Choose the correct pH of the lachrymal fluid

a) 8.0
c) 7.4
b) 6.2
d) 9.0

10 Which one of the following is used as isotonicity adjuster

a) Dextrose
c) Nacl
b) Boric acid
d) All of the above

11 Viscosity enhancer in ophthalmic preparation is

a) Carbomers
c) Dextran
b) Polyvinyl alcohol
d) Povidone

Q. II: Very Short Answer Questions **2 Marks**

1. Role of viscosity modifiers in ophthalmics.
2. Stabilizing agents used in eye drops.
3. Name any four preservatives used in ophthalmic preparations.
4. Name sterilization methods for eye ointment.
5. Preservation for ophthalmic preparations.
6. Standards for ophthalmic preparations.

Q. III: Short Answer Questions **5 Marks**

1. Discuss the formulation of an eye ointment.
2. Write a note on evaluation of an eye ointment.
3. Write a note on evaluation of eye drops.
4. Explain the formulation of eye drops.
5. Explain the requirements for the ophthalmic preparations.
6. Define and classify ophthalmic products. Explain in brief the sterilization of eye drops.
7. Explain sterility test for opthalmic preparation.
8. Explain the manufacture of ophthalmic ointments.

Q. IV: Long Answer Questions **10 Marks**

1. Add a note on different types of ophthalmic preparations. Write formulation of eye ointment.
2. Discus in detail formulation requirements and method of preparation of eye lotions.
3. Explain about the formulation of ophthalmic drops with all necessary details.
4. Describe the factors to be considered for the formulation of ophthalmic preparations.

UNIT-V

CHAPTER 8

COSMETICS

INTRODUCTION

Cosmetics are articles intended to be rubbed, poured, sprinkled, or sprayed on, introduced into, or otherwise applied to the human body or any part thereof for cleansing, beautifying, promoting attractiveness, or altering the appearance without affecting structure or function.

Among the products included in this definition are skin moisturizers, lipsticks, nail polishes, eye and facial makeup products, shampoos, permanent waves, hair colouring products and deodorants as well as any material intended for use as a component of a cosmetic product.

The term cosmetic is derived from a Greek word which means to 'adorn' *i.e.,* adding something decorative to a person or a thing.

Nowadays, cosmetics are considered essential components in life. They not only attract the people towards it but also impart psychological effects. It has gained popularity in the last 3-4 decades and its use has been increased exponentially both in males and females.

Even in earlier days, men and women used to decorate their bodies for improvement of appearance. Men used leaves of vegetables and parts of animals whereas women used to wear coloured stones and flowers around their neck and wrist. Gradually, they started using coloured earth and ointments on their face and body. Even bangles and necklaces made of baked earth materials became very common among the people.

Applications of Cosmetics

1. Cosmetics enhance the attractiveness of the body
2. Cosmetics used as a cleansing, moisturising and beautifying agent
3. They help in altering the appearance of the body without affecting its functions
4. Sunscreen products help in protecting the body from UV rays and treating sunburns
5. Acne, wrinkles, dark circles under eyes and other skin imperfections are treated by cosmetics
6. Cosmetics help in treating skin infections

Classification of Cosmetics

Based on part or organ of the body on which they are applied cosmetics are classified as:

a) Cosmetics used for the hair

   Examples: Shampoos, hair dyes, tonics, hairdressing and brilliantines, hair waving preparations, beard softeners, shaving media, depilatories etc

b) Cosmetics applied on the skin

   Examples: Cold cream, vanishing cream, sunscreens, lotions, deodorants, make-up preparations, powders, bath and cleansing preparations etc.

c) Cosmetics for the teeth and mouth

   Examples: Toothpaste, lipsticks, mouthwashes etc.

d) Cosmetics for the nails

   Examples: Nail polishes, nail polish removers, manicure preparations etc.

e) Cosmetics for the eye

   Examples: Eyeshadow, mascara, eyeliner etc.

Some cosmetic preparations are discussed below:

LIPSTICKS

Lipsticks may be basically defined as a dispersion of the colouring matter in a base consisting of a suitable blend of oils, fats and waxes with suitable perfumes and flavours moulded in the form of sticks to impart attractive gloss and colour, when applied on lips.

Lipsticks provide the moist appearance to the lips accentuating them and disguising their defects.

Ideal characteristics of good lipsticks:

1. It should be safe and non-irritating to the lips.
2. It should efficiently cover lips with colour and impart a gloss which would last longer.
3. It should be able to adhere firmly to the lips and should not provide any greasy appearance.
4. The lipstick should possess a pleasant fragrance and a good flavour.
5. It should possess good thixotropic property so as to deposit the colour with minimum pressure.
6. It should possess required plasticity and be able to maintain all the properties throughout the storage period.
7. It should be easily dried after application but should not result in blooming or sweating of the lips
8. The stick should possess even firmness and should maintain its strength at varying temperatures up to 55°C.
9. The stick should not dry or crumble easily on storage.

Formulation of lipsticks

Lipstick base is made by mixing the oils and waxes in varying proportions in order to obtain a desirable viscosity and melting point.

The raw materials involved in the formulation of the lipsticks are given in Table 8.1 and details of the raw materials used for formulation of lipstick are given in Table 8.2.

1. *Solid components/waxes:* The solid components are responsible for the final structure of the product by solidifying the liquid matrix. The materials required for attaining a reasonable body, hardness, melting point and shrinkage necessary for the easy release of the mould are together referred to as natural waxes.

2. ***The liquid components:*** The liquid components are mostly constituted by the oils such as mineral oil, vegetable oil, castor oil, alcohol etc. the properties of the oils should be as follows:

i) It should possess good dissolution properties in order to dissolve all the bromo acids.
ii) It should possess an optimum viscosity range.
iii) It should be colourless, odourless and tasteless.
iv) It should be non-toxic and non irritating.
v) It should be easily compatible and stable.

Table 8.1: Common ingredients used for formulation of the lipsticks

Ingredients	*Examples*
The solid components /waxes:	
(a) The hydrocarbon waxes	White beeswax
(b) The mineral waxes	Ozokerite wax, ceresine wax.
(c) Hard waxes	Carnauba wax, candelilla wax, hard paraffin.
(d) Microcrystalline waxes	
The liquid components	Mineral oils, vegetable oils (*e.g.,* castor oil) Butyl stearate, glycol, water, silicone-fluids, IPM (isopropyl maleate)
The softening agents	Anhydrous lanolin, lanolin, cocoa butter, lecithin, petrolatum
The colouring agents	Carmine, dyestuff stain, pigmented stain, lakes etc.
Pearlescent pigments	Guanine crystals, bismuth oxychloride
Opacifying agents	Titanium dioxide
Perfumeries	Rose oil, cinnamon oil, lavender oil etc.
Miscellaneous agents:	
(a) Preservatives	Parabens
(b) Antioxidants	BHA, BHT, tocopherol etc.
(c) Flavouring agents	Cinnamon oil, spearmint oil etc.

The most commonly used liquid components may be as follows.

Mineral oils: These are used in concentrations of less than 5% and are not rancid. Mineral oils consist of a blend of hydrocarbons obtained from a petroleum source. They may be available as either light mineral oils or heavy mineral oils. They are mostly used in order to impart gloss to the product rather than their solvent property.

Table 8.2: Details of the solid components /waxes used in formulation of the lipsticks.

Ingredients	*Source*	*Melting point*	*Concentration*	*Advantages*	*Disadvantages*	*Uses*
A) Hydrocarbon waxes						
White Beeswax	Obtained from honeycombs of the honey bee *Apis mellifera*	62–65°C	3 – 10%	It is compatible with vegetable minerals and animal waxes. It can be moulded into the required form.	When it is used at a concentration of more than 20%, it forms a dull film on the surface of the lips.	1. It has good plastic property and can be readily deformed when it is warmed. 2. It is a stiffening agent for lipsticks. 3. It forms a good base in the formulation of moulded products
B) Mineral waxes						
1. Ozokerite wax	Obtained naturally from bituminous products	56–82°C	5–10%	It is easily available in various grades.	It may be subjected to adulteration	1. It is used to increase the melting point of the base. 2. It ensures the maximum retention of the oil matrix. 3. It can be easily transformed into various grades.
2. Ceresine wax	Obtained naturally from the bituminous products like the ozokerite wax	60–75°C	5–10%	It is easily available in various grades.	It may be subjected to adulteration	1. It is used as stiffening agents to provide firmness to the finished product. 2. It is used to increase the melting point of the base.

Table 8.2: *(Contd...)*

Ingredients	*Source*	*Melting point*	*Concentration*	*Advantages*	*Disadvantages*	*Uses*
C) Hard waxes						
1. Candelilla wax	Obtained from Euphorbiaceae plants (*Euphorbia cerifera, Euphorbia antisyphilitica*)	65–75°C	5–10%	It adds glossy and lustre look to the lips	It makes preparation hard	It is used to increase the hardness and melting point of the product either alone or in combination with carnauba wax.
2. Carnauba wax	Obtained as an exudate from the pores of the leaves of the Brazilian wax palm tree *Copernicia prunifera*	80–90°C	5–10%	It produces translucent or various shades of opacity	It is not miscible with the other waxes and remains as a separate solid phase due to its high melting point.	1. It is used to provide rigidity to the stick. 2. It is used in a modest proportion in order to ensure high melting points. 3. It helps in moulding by shrinking the stick away from the surface of the mould in order to aid easy removal.
3. Hard paraffin	It may be present as a purified blend of several solid hydrocarbon bases that are obtained from petroleum	55–65°C	0.5–2%	Imparts rigidity to the product Improve the gloss of the finished products.	It has limited solubility in the castor oil and hence doesn't dissolve and may provide a greasy look	1. It is occasionally used in minor quantities to improve the gloss of the finished products. 2. Imparts rigidity to the product.
D) Microcrystalline waxes						
Microcry-] stalline waxes	These are the hydrocarbons containing a long carbon chain.	60–120°C	1–5%	The shape of the lipstick is maintained	They possess low solubility in the castor oil	1. They help in maintaining the crystal structure of the lipstick and hence may prevent the sweating

Vegetable oils: The vegetable oils used may be sesame oil and olive oil, they have low solubility towards staining dyes and hence less commonly used.

Castor oil: It is obtained from the seeds of the castor plant, *Ricinus communis*. It forms a most valuable lipstick base and used in a concentration of 40-50% of the total formulation. Castor oil has high viscosity, good dissolving power, possess stability towards oxidation and it is widely compatible with other ingredients. The high viscosity may avoid smearing off of the lipsticks.

Butyl stearates: They are useful for the dispersion of colour though they possess less solubility. Butyl stearates can readily wet the colouring pigments. They are odourless and free from rancidity.

Propylene glycol: It is non-toxic and possesses a sweet taste. Propylene glycol has good wetting property towards high colouring stains. It is always used in combination with other monoesters of propylene glycol.

Water: It is not used as a solvent but may be used in minor quantities in order to dissolve the colour.

Silicone fluid: It is used in minor quantities mostly to aid in mould release and prevent the rub-out of the wax.

Isopropyl maleate (IPM): It is used in a concentration of 2-3% to increase lip gloss. It acts as a co-solvent along with mineral oil and helps in increasing lip gloss.

3. *Softening agents:* They are used to increase the spreadability by softening the lipstick. The most commonly used softening agents include.

Anhydrous lanolin: It is also known as wool fat or wool wax. It is used at a low concentration of about 0.25% in order to impart gloss, softness, emolliency and protection of the lips. The melting point ranges between 36-42°C.

Lanolin: It is also referred to as hydrous wool fat. It is used in minor quantities in order to improve the covering properties of the film. It contains 25-30% of water and may result in sticky and greasy products. It aids in the dispersion of coloured pigments.

Lanolin derivatives: They include ethers, esters and lanolin oils. They are almost non-drying and thus provide a non-greasy look to the film. They are also used as blending agents or plasticizers.

Cocoa butter: It was used in the past due to its good emollient property. The usage has been stopped due to rancidity and surface crystallization. It provides oily look on the lips and hence imparts good gloss.

Petrolatum: It is a hydrocarbon obtained from petroleum. It is odourless and tasteless. It is added mainly to enhance the gloss.

Lecithin: It is used in minor quantities to impart smoothness and emollient effect. It increases the ease of application.

4. *Colouring agents:* Colour may be imparted to the lips either by staining the lip with a dyestuff colour or by covering the lips with colouring layers. The colours used in the formulation of lipsticks are of 2 types.

- *(a) Soluble colours*: They are dyestuff agents which are easily soluble in oil, water and alcohol.
- *(b) Insoluble colours*: They are organic or inorganic pigments which are insoluble.

Properties of colouring agents

1. They should impart good opacity to the lips by imparting good colour.
2. They should be easily and uniformly miscible with the oils used.
3. The colours must be certified with the F, D & C grade.
4. They should possess very low content of impurities such as arsenic, lead etc.

The commonly used colourants for lipstick are:

Carmine: It was extensively used in the past and is obtained as carminic acid from the cochineal insects by extracting the insects with ammonia, the carminic acid obtained is precipitated with alum and is dried and used.

Dyestuff stains: They include eosin dyes and provide a long-lasting effect on the lips by retaining the colour on the lip cells. They are a) Eosin dye: it is used to impart orange-red colour to the lips. b) Acid eosin dye: it has an orange colour and may change to intense red colour at acidic pH of 4.

Pigmented stains: They form a dispersion in the solvent base. They may be either organic or inorganic. They are used in combination with metallic lakes in order to improve the intensity of the colour.

Lakes: They are potential pigments of many of the D and C colours. They may be adsorbed on the aluminium hydroxides, barium oxides, calcium oxides etc. Examples: aluminium lakes, barium or calcium lakes, strontium lakes. They are used at concentrations of about 8-10%.

4. *Pearlescent pigments:* They are used to impart nacreous or a pearl-like appearance to the product when applied on the lips. The natural pearlescent pigments may be guanine crystals obtained from fish scales. Bismuth oxychloride in 70% castor oil may also provide a lustrous look.

5. *Opacifying agent:* It is used for opacifying or whitening of lipsticks, *e.g.,* titanium dioxide. It can also alter the basic shade of the pigment. Various shades can be obtained by varying the proportions.

6. *Perfumeries:* Light floral fragrances can be used in lipsticks. They include rose oil, cinnamon oil, lavender oil etc. The fruity flavours that cover fatty odour of the oily waxes may also be used. They should be tasteless, non-irritating and compatible.

7. *Miscellaneous agents:* They include the following -

(a) Preservatives: They are used to increase the life period of the product by reducing the microbial growth. Though they are anhydrous preparations, preservatives such as methylparaben and propylparaben may be commonly used. The concentration of the preservatives should not exceed 0.1%.

(b) Antioxidants: The ingredients used in the formulation may be susceptible to oxidation. This may result in the degradation of the product. Thus, antioxidants are added in order to prevent oxidation of the ingredients. The commonly used antioxidants are butylated hydroxyanisole (BHA), butylated hydroxytoluene (BHT), tocopherol, propyl gallate, butylated hydroxy quinones etc.

(c) Flavouring agents: They are included in order to impart good flavour to the product. They may include the spearmint oil, cinnamon oil etc.

Alone with or with colouring agents like sodium saccharin and the ammonium glycyrrhizate may also use in order to improve the taste.

Preparation of lipsticks

Successful preparation of lipstick shades depends upon the adequate dispersion of the lake colours in the lipstick mass. It is advisable to prepare the dispersion of lake colours in castor oil. Dispersions are generally prepared by milling about 25% concentrations of lakes in castor oil.

Method of preparation

1. Bromo acid solution is first prepared and set aside until required.
2. If commercial colour pastes are not being used, then lake colours are first dispersed by mixing with a suitable quantity of castor oil.
3. The colour paste obtained is passed through a triple roller mill until it becomes smooth and free from agglomerates and gritty particles.
4. The colour mixture is then mixed with the bromo acid mixture.
5. All the ingredients of the base are added and melted in increasing order of their melting points.
6. This mixture is re-milled until it is perfectly smooth.
7. Preservatives and anti-oxidants are dissolved in remaining oil and are added to the mixture.
8. Finally, the perfume is added and the mass is stirred thoroughly, but gently to avoid entrapment of air.
9. Automatic ejection mould is preferred for the large-scale production.
10. The mould is lubricated with liquid paraffin or isopropyl myristate before pouring the mass into the mould.
11. It is important to prevent settling down of the colouring mass when the moulds are chilled.
12. Lubrication facilitates easy removal of sticks.

SHAMPOOS

A viscous cosmetic preparation with synthetic detergents used for washing hair is called shampoo. Its principle function is to clean the scalp such that it should become free from sebum and foreign substances. Shampoo also makes the hair lustrous and good looking. In olden days detergent soaps were used for washing hair, but nowadays it has been replaced by shampoo. Today shampoo has become an important hair cosmetic for both men and women. However, the detergent and other raw materials selected for shampoo preparation should be non-toxic to the scalp, eyes etc. apart from cleaning, shampoo may also be used for medicinal purpose (*i.e.,* medicated shampoo) after preparation, each and every shampoo must be evaluated.

Ideal properties of shampoos

1. It should have an optimum viscosity such that it facilitates ease during application.
2. It should have good spreading properties and it should produce sufficient lather after application.
3. It should be able to remove waste material such as debris, soil, sebum, dead cells, salts (due to sweat) etc., from the scalp.
4. It should rinse out completely after washing and provide lustre to the hair.
5. After drying, the hair should not give rough appearance and should not form any kind of film on the scalp.
6. It should facilitate ease of combing after shampooing.
7. It should produce good odour both before and after shampooing.
8. It should not produce any kind of irritation or itching to the scalp.
9. It should not support any microbial growth.
10. It should be stable and have a shelf life of about 2 to 3 years.

Different types of shampoos and their formulation aspects are given in Table 8.3.

Formulation of shampoo

The various ingredients contain in the shampoo are given in Table 8.4.

1. *Surfactants:* The main use of a surfactant is to cleanse and to produce foam. They are generally, categorized into four types.

(a) Anionic surfactants
(b) Non-ionic surfactants
(c) Cationic surfactants
(d) Amphoteric surfactants

Anionic surfactants: These surfactants have good foaming property, hence they are used as principle surfactant. They are considered as the main ingredient of shampoo formulation.

Some commonly used anionic surfactants are:

(i) Alkyl sulphates: When fatty acids are subjected to catalytic reduction, it results in formation of long-chain sulphated derivatives called as alkyl sulphates. Example: lauryl sulphate, myristyl sulphate.

Table 8.3: Different types of shampoos and their formulation aspects.

Type of shampoo	***Description***	***Ingredients for 100 g)***
Clear liquid shampoos	These are clear liquid preparations, usually made by using detergents of low cloud point. Alkanolamides can also be used in these preparations. Some of these shampoos may be transparent.	Surfactant - Triethanolamine lauryl sulphate: 50 g Foam booster - Lauric isopropanolamide : 2 g Water : 48 g Preservative, Perfume, Colour : q.s.
Liquid cream shampoos	These are also called as lotion shampoos which are a modification of clear liquid shampoos. Addition of opacifier such as glyceryl monostearate, glycol stearate etc. to the clear liquid shampoo yields liquid cream shampoo. Solubilising agents such as magnesium stearate is also used to dissolve the added opacifier.	Surfactant - Triethanolamine lauryl sulphate : 35 g Opacifier - Glyceryl monostearate : 2 g Stabilizer- Magnesium stearate : 1 g Preservative, perfume, colour : q.s. Water : 62g
Cream shampoos	These shampoos have a paste-like consistency and are packed in a collapsible tube or wide mouth jar. They find great use in hair salons. The paste consistency is developed by addition of alkyl sulphates. Also,	Surfactant- Sodium lauryl sulphate : 38 g Builder - Cetyl alcohol : 7 g Preservative, perfume, colour : q.s.

Table 8.3: *(Contd...)*

Table 8.3: *(Contd...)*

Type of shampoo	***Description***	***Ingredients for 100 g)***
	cetyl alcohol is added, which serves as a builder.	Water : 55 g
Gel shampoos	These are transparent and thick usually made by incorporating a gelling agent (*e.g.*, cellulose) they are of great use in hair salons and beauty parlours. The principle ingredient is detergent which can be used either alone or in combination with soap by altering the proportion of detergent; gel of required consistency can be obtained. Addition of methyl cellulose to clear liquid shampoo and its subsequent thickening also gives rise to gel shampoo.	Alkyl dimethyl benzyl ammonium chloride : 15 g Surfactant- Triethan olamine lauryl sulphate : 28 g Coconut diethanolamine : 7 g Hydroxypropyl methylcellulose : 1 g Preservative, perfume, colour : q.s. Water : 49 g
Powder shampoos	As name suggests, it is available in the form of dry powder. Initially, it was prepared from dry soaps. But now a days dry synthetic detergents are used for their preparation. Powder shampoo is prepared, where the addition of water or other solvent reduces the activity of the components, especially in case of medicated shampoo.	Surfactant- Sodium lauryl sulphate : 20 g Sodium sulphate : 65 g Sarcoside : 5 g Sodium bicarbonate : 10 g Perfume : q.s.
Dry shampoos	Dry shampoo is also a type of powder shampoo. Initially, they are applied on to head and then removed by brush. It doesn't involve the use of water. They are usually preferred, when the hair are greasy. This formulation usually includes adsorbents.	Adsorbent - Starch : 15g Adsorbent - Talc : 45 g Adsorbent - Kieselguhr : 40 g Perfume : q.s.
Aerosol shampoos	They are called aerosol shampoos because they are packed in aerosol containers. Their formulation, preparation and packing is complicated as an additional propellant is included. The propellant added must be compatible and should not reduce the activity of shampooing ingredients.	Surfactant - Triethanolamine lauryl sulphate : 60 g Coconut Diethanolamide : 2 g Propellant : 10 g Water : 28 g Preservative, perfume, colour : q.s.
Special shampoos: These shampoos which are meant for a special purpose		
a) Medicated shampoos	These shampoos contain medicinal agents. These agents treat the disor-	Surfactant- Triethanolamine lauryl

Table 8.3: *(Contd...)*

Table 8.3: *(Contd...)*

Type of shampoo	*Description*	*Ingredients for 100 g)*
	ders of the scalp or hair. Examples of medicated shampoos are Anti-lice shampoo, anti-dandruff shampoo, anti-baldness shampoo etc. The medicinal agent added should not irritate the sebaceous glands, it should not sensit-sensitize the scalp, the degree of itching and scaling should also be reduced. Among all, anti-dandruff type of medicated shampoo is most widely used.	sulphate : 60 g Anti-dandruff - Thymol : 0.1 g Counter-irritant - Camphor : 0.1 g Water : 38.8 g Preservative, perfume, colour : q.s.
b) Conditioner shampoos	These shampoos serve for hair conditioning .initially they clean the hair (and scalp) and keep them in smooth and lustrous condition. They also prevent sticking of hairs. Conditioner shampoo nowadays is widely used by both men and women. Most of the conditioners are made from quaternary ammonium compounds. These compounds have the property of reducing electric charges between the hair, as a result, hair become lustrous easily manageable. These compounds can also exhibit a bactericidal effect.	Stearyl dimethyl benzyl ammonium chloride: 5.5 g Ethylene glycol monostearate : 2 g Cetyl alcohol : 2.5 g Preservative, perfume, colour : q.s. Water : 90 g

(ii) *Alkyl polyethylene glycol sulphates*: These anionic surfactants exhibit good cleaning as well as good foaming property. They are alkyl ether sulphates which form water-soluble sodium salts. The solubility of this salt is greater than sodium lauryl sulphate, hence also serves as a solvent for non-polar ingredients.

(iii) *α-olefin sulphate*: It is an alkyl sulphonate obtained by sulfonation of linear olefin. It produces an excellent foam and the property of foaming is unaffected by sebum and hard water. It produces a mild detergent effect without harming the scalp. It is stable at both acidic and basic pH and widely used to prepare low pH shampoo. It has a low cloud point hence, also used to prepare clear liquid shampoo.

Apart from the above, other anionic surfactants such as sulfosuccinates, acyl lactylates etc, are also used.

Table 8.4: Formulation table for shampoos

Ingredients	***Examples***
Surfactants	
(a) Anionic surfactants	Alkyl sulphates, alkyl ether sulphate
(b) Non-ionic surfactants	Alkanolamides
(c) Cationic surfactants	Alkyl amines, alkyl imidazolines
(d) Amphoteric surfactants	Alkyl amino acid
Foam boosters	Monoethanolamides, lauramide DEA, cocamide DEA etc.
Germicide and anti-dandruff agents	Benzalkonium chloride, cetrimide, selenium sulphide, cadmium sulphide.
Conditioning agents	Lanolin, egg, amino acids
Pearlescent agents	Methyl-7diethylamino coumarin, 4-methyl-5, 7-dihydrocoumarin.
Sequestrants	EDTA, citric acid
Thickeners	Alginates, polyvinyl alcohol, methyl cellulose
Perfuming agents	Herbal fruits or floral fragrances
Preservatives	P-hydroxy benzoic acid, phenyl mercuric nitrate
Colour	FD & C dyes.

Non-ionic surfactants: These are considered as secondary surfactants. They are not used to produce foam but used as foam boosters, viscosity inducers, emulsion stabilizers and opacifiers (pearlescent agent). This is because they have less foaming power. Even though they have good cleaning property, they are not used as principle surfactant.

Some commonly used non-ionic surfactants:

(i) Polyalkoxylated derivatives: These are ethoxylated alcohols and phenols, block polymers, sorbitol ester (polyethoxylated) and polyglyceryl ethers. These derivatives are obtained when hydrogen (labile) containing hydrophobic compound is subjected to polyaddition reaction with either ethylene or propylene oxide. They are stable at a wide range of pH. They have stabilizing, emulsifying, pearlscent and foaming properties they are available at low cost and cause irritation to eye mucosa. However, they are used as mild detergents and impart a good rinsing property.

(ii) Fatty acid alkanolamides: These include monoalkanolamides and diethanolamides etc. monoalkanolamides are made from long chain

fatty acids they are insoluble in water due to their waxy nature. Hence, they are added directly to the detergent solution and dissolved by gentle warming. Initially, the detergent solution is made by using principle surfactant to which various ethanolamides are added to serve as solubilising agent (lauric monoethanolamide), a viscosity inducing agent (lauric monoethanolamide), pearlescent and thickening agent (stearic ethanolamide), softening and hair conditioning agent (oleic ethanolamide) and foam boosters.

However, the ratio of detergent solution to the monoethanolamide must be 100:15 and more than this ratio may be harmful to scalp and hair.

(iii) Amine oxides: Amine oxides are obtained by the oxidation of tertiary aliphatic amine with hydrogen peroxide. These compounds possess strong polar linkage between nitrogen and oxygen hence, they are also called as polar non-ionic surfactants. They constitute a major group of synthetic surfactants. They are water soluble and compatible with various surfactants. They are added as secondary surfactants because of their conditioning, foam boosting and anti-static property. Coconut and dodecyl dimethylamine oxides are most commonly used for this purpose.

Cationic surfactants: Surfactants that contains positive charge on their hydrophobe are called as cationic surfactants. They are used as both principle and secondary surfactants. These surfactants are used in low concentration because they are toxic to the eye. Hence, they are considered as secondary surfactants. They have good foaming and partly cleaning properties. Hence, they are also used as principle surfactants in conditioner shampoos.

Some commonly used cationic surfactants:

(i) Alkylamines: They constitute a major group of cationic surfactants. They are used in combination with hydrophilic surfactants in order to provide conditioning and anti-static property to the shampoo. However, they precipitate when combined with anionic surfactants. Usually, they are used in the form of water-soluble salts.

(ii) Ethoxylated amines: These are nitrogen-containing surfactants which are obtained by ethoxylation of long-chain alkylamines. They are waxy in nature with a low melting point. Because of their waxy

nature, they are also used as viscosity inducer. However, their main function is emulsification and hair conditioning, sometimes, they are also used as foam boosters. Due to their emulsifying property, complete dispersion of various ingredients is achieved.

(iii) Alkyl-betaines: These classes of cationic surfactants are obtained from N-dimethylglycine. They are readily compatible with the majority of surfactants. These surfactants i) Enhance the efficiency of foam (foam booster); ii) Contain conditioning and anti-static property; iii) Have viscosity inducing property; iv) Non-irritant to skin and eye.

Because of the above properties, alkyl betaines are considered as secondary surfactants. They are also used as principle surfactant in baby shampoo and often used a combination with ionic surfactants.

Amphoteric surfactants: The surfactants which possess both cationic and anionic charges with respect to acidic and basic media are called as amphoteric solvents. They form zwitterions when the pH of media is neutral. These agents produce a mild action and show compatibility with surfactants. They possess excellent hair conditioning property and hence used as secondary surfactants.

Some commonly used amphoteric surfactants:

(i) Dialkyl ethylene diamines: These surfactants are soluble in water and compatible with surfactants. They are used as detergents and to a lesser extent as an emulsifier. They are usually prepared as an aqueous solution or paste into which remaining shampoo ingredients are added. These agents are combined with anionic surfactants in order to minimise the irritation caused by them. These agents neither enhance nor inhibit the foaming property of the principle surfactant. They are most widely used an anti-irritating agent when anionic compounds are used as principle surfactant (anionic surfactants are irritant to the eye). These agents also possess conditioner and anti-static property as a result of which the hair becomes smooth and soft. However, the pH of the shampoo prepared by using these surfactants must be neutral (*i.e.,* in between 6.5 to 7.5).

(ii) N-alkyl amino acids: The important compounds of this class are derived from b-amino acids and asparagines. A compound called N alkyl–beta iminopropionate is derived from β-amino acid and it exhibits good foaming property, possesses slightly alkaline pH. By changing

the pH to acidic range, the manageability of hair is improved. Whereas, the derivatives of asparagine are well compatible with both anionic and cationic surfactants. It also possesses the properties like foaming, cleaning and condition, depending upon the pH, these compounds change their nature *i.e.,* they become zwitterions at pH 6 and at neutral pH, they become amine. The solubility of N-alkyl amino acids is greater when they are in the form of sodium salts, whereas the solubility decreases with zwitterionic form. The foaming property of these agents decreases with a decrease in pH. This is because at low pH they become cationated (*i.e.,* cationic form), these agents are highly stable and sometimes also employed as emulsifiers.

2. *Foam boosters:* The surfactants used in the preparation also serves as foaming agents. They form rich lather *i.e.,* foam which is stabilized or strengthened by using a substance called foam boosters. The substances like fatty acid alkanolamides, amine oxides are used. They make the foam dense and allow it to remain for the long duration. Usually, they are added in quantity of about 2 to 5 %. Fatty acids and fatty alcohols when added in a range of 0.25 to 0.50% concentrations, they also act as foam boosters.

3. *Germicide and anti-dandruff agents:* Germicides are the agents which prevent the growth of micro-organism on the scalp whereas anti-dandruff agents are used to eliminate dandruff from the scalp.

Quaternary ammonium compounds (benzalkonium chloride, cetrimide), phenol derivatives and tetramethyl thiuram disulphide etc. commonly used germicides. Selenium sulphide and cadmium sulphide are the examples of anti-dandruff agents.

4. *Conditioning agents:* These agents improve the condition of hair. These agents have the property of reducing electric charges between the hair, as a result, hair becomes lustrous and hence easily manageable. These agents also exhibit a bactericidal effect. They make the hair silky and shiny. Most commonly used conditioning agents are lanolin, oils, herbal extracts, egg, amino acids etc. among the above, amino acids give an efficient conditioning effect.

5. *Pearlescent agents:* These agents are usually added as adjuvants to the conditioning agents. They improve the conditioning property. Addition of this agent also imparts brightness to hair. They make the preparation transparent or opaque, hence they are also called as opacifying agents. The commonly used pearlescent agents are alkanolamides and coumarins like 4-methyl-7 diethyl amino coumarin, 4-methyl-5,7 dihydrocoumarin etc. also alcohols and phosphates improves transparent solubilization.

6. *Sequestrants:* These are complex forming agents. They form complex with metal ions like calcium and magnesium. The surfactant is liable to form a complex with the metals present in water *i.e.,* calcium and magnesium. Hence, the addition of sequestrants prevents complex formation between metal and surfactant. The sequestrant itself forms a complex with the metal ions. Thus, it prevents the formation of a film on the scalp *i.e.,* the film formed by surfactant and metal ions. The commonly used sequestrants are EDTA, citric acid etc.

7. *Thickening agents:* These agents are usually added to make the preparation thick *i.e.,* viscous. Such viscous preparation facilitates ease of handling. Also, they prevent wastage during application. Already the addition of various agents, such as surfactants, foam boosters etc makes the preparation viscous even though the thickening agent is added. Substances like methylcellulose, alginates polyvinyl alcohol, polyethylene glycol (macrogols) etc are commonly used to adjust the viscosity of a shampoo.

8. *Perfumes:* Addition of these agents imparts good fragrance to the shampoo. It also neutralises the undesirable odour of other ingredients of formulation especially surfactants. Nowadays it has become an important factor for consumer satisfaction. The selected perfumes must be such that they should retain good smell for a fixed period of time even after shampooing. The added perfumes should not affect the solubility and stability of the preparation. They are usually obtained from natural sources such as flowers, fruits, herbs etc.

9. *Preservatives:* These agents have the ability to prevent the growth of microorganisms. They are usually added to maintain the stability of the preparation for a desired period of time. The shampoo is a wet preparation that provides a media for the culture of various micro-organisms hence, addition of preservative is essential. The preservative used should not cause any irritation to the scalp. Para-hydroxy benzoic acid and phenylmercuric nitrate are commonly used preservatives.

10. *Colour:* Addition of colour gives a pleasant appearance to the preparation. Various FD & C dyes are used for colouring the preparation. The added colour must be water soluble and it should not impart any colour to hair or scalp.

Preparation of shampoo

A simple procedure is involved in the preparation of shampoo. Initially only one method available for the preparation of shampoo, but later the basic method was modified in order to obtain different types of shampoo like cream, gel, aerosol etc.

A general method for preparation of shampoo

The liquid shampoo is usually prepared by this method which involves the following steps:

1. Initially, the detergent is converted into a solution form or a detergent solution may be directly obtained from the manufacturer.
2. Take about half of the detergent solution into a separate container. To it, add the total amount of secondary surfactant *i.e.,* alkanolamide.
3. Dissolve the alkanolamide with stirring. Sometimes, gentle heat is also applied.
4. To the remaining half of the detergent solution add a suitable amount of perfume and dissolve it.
5. The perfume solution is then added to the alkanolamide solution.
6. Colour and preservatives are dissolved separately in sufficient volume of water and then added to the main solution.
7. The whole solution is mixed well by gentle stirring and excessive stirring may lead to bubble formation.
8. The final volume of the preparation is usually adjusted by the addition of clear sterile water. This gives clear liquid shampoo.
9. However, when the preparation contains lauryl alcohol ether sulphate. It is required to adjust the viscosity of the shampoo.
10. Viscosity adjustment is done by using an electrolyte solution. Usually, a solution of sodium chloride is added subsequently with constant stirring. Care must be taken to prevent the excess addition of sodium chloride.

The methods of preparation of various types of shampoos are a modification of the general method of preparation of shampoo.

(a) Preparation of cream shampoo: Certain formulae of cream shampoo may include glycol stearate or waxes. Usually, glycol stearate is used as an opacifier and preparation method of such formulation is similar as discussed above. But when wax is included in the formula, the process involves the following steps.

1. Initially, a solution of detergent and water are heated to about 80°C.
2. The wax is heated separately in a container at 80°C which facilitates the melting of wax.
3. Both the solution are kept at 80°C and mixed. Uniform mixing is achieved by constant and gentle stirring.
4. The solution is allowed to cool to about 40-45°C. After which the remaining ingredients, such as additives, colours, perfume and preservatives are added and stirring is continued.
5. Finally, under warm conditions, the mixture is transferred into a suitable container and packed.

(b) Preparation of gel shampoo: The method involved in the preparation of gel shampoo is similar to that of clear liquid shampoo. After preparation, the liquid shampoo is usually treated with a suitable thickening or gelling agent such as hydroxypropyl methylcellulose. This gives a gel-like consistency. Addition of appropriate amount of anionic and amphoteric surfactants also leads to the formation of gels.

(c) Preparation of aerosol shampoo: These types of shampoo are initially prepared by using (earlier discussed) general method. The prepared shampoo is then incorporated with a suitable propellant. The whole mixture is packed in an aerosol container. The propellant creates a pressure within the container due to which spraying action is achieved and the product (shampoo) is sprayed in the form of foam. Here packing plays an important role and the propellant used should not react with the shampoo.

(d) ***Preparation of powder shampoo:*** Powder shampoo is prepared by simple blending. Here, all the ingredients are taken. They are powdered to a suitable degree of fineness. The powdered ingredients are blended by using a suitable blender. Two separate solutions of perfume and colour are prepared by using alcohol or water as solvents. The prepared solutions are then sprayed onto the blended mixture. The wet mixture is dried and packed. Otherwise, the ingredients are internally soaked into the solutions of colour and perfume. The wet mass is dried and then subjected to blending.

COLD CREAMS

Cold creams are water-in-oil type of emulsions produce cooling sensation by the evaporation of water, after application of cream to the skin. They should possess emollient action and the layer left on the skin after application should be non-occlusive.

A simple cold cream consists of ingredients like beeswax, mineral oil (light liquid petrolatum), water, and borax. Beeswax consists of mainly free cerotic acid and myricylpalmitate with small quantities of other highest fatty acids and alcohols and about 10% of hydrocarbons. Borax in water hydrolyses to form NaOH and H_3BO_3. The reaction of cerotic acid from beeswax and NaOH forms a soap called sodium ceroate which then forms water-in-oil emulsion. Example for formulation of cold cream is given in Table 8.5.

Table 8.5: Formulation table of cold cream

Ingredients	*Quantity for 100 g*
White beeswax (emollient)	20 g
Mineral oil (Lubricant)	50 g
Distilled water (vehicle)	28.8 g
Borax (*In-situ* emulsifier)	0.7 g
Perfume (odour)	0.5 g

Method

1. Beeswax is a melted in a container by using a water bath to a temperature of about 70°C.
2. Then mineral oil is added to the melted beeswax. This is mixture A.
3. In another container, water is heated to a temperature of about 70°C and borax is dissolved in it. This is mixture B.

4. Mixture B (aqueous phase) is added slowly to mixture A (oily phase) along with stirring. Stirring is carried out until a creamy emulsion is formed.
5. Finally, perfume is added to the preparation when it attains a temperature of about 40°C.

VANISHING CREAMS

Vanishing creams are oil in water type of emulsion, when applied on the surface of the skin, they spread as thin oil less film which is not

Table 8.6: Formulation of vanishing cream

Ingredients	*Uses*
1. Main ingredient	It governs the consistency of the cream and imparts pearlescent property to the cream by forming crystals. *e.g.,*: Stearic acid
2. Humectants	Humectants retain the moisture content of the preparation. *e.g.,*: Glycerin, sorbitol, Propylene glycol
3. Alkalies	
(a) Potassium hydroxide	It imparts fine texture and consistency without providing harshness.
(b) Sodium hydroxide	It is used in combination with potassium hydroxide because it forms a hard cream when used alone.
(c) Carbonates *i.e.,* potassium and sodium carbonate.	They are not widely used, because they liberate carbon dioxide. Due to this, creams become spongy.
(d) Ammonia	It is effective, but difficult to handle because of odour and volatility. It also makes creams yellow in colour with age.
(e) Borax	It is used in combination with potassium hydroxide to produce a white emulsion.
4. Emulsifying agents	Triethanolamine soap, amino glycol soap or glyceryl monostearate
5. Purified water (*i.e.,* distilled and de-ionized water)	It provides stability to the cream. If hard water is used, it leads to the formation of soaps of lime and magnesium, which causes inversion of emulsion and hence stability is reduced.
6. Preservatives	They prevent deterioration caused by bacteria or fungi. *e.g.,*: Methylparaben and propylparaben
7. Perfume should be added when the cream attains a temperature of about 40°C.	It provides odour to the cream and also has aesthetic value. *e.g.,*: Geranium, sandalwood, lavender oil, terpineol etc.

visible to the naked eye. Hence, they are called vanishing creams. They are used to hold powder on the skin as well as to improve adhesion. Formulation of vanishing cream is given in Table 8.6.

Properties of ingredients:

1. It should have a high melting point.
2. It should be pure white in colour
3. It should possess very little odour.
4. It should have less iodine number.

Example for preparation of vanishing cream is given in Table 8.7.

Table 8.7: Formulation table of vanishing cream

Formula	*Quantity for 100 g*
Stearic acid (main ingredient)	24 g
Potassium hydroxide (softening agent)	1 g
Water (vehicle)	64 g
Glycerin (humectant)	10 g
Perfume (odour)	0.5 g

Method

1. Stearic acid is melted in a container by using a water bath.
2. Potassium hydroxide is dissolved in water and then glycerin is added. This mixture is heated to a temperature of about 75°C. This is an aqueous phase.
3. Slowly aqueous phase is added to melted stearic acid with continuous stirring.
4. Perfume is added to the preparation when it attains a temperature of about 40°C.

Note: During cooling, care should to be taken, as the cream passes through two transformations *i.e.,* softening and hardening. Then cream attains its desired form. Even formation of crust on the top surface of cream should be avoided by stirring to prevent lump formation.

TOOTHPASTE

Dentifrices such as toothpaste, tooth powders and tooth gels are meant for the cleaning the surface of the teeth by removing the food debris and plaque adhered to the surface of the teeth.

The general requirements for a dentifrice are as follows:

1. It should be capable of cleaning the teeth adequately by removing food debris, plaque and stains efficiently.
2. It should leave a pleasant, cool and refreshing sensation in the mouth.
3. It should be harmless, non-toxic and should not cause irritation in the mouth or any ulcers in the buccal cavity.
4. It should be able to maintain its flow properties all through its commercial period of storage.
5. The abrasive character of the dentifrice should be under the limits of the standards and should not be harsh on the enamel and the dentine.
6. It should conform to the standards of the cosmetic directive which states that it is not liable to cause damage to human health when used under normal conditions.
7. The assessment of any claims shall be certified based on properly conducted clinical trials.
8. Most of all it should be economical to purchase in order to encourage regular and frequent use by common people.

Formulation

Toothpaste is the most popular form of dentifrices. They include the following ingredients which determine the quality and efficiency of toothpaste, these are given in Table 8.8.

1. ***Polishing agents/abrasive agent:*** The abrasives or the polishing agents are used to polish the teeth and remove food debris adhered to the surface of the teeth. They are used in a concentration of about 20-50% of the total formulation. The abrasives agents: i) should not produce any gritty sensation in the mouth. ii) should possess good abrasive properties. iii) should not lead to any incompatibilities and should be compatible with the other ingredients. iv) should be harmless to the

Table 8.8: Ingredients for toothpaste formulation

Ingredients	*Examples*
Agents responsible for the cleansing action	
1. Polishing agents /abrasive agents	(a) Precipitated calcium carbonate
	(b) Phosphates of calcium
	(c) Dental graded silica/polymers of silica $(SiO_2)_n$
	(d) Trihydrated alumina
2. Foaming agents /surfactants	(a) Sodium lauryl sulphate
	(b) Sodium lauroyl sarcosinate.
Agents responsible for the formation of toothpaste	
1. Humectants	(a) Sorbitol
	(b) Glycerine
	(c) Propylene glycol.
2. Gelling agents/binding agents	(a) Sodium carboxymethyl cellulose
	(b) Cellulose derivatives
Agents responsible for the improving palatability	
1. Sweetening agents	(a) Sodium saccharin
	(b) Sucrose
2. Flavouring agents	(a) Cinnamon oil
	(b) Spearmint oil etc.
Miscellaneous agents	
1. Colouring agents	
2. Whitening agents	
3. Preservatives	
4. Therapeutic agents	

enamel and the abrasive property should be under limits. v) should provide a good shine to the enamel.

The most commonly used abrasive agents are:

Precipitated calcium carbonate ($CaCo_3$): It is also known as precipitated chalk and is available in a number of grades. The crystalline form of the precipitated chalk *e.g.,* calcite (rhombohedral crystals-stable polymorph of calcium carbonate), aragonite (orthorhombic crystals of calcium carbonate).

Phosphates of calcium: A large variety of insoluble calcium phosphates are used as abrasive agents. *e.g.,* Dicalcium phosphate (DCP) dihydrates ($CaHPO_4$ $2H_2O$): It is a commonly used abrasive agent among the phosphates of calcium.

Dental grade silica /polymers of silica ($(SiO_2)_n$): They are polymers of silica that are commonly used as abrasive agents in the formulation of toothpaste gels in large quantities. They are available in two forms:

i) Abrasive silica: They are also referred to as xerogels, possess the good abrasive property and are used in low concentration. They have the least effect on the consistency of the finished product.

ii) Thickening silica: They are referred to as aerogels. The particles are small in size and possess a greater surface area. They have the ability to swell and provide a thickening effect to the pastes.

Trihydrated alumina ($A1_2O$-$3H_2O$): It is available in suspension or as a crystalline powder.

2. ***Foaming agents/surfactants:*** They are also known as wetting agents. The mechanism of cleansing action is by reducing the surface tension at the interface of the adhered material and enamel of the teeth. They aid in abrasive action by wetting the surface of the teeth. They help in the diffusion of cleansing agents into narrow spaces, thus enhancing the cleansing action. The most commonly used surfactants are sodium lauryl sulphate (0.5 to 2%) and sodium lauroyl sarcosinate.

The ideal properties of the surfactants are:

(a) It should be compatible with other ingredients of the formulation.
(b) It should possess good surface active property.
(c) It should be non-toxic and non-irritant to the oral mucosa of the buccal cavity.
(d) It should be tasteless.

3. ***Humectants:*** These are added to prevent the rapid drying of toothpaste. They prevent excessive moisture loss from the product by hydrogen bond formation. These may additionally impart plasticity to the final product. Examples: Sorbitol, glycerol, polyethylene glycol, propylene glycol etc. The concentration of the humectants used in the formulation may vary from 20 to 40%.

Sorbitol 70: It consists of 70% w/v concentration of the sorbitol in the solution. It has good compatibility with other ingredients. It enhances sweetening property and imparts cooling sensation in the mouth. It has high viscosity and can produce stiff toothpaste. It is less expensive than glycerin.

Glycerin: It can be used in the concentration range of 5 to 10%. Glycerin has several advantages as it is easily available from both natural and synthetic sources. It is stable, compatible and safe with other ingredients. It provides good shine and gloss to the product.

4. ***Gelling or Binding agents:*** Binding agents are used in order to hold the solid and liquid components together to form a smooth paste and maintain its property, particularly during storage. These also prevent bleeding from the paste and add up viscosity of the final formulation. The most commonly used binding agents are cellulose derivatives such as carboxymethyl cellulose (CMC), sodium carboxymethyl cellulose (Na-CMC), hydroxyethyl cellulose, cellulose ethers etc.

5. ***Sweetening agents:*** Sweetening agents are added in order to improve the sweetening properties and cover the bitter taste of the ingredients like binders, surfactants etc. They also help in promoting the acceptance of the product when administered orally.

The most commonly used sweetening agents are aspartame, sodium saccharin (0.05 to 0.31%), cyclamates, mannitol and potassium acesulfame.

6. ***Flavouring agents:*** Flavoring agents are an important part of the formulation of toothpaste. These are generally a mixture of edible volatile oils consisting of spearmint and peppermint oil as major components. The other components included may be thymol, menthol, eucalyptus oil, anise oil, oil of wintergreen etc. Flavouring agents are used in the concentration of about 0.5 to 1.5%. They may react with other components of the formulation which may result in incompatibility.

7. ***Colouring agents:*** Coloring agents adds visual appeal to toothpaste. Examples of colouring agents are red, green (D&C #5), and blue. Titanium dioxide imparts a white colour to the toothpaste.

8. ***Preservatives*:** Preservatives basically prevent the growth of microorganisms in toothpaste and these are used in the formulation in order to maintain the properties of the product throughout the storage

period. Common preservatives include sodium benzoate, methylparaben and propylparaben etc.

9. *Therapeutic agents:* The therapeutic agents may be incorporated in toothpaste are anticaries agents (fluoride derivatives like NaF, Na_2FPO_3), anti-plaque agents (chlorhexidine, triclosan), bleaching agents (H_2O_2, sodium peroxide) etc. example for toothpaste is given in Table 8.9.

Table 8.9: Formulation table for toothpaste

Ingredients	*Quantities for 100 g*	*Role of ingredients*
Calcium carbonate	28 g	Abrasive agent
Sodium lauryl sulphate	0.5 g	Surfactant
Gum tragacanth	0.75 g	Binding agent
Glycerine	11 g	Humectant
Sodium saccharin	0.05 g	Sweetening agent
Water	9.7 g	Liquid phase
Flavour	q. s.	Flavouring agent
Preservatives	q. s.	

Method

i) All the solids ingredients of the formulation except surfactants are mixed together in a mortar.

ii) The liquid components such as humectants and water are gradually added to the dry mix.

iii) The trituration process is carried out by pestle until a smooth paste is formed.

iv) The remaining ingredients like surfactants, flavouring agents and preservative are added to the paste mixture.

HAIR DYES

Hair dye is one of the oldest known beauty preparations and was used by ancient cultures in many parts of the world. Records of ancient Egyptians, Greeks, Hebrews, Persians, Chinese and early Hindu peoples all mention the use of hair colourings. Early hair dyes were made from plants, metallic compounds, or a mixture of the two. Rock alum, quicklime and wood ash were used for bleaching hair in Roman times and herbal preparations included mullein, birch bark, saffron, myrrh and turmeric. Henna was known in many parts of the world; it produces a reddish dye.

Many different plant extracts were used for hair dye in Europe and Asia before the advent of modern dyes. Indigo, known primarily as a fabric dye, could be combined with henna to make light brown to black shades of hair dye. An extract of the flowers of the chamomile plant was long used to lighten hair and this is still used in many modern hair preparations. The bark, leaves, or nutshells of many trees were used for hair dyes. Wood from the brazilwood tree yielded brown hair dyes and another hair dye known in antiquity as fustic was derived from a tree similar to the mulberry. Other dyes were produced from walnut leaves or nut husks and from the galls, a species of oak trees. Some of these plant-derived dyes were mixed with metals such as copper and iron, to produce more lasting or richer shades.

Hydrogen peroxide was discovered in 1818, but it was not until 1867 that it was exhibited at the Paris Exposition as an effective hair lightener. A London chemist and a Parisian hairdresser began marketing a 3% hydrogen peroxide formula at the Exposition *as eau de fontaine de jouvence golden* (golden fountain of youth water) and this was the first modern chemical hair colourant.

Advances in chemistry led to the production of more hair dyes in the late nineteenth century. The first synthetic organic hair dye developed was pyrogallol, a substance that occurs naturally in walnut shells. Beginning in 1845, pyrogallol was used to dye hair brown and it was often used in combination with henna. So-called amino dyes were developed and marketed in Europe in the 1880s. The earliest was p-phenylenediamine, patented in Germany by E. Erdmann in 1888 as a dye for fur, hair and feathers. To dye hair with p-phenylenediamine and related dyes, a weak solution of the chemical, mixed with caustic soda, sodium carbonate, or ammonia, was applied to the hair. Then hydrogen peroxide was applied, which brought out the colour. The amino dyes produced a more natural-looking black than previous dyes and could make shades of red and brown as well.

A French hairdresser, Gaston Boudou, first marketed a standardized range of hair dyes in 1910. Whereas earlier hair colours had been mixed on the spot by hairdressers and the colours produced were variable, Boudou's dyes produced a predictable colour. Sold in a range of 18 colours, from black to light blond, these became very popular.

The amino dyes, however, caused allergic reactions in a significant portion of users. Researchers in the United States is credited with creating a modified, less toxic amino-based hair dye, for standardizing the method of applying the dye, and for establishing strict specifications for the purity and strength of the raw materials. Further advances in hair dye chemistry were made by the makers of Clairol. Clairol produced the first one-step hair dye in 1950. This eliminated the time-consuming preliminary shampoo and pre-lightening that was the established hair-dying protocol.

Classification of hair dyes

1. Temporary hair colourants.
2. Semi-permanent hair colourants/ Direct dyes
3. Oxidative dyeing systems
   a) Semi-permanent hair colourants
   b) Permanent hair colourants
4. Gradual hair colourants
5. Natural dyes

Formulation

Most commercial hair dye formulas are complex, with dozens of ingredients and the formule differ considerably from manufacturer to manufacturer. In general, hair dyes include dyes, modifiers, antioxidants, alkalizers, soaps, ammonia, wetting agents, fragrance and a variety of other chemicals used in small amounts that impart special qualities to hair (such as softening the texture) or give a desired action to the dye (such as making it more or less permanent). The dye chemicals are usually amino compounds and show up on hair dye ingredient lists with such names as 4-amino-2-hydroxytoluene and m-aminophenol. Metal oxides, such as titanium dioxide and iron oxide, are often used as pigments as well.

Other chemicals used in hair dyes act as modifiers, which stabilize the dye pigments or otherwise act to modify the shade. The modifiers may bring out colour tones, such as green or purple, which complement the dye pigment. One commonly used modifier is resorcinol, though there are many others. Antioxidants protect the dye from oxidizing with air. Most commonly used is sodium sulfite. Alkalizers are added to change the pH of the dye formula because the dyes work best in a highly alkaline composition. Ammonium hydroxide is a common alkalizer. Beyond these basic chemicals, many different chemicals are used to impart special qualities to a manufacturer's formula. They may be shampoos, fragrances, chemicals that make the formula creamy, foamy, or thick, or contribute to the overall action of the formula.

Hair dyes are usually packaged with a developer, which is in a separate bottle. The developer is most often based on hydrogen peroxide, with the addition of small amounts of other chemicals depending on the manufacturer. Example of hair dye formulation is given in Table 8.10.

Table 8.10: Formula for preparation of semi-permanent hair dye

Ingredients	*Quantity (%)*
Quatenary ammonium compound (colour)	10–12
Surfactants (anionic surfactants)	8–10
Buffer	6–8
Surfactant (alkanolamide)	4–6
Colour (dye stuff)	1–2
Water (solvent)	q.s. upto 100

Method of preparation

A mixture of alkanolamide and anionic surfactant is prepared. Dye is added to the above mixture and is dissolved. Buffer and quaternary ammonium compounds are dissolved in water. This aqueous solution is added to the solution of dye with stirring. This dye is investigated for the effect of quaternary ammonium compound, pH, aldehydes and alcohol additions. Now the viscosity of the dye is adjusted by adding hydrophilic colloids like methyl cellulose, natural gum etc. viscosity of the colourant is increased by the addition of non-ionic thickener in its composition. Addition of amphoteric surfactant in the colourant accompanied by basic dyes.

SUNSCREENS

The sun produces a wide range of electromagnetic radiation. Although we are most aware of the visible light from the sun, the only light we can see with the unaided eye, there are a number of types of light we cannot see. One of these is infrared light, which is responsible for heating our planet. Another is ultraviolet light which is responsible for sunburn and suntan and increases the risk of basal cell carcinoma and malignant melanoma. Ultraviolet light is artificially divided into three ranges:

UVA is radiation in the 320-400 nm range

UVB is radiation in the 290-320 nm range

UVC is radiation in the 100-290 nm range

UVC is totally blocked by the ozone layer in the upper atmosphere of the Earth. The ozone layer blocks some of the UVB and all of the UVA passes through the ozone layer. Generally, UVB has been blamed for sunburn, but some studies indicate that UVA may also cause skin damage. Mild sunburn is a first-degree radiation burn which produces reddening of the skin with accompanying pain. Generally, as the skin heals, redness may persist and the outer layers of the epidermis will peel within a week with accompanying itching. Prolonged exposure can result in a second-degree burn which is characterized by blistering of the skin and more severe pain. Third-degree sunburn is rare.

One of the body's defences against UV radiation is the production of melanin, a pigment that results in darkening of the skin. An individual's response to UV radiation and melanin production is dependent on skin colour and other genetic factors. Even if an individual has dark skin, or whose skin readily produces melanin when exposes to UV radiation, may still experience sunburn as a result of the high intensity of UV radiation and an extended length of exposure.

Sunscreens are cosmetic formulations that block UV rays. Sunscreens are assigned sun protection factors, or SPF, ratings that are supposed to indicate the level of protection from UV radiation. The SPF rating is a multiplier that tells how long one can safely remain in the sun. For example, if an individual whose unprotected skin becomes sunburned in 5 min, then an SPF15 sunscreen should allow that individual to stay in the sun for 15 times of 5 min or 75 min, without burning.

Some active ingredients in sunscreens are:

Benzyl salicylate and salicylate derivatives. One of the first sunscreen agents. It provides UVB protection, but not UVA. It is not soluble in water and can be used in waterproof formulations. It is often used in combination with other ingredients. One of the derivative compounds is known as homosalate.

Benzyl cinnamate and cinnamate derivatives. Another early sunscreen agent. It is an effective UVB blocker but is not waterproof. Often found in combination with other ingredients.

PABA (p-aminobenzoic acid) was extensively used in many formulations, however, it was not water soluble and needed to be used in alcohol-based solutions, it would discolour fabrics, and many individuals experienced or developed allergic reactions to it. Most sunscreen lotions are now PABA free Butyl methoxydibenzoylmethane and related compounds.

Zinc oxide and titanium dioxide are two inorganic compounds that are insoluble in most liquids. These block the UV radiation because their preparations are opaque to light. Sunscreen lotions containing these are normally white opaque ointments on the skin.

Each of the active ingredients provides an SPF factor related to its concentration in the sunscreen. Increasing the concentration of the ingredient should also increase the SPF rating of the sunscreen. Example for sunscreen cream and sunscreen lotion are given in Table 8.11 and Table 8.12 respectively.

Table 8.11: Formulation table for sunscreen cream.

Ingredients	*Quantity (%)*
Benzyl salicylate	14
Borax	1.8
White mineral oil	20
Beeswax	20
Petrolatum	15
Perfume	0.5
Water	28.7

Method

i) Heat the water and dissolve the borax in it.
ii) Melt the borax, petrolatum and mineral oil together.
iii) Add the liquids to fats with constant stirring.

iv) When the temperature drops to about 45°C. add the perfume
v) Transfer the preparation into container, label and label it.

Table 8.12: Formulation table for Sunscreen lotion.

Ingredients	***Quantity (%)***
Benzyl salicylate	11.5
Alcohol	10
Glycerin	5
Perfume	0.25
Water	73.25

Method

i) Dissolve the benzyl salicylate in alcohol
ii) Add perfume, glycerin and water
iii) Filter the preparation and transfer into the container and label it.

Glossary

Cosmetics	Means; adding something decorative to a person or a thing
Wool fat	Anhydrous lanolin
Lanolin	Hydrous wool fat
Carmine	It is obtained as the carminic acid from the cochineal insects by extracting the insects with ammonia
Surfactants	Main use of a surfactant is to cleanse and to produce foam
Foam boosters	Produced foam is stabilized or strengthened by using a substancc called foam boosters
Pearlescent agents	They improve the conditioning property and also imparts brightness to hair
Sequestrants	These are complex forming agents and form complex with metal ions like calcium and magnesium
Thickening agents	These agents are usually added to make the preparation thick *i.e.*, viscous
Preservatives	These agents have the ability to prevent the growth of microorganisms
Vanishing creams	When applied on the surface of the skin, they spread as a thin oil less film which is not visible to the naked eye
Cold creams	These types of creams are the water-in-oil type of emulsions. They produce cooling sensation by the evaporation of water, after application of cream to the skin. Hence, they are known as cold creams
Stearic acid	It governs the consistency of the cream and imparts pearlescent property to the cream by forming crystals

Humectants	Humectants retain the moisture content of the preparation
Abrasive agents	Abrasive agents polish the teeth and remove food debris adhered to the surface of the teeth
Surfactants	The mechanism of cleansing action is by reducing the surface tension at the interface of the adhered material and enamel of the teeth.
Therapeutic agents	Therapeutic agents may be incorporated in toothpaste are anticaries agents
Sunscreens	Sunscreens are cosmetic formulations that block UV rays. Sunscreens are assigned sun protection factors, or SPF, ratings that are supposed to indicate the level of protection from UV radiation
Sun protection factor (SPF)	A measure of how well a sunscreen preparations will protect skin from UVB rays.

QUESTION BANK

Q. I: Multiple Choice Questions

1 A commonly used antioxidant for oil system is
- a) Butylated hydroxyl toluene
- b) Ascorbic acid
- c) Sodium metabisulfite
- d) Thyoglycol

2 A synthetic sweetening agent which is approximately 200 times sweeter than sucrose and has no aftertaste is
- a) Saccharin
- b) Aspartame
- c) Cyclamate
- d) Sorbitol

3 Surfactants are characterized by the presence of
- a) Water-soluble groups alone
- b) Fat solubilising groups alone
- c) water and fat solubilizing groups in the same molecule
- d) Groups with a positive charge

4 Benzyl peroxide is
- a) An astringent
- b) An emollient
- c) A preservative
- d) A keratolytic

5 HLB system is used to classify
- a) Surfactants
- b) Preservative
- c) Antioxidants
- d) Sequestering agent

6 In cosmetic preparation, an antioxidant used in an aqueous system is
- a) Sodium formaldehyde sulphoxylate
- b) Phenol
- c) α-tocopherol
- d) Methylparaben

7 A plasticizer and high boiling point solvent used in the preparation of nail lacquers are

P) Butyl stearate
R) Ethyl alcohol
Q) Ethyl lactate
S) Acetone

a) P, Q
b) Q, S
c) R, S
d) Q, R.

8 Candelilla wax having melting point______ is used in lipstick formulation

a) 80-90
b) 36-42
c) 65-75
d) 38-60

9 Commonly used preservative in shampoo

a) Benzalkonium chloride
b) Methylparaben
c) PABA
d) Ethylparaben

10 All-purpose creams are also known as _____creams

a) Vanishing
b) Sports
c) Foundation
d) Cleansing

11 What is the use of stearic acid in vanishing cream?

a) Increases consistency
b) Increases white shining
c) Increases transparence
d) Maintains stiffness

12 Which vegetable oil is mostly used in lipstick?

a) Peanut oil
b) Liquid paraffin
c) Almond oil
d) Castor oil

13 Which of the following step is involved in the preparation of lipstick?

a) Mixing
b) Moulding
c) cooling
d) All of the above

14 The rate of creaming is determined by

a) Stoke's law
b) Dalton's law
c) Hallsher's law
d) Raoult's law

15 _____ cream used to remove facial make up

a) Vanishing
b) Cold
c) Cleansing
d) None of the above

16 Vanishing cream is _____ type of emulsion

a) Water in oil
b) Oil in water
c) oil in water in oil
d) None of the above

Q. II: Very Short Answer Questions **2 Marks**

1. Define and classify cosmetic preparations
2. Add a note on sun protection factor
3. List out the components of toothpaste with their use.
4. What are the functions of essential ingredients in toothpaste?
5. Give the ideal properties of shampoos.
6. Give the composition of shampoo.
7. Give typical formula of toothpaste.
8. What are the conditioning agents used in a shampoo?

Q. III: Short Answer Questions **5 Marks**

1. Explain the preparation of vanishing cream.
2. Add a note on the preparation of cold cream
3. List out the ideal properties of lipsticks. Add a note on different bases used in lipsticks.
4. Discuss in detail the formulation of toothpaste.
5. Write a note on lipsticks.
6. Explain the manufacture of shampoo.
7. Give the steps involved in the preparation of lipstick.
8. Add a note on the formulation of hair dyes.
9. Add a note on the formulation of sunscreens.

Q. IV: Long Answer Questions **10 Marks**

1. Discuss the formulation of cold cream and vanishing cream.
2. Describe in detail formulation of lipsticks.
3. Explain the formulation of sunscreen and hair dyes.
4. Discuss in detail formulation aspects of Shampoos.

CHAPTER 9

PHARMACEUTICAL AEROSOLS

INTRODUCTION

Pharmaceutical aerosols are pressurized dosage forms that upon actuation emit a fine dispersion of liquid and/or solid materials containing one or more active ingredients in a gaseous or liquid medium.

Aerosol products are meant for topical, systemic and oral administration and they may be designed to expel the contents as a fine mist, a coarse wet or dry spray, a steady stream or stable or fast-breaking foam.

Various types of aerosol products are dry powder inhalers, metered dose inhalers (MDI), nebulizers, sublinguals, skin and dental sprays.

Advantages of Aerosol Packaging:

1. Administration of drug by aerosol is easy, rapid and convenient
2. The drug can be directly delivered to the affected area, hence systemic side effects are reduced
3. It protects the drug from gastrointestinal degradation and first pass metabolism
4. The desired dose can be removed without affecting the remaining quantity of the container
5. It provides minimum contamination hence, sterility of the dose can be maintained

6. Product is protected from light and oxidation, hence stability is increased
7. It helps in reducing the skin or mucous membrane irritation and has a cooling effect
8. Aerosol system can be used in the treatment of respiratory illness like asthma or chronic obstructive pulmonary disease (COPD).
9. Aerosols are easy to control the physical form, particle size, dose etc.
10. Aerosols are used for both systemic and local application.

Disadvantages of Aerosol Packaging:

1. The cost of aerosol system is high
2. Valve clogging may take place which leads to wastage of the aerosol product
3. It leads to inhalation toxicity if exposed to vapours of aerosols for longer periods of time
4. Pressure of the aerosol container drops rapidly after dispensing the product. This is seen especially in case of compressed gas propellants. This result in variation in the amount of product applied or used, thereby decreasing its efficacy.

Components of Aerosol Systems

Following are the different components of aerosol system

1. Propellant
2. Container
3. Valve
4. Actuator
5. Product concentrate

Propellants for aerosol systems

The propellants are considered as an important element in the formulation of aerosols. It is responsible for the development of pressure within the container, supplying the necessary force to expel the product when the valve is opened. Propellants help in maintaining proper pressure in the container. Different types of propellants used in the formulation of aerosols are classified into:

1. Liquefied gases
2. Compressed gases

Liquefied gases

Liquefied gases have been widely used as propellants for most aerosol products. These liquefied propellants are actually gases which exist as a liquid under pressure. Some part of the liquefied propellants also exists as gas and occupies the head space in the container. When the product is dispensed from the container, the part of liquefied propellant turns into a gas and occupies the headspace. In this way, the headspace is always occupied by gas which maintains the constant pressure and even performance of the spray is also maintained.

Liquefied gases are widely used in the formulation of aerosols because they are capable of dispensing active ingredients in the form of fine mist. Apart from that, they are inert and non-toxic in nature. Liquefied gases are of three types: (a) Chlorofluorocarbons, (b) Hydrofluorocarbons, (c) Hydrocarbons

(a) Chlorofluorocarbons

Chlorofluorocarbons are of various types, such as:

1. Trichloromonofluoromethane or propellant 11.
2. Dichlorodifluoromethane or propellant 12.
3. Dichlorotetrafluoroethane or propellant 114.

Vapour pressure of the propellant is one of the important physicochemical property. The desired range of vapour pressure can be obtained by blending various propellants like propellant 11 and 12 or propellant 12 and 114 together respectively. But this vapour pressure obtained should be within the limits of the vapour pressure of the individual propellant.

The ideal system can be achieved if mole fraction of one component is small compared to the other component in a system. This is because the mole fraction in a smaller quantity does not affect the vapour pressure of the aerosol.

The physicochemical properties of the propellants are considered important in the formulation of pharmaceutical aerosols. The power of the solvent, stability of the formulation and the rate of reaction of the

Table 9.1: Properties of chlorofluorocarbons

Propellant	*Molecular formula*	*Molecular weight*	*Vapour pressure (psia) at 70°F*	*Boiling point °F (1 atm)*
Trichloromonofluoromethane (propellant 11)	CCl_3F	137.28	13.4	74.7
Dichlorodifluoromethane (propellant 12)	CCl_2F_2	120.93	84.9	–21.6
Dichlorotetrafluoroethane (propellant 114)	$CClF_2\ CClF_2$	170.93	27.6	38.4

propellants can be determined through these properties. Properties of chlorofluorocarbons are given in Table 9.1.

Physical properties of chlorofluorocarbons

1. Propellants (such as 11, 12, 114) are non-polar compounds.
2. They are miscible with non-polar solvents at desired temperature and have the ability to dissolve many substances.
3. They are immiscible with water.
4. In order to make them miscible with water, co-solvents such as ethanol, 2-propanol or DMF is added.
5. Instead of adding co-solvents, emulsions of aerosols can be formed for topical administration.

Chemical properties of chlorofluorocarbons

1. They are non-toxic in nature.
2. They are non-flammable.
3. They are chemically inert.
4. Propellant 11 undergoes hydrolysis, hence it is not preferred in the formulation of an aerosol of aqueous product. Propellant 11 forms hydrochloric acid after undergoing hydrolysis.
5. The addition of fluorine atom to carbon present in the propellant increases stability.

(b) Hydrofluorocarbons

Hydrofluorocarbons break down in the atmosphere at a faster rate than CFCs resulting in a lower ozone layer depleting effect.

Hydrofluorocarbons are non-flammable, less expensive and they are environmentally acceptable hence, used in the formulation. Properties of hydrofluorocarbons are given in Table 9.2.

Table 9.2: Properties of hydrofluorocarbons

Propellant	***Number***	***Formula***	***Liquid density***	***Vapour pressure (psia) at 70°F***
Difluoroethane	152a	CH_3CHF_2	0.91	76.4
Chlorodifluoromethane	22	$CHClF_2$	1.21	–135.7
Trifluoromonofluoroethane	134a	CF_3CH_2F	1.21	85.8
Chlorodifluoroethane	142b	CH_3CClF_2	1.12	43.8

(c) Hydrocarbons

Hydrocarbons are preferred to chlorofluorocarbons in formulating topical aerosol, due to the following reasons.

1. They are chemically stable.
2. They have a density of less than 1.
3. They have a low order of toxicity.
4. A wide range of solubility
5. They are light in weight than water. Therefore, the layer of hydrocarbons remains on top of the aqueous layer and this helps in expelling the contents from the container.
6. Hydrocarbons are blended according to the final pressure obtained, but not on the proportion of hydrocarbons used. This is because the pressure of the hydrocarbons depends on its purity.
7. Hydrocarbons do not undergo hydrolysis. Hence, these are used in the formulation of water-based aerosols.
8. They are used in metered dose inhalers as well as for topical administration.
9. They do not contain halogenated atoms, hence their solubility is more compared to fluorinated hydrocarbons.

Properties of some of the hydrocarbon propellants are given in Table 9.3.

Table 9.3: Properties hydrocarbon propellants

Propellants	*Number*	*Formula*	*Liquid density (g/ml)*	*Vapour pressure (psia) at 70°F*
Butane	A-17	C_4H_{10}	0.58	31.6
Propane	A-108	C_3H_8	0.50	122.8
Isobutane	A-31	C_4H_{10}	0.56	45.8

Compressed gases

Propellants like nitrogen, oxygen and carbon dioxide are used as compressed gases. The compressed gases help in dispensing the product in the form of mist, foam or semisolid. The product formed after dispensing depends on the nature of the formulation and valve design of the container. They are also capable of producing fairly wet spray and foams if expansion power is present but foams produced by compressed gases are less stable compared to liquefied gas foams. Properties of some compressed gases is given in Table 9.4.

Table 9.4: Compressed gases as propellants

Propellants	*Molecular formula*	*Molecular weight*	*Vapour pressure (psia) at 70°F*	*Boiling point °F*
Nitrogen	N_2	28	492	–320
Carbon dioxide	CO_2	44	852	–109
Nitrous oxide	N_2O	44	735	–127

Compressed gases are used in:

1. Dispensing food and non-food products in its original form *i.e.,* semisolid.
2. Dental creams, hair preparations, ointments and antiseptics.
3. Saline solutions which are used as contact lens cleaner and in barrier systems.

Advantages

1. They are chemically inert.
2. They are non-toxic in nature.
3. They are non-flammable.

4. They are non-polar compounds which have the ability to dissolve many substances.
5. The addition of fluorine atom to a carbon present in the propellants enhances the stability.

Disadvantages

1. They are immiscible with water; hence co-solvents are added to make them miscible.
2. They are responsible for depleting the ozone layer which can lead to skin cancer.

Containers for aerosol systems

Containers used for aerosol systems must withstand the pressure as high as 140 to 180 psig (pounds per sq. inch gauge) and temperature of about 54.44°C (130°F). Various types of materials used in the manufacture of aerosol containers are:

1. *Metal*
   a. Tin-plated steel
   b. Aluminium
2. *Glass*
   a. Plastic-coated Glass
   b. Uncoated glass

Metal as the material for aerosol containers:

Tin-plated steel containers

1. They are light in weight.
2. They are available as thin sheets.
3. They help in the large-scale production of aerosol containers.
4. If additional protection is required, then metal containers are coated with organic materials
5. They provide sufficient protection to certain products without any treatment on the inner side of the container.

Procedure: Thin lithographed sheets are cut into pieces to make the body, top and bottom of the container. They are fabricated so that the desired shape can be obtained. The body of the sheet can be made into cylindrical shape through flanging and soldering operation where the top and bottom are attached to the cylindrical body. This process is slow and expensive hence, a new welding method is developed. This method includes two processes such as (a) soudric system and (b) conoweld system.

Soudric system: In this method, the rounded bodies are first welded. Then they are passed to a conventional line where the rounded bodies are flanged with the top and bottom pieces.

Conoweld system: In this method, the folded body are passed through two electrode rings which are in the rotation. Then the top and bottom pieces are attached.

The advantages of using soudric and conoweld system are:

1. The interaction between the product and the container is reduced.
2. This method eliminates the use of soldering operation.
3. It reduces the time required for manufacturing.

Aluminium containers

Aluminium aerosols containers are:

1. Produced by an impact extrusion process in order to obtain a container which in seamless (no line of joining in the container).
2. Used in most of the metered dose inhalers and pharmaceutical aerosols
3. Able to withstand high pressures.
4. Compatible in nature.
5. Provide more resistance to corrosion.
6. Available in different sizes ranges.
7. Less reactive in nature.
8. The inside of the aluminium container is coated with organic materials like epoxy, vinyl, phenolic or polyamide resins to provide additional resistance.

Glass as the material for aerosol containers:

Glass containers have fewer problems with respect to chemical compatibility with the formulation than do metal containers and it is not subject to corrosion. Glass is also more adaptive to creativity in design.

Plastic-coated glass containers: These containers help in preventing the glass from breaking into small pieces at the time of breakage. These plastic coated glasses are used as containers in topical and MDI aerosols.

Uncoated glass containers: Their cost is low and they provide more clarity by which all the contents of the container can be viewed.

Valves for aerosol

Valves are the important and basic part of aerosol containers permit expulsion of the contents of the can in the desired form, at the desired rate. In addition, in the case of metered valves proper amount or dose can also be regulated. The performance of the aerosol depends on both types of formulation and valve.

The pharmaceutical aerosol value consists of different parts made up of plastic, rubber, aluminium and stainless steel. The different parts of the valve assembly include mounting cup (ferrule), valve body, stem, gasket, spring and dip tube. Different components of valve assembly are shown in Fig. 9.1.

Mounting cup (ferrule): Mounting cup is made up of tin-plated steel or aluminium connects the valve properly to the container. Mounting cup is exposed to the contents and oxygen in the headspace of the container hence; the corrosion is avoided by applying a single or double coat of epoxy or vinyl to the underside.

Whereas ferrules are used in case of either glass bottles or small aluminium tubes. Ferrules are made up of aluminium or brass. Ferrules end are rolled under the lip of the bottle for attachment purposes.

Valve body: Valve body is made of nylon and which contains two openings of about 0.013-0.080 inch in size one is present at the point of attachment of the dip tube and another opening is known as vapour tap which helps in the following way.

1. It allows the escape of vaporized propellant and liquid product.
2. It helps in producing a fine particle size of the products.

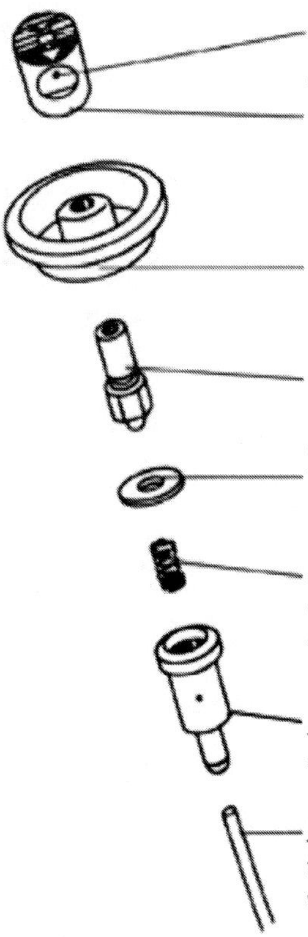

Fig. 9.1: Different components of valve assembly.

3. Insoluble materials may be present in the products which lead to valve clogging. This can be prevented with the help of vapour tap.
4. Even if the container is in an inverted position, then vapour tap assist in proper dispensing of the product.
5. The chilling effect on the skin due to propellants is reduced.
6. The flame extension due to hydrocarbon propellant is reduced by these vapour taps.

Stem: Stem is also made up of nylon or metals such as brass and stainless steel. Stem supports the actuator and delivers the formulation in the proper form to the chamber of the actuator. The stem consists of one or many orifices. One orifice range from 0.013-0.030 inch in size while other orifices are about 0.040 inches in sizes.

Gasket: Gasket is made from rubbers such as Buna-N and Neoprene. It helps in sealing the stem orifice when the valve is closed.

Spring: It is made from stainless steel. It holds the gasket and brings back the valve in its closed position after the actuator is pushed or depressed.

Dip-tube: Dip-tube is the tube with an inner diameter of about 0.120-0.125 inch made from polyethylene or polypropylene materials. In the case of highly viscous products, the inner diameter of the dip tube can be as large as 0.195 inches. The inner diameter of the dip tube is selected based on the viscosity of the product and the desired delivery rate.

Actuators of aerosol

Actuators are specially designed buttons placed on the valve stem, which helps in easy opening and closing of the valve. Actuators provide rapid and proper release of the products from the container. The desired form of product *i.e.*, spray, wet stream, foam or solid stream can be achieved by using different types of actuator, these include:

1. Spray actuators
2. Foam actuators
3. Solid stream actuators
4. Special actuators

Spray actuators: The stream of propellants and product concentrate are dispensed in the form of small particles through orifices present. These orifices are usually one to three in number in the diameter range of 0.016-0.040 inch. Large orifices are used in case of a high percentage of propellant blends which contain propellant 12 (have a low boiling point) and propane. The spray actuators are used for topical administration purposes. For *e.g.,* spray-type, bandages, antiseptics, local anaesthetics and foot preparations.

Foam actuators: The orifices are large in size having the diameter in the range of 0.070-0.125 inch. The opening present in the aerosol allows the product to move to a larger chamber. In this chamber, the product expands and dispensed from the large orifice in the form of foams.

Solid stream actuators: These actuators are used to dispense semisolid type of preparation such as ointments. They are similar to foam actuators where a large opening allows the product to pass through the valve stem and then finally into the actuator where the product gets dispensed.

Special actuators: These actuators are specially designed to deliver the medicaments on specific sites such as throat, nose, eye, vagina etc.

Metered dose inhalers (MDI)

Metering values are used when the formulation is potent medicament and measured the amount of product need to be expelled from the container. MDI's are convenient to use compared to nebulizers or atomizers.

MDI's have become a popular choice for delivering drugs to the lungs either in the form of solutions or suspensions; they can deliver the medicament of required dose with appropriate particle size.

Advantages of MDI's

1. A close regulation on the drug dose can be achieved using MDIs.
2. Steroidal drugs can be administered using MDIs.
3. Potent drugs can be delivered through MDIs.
4. Wastage of drug is minimized by using MDIs

Product concentrate

Product concentrate of aerosol system consists of active ingredients or a mixture of active ingredients along with surfactants, antioxidant and solvents constitute the product concentrate.

Principle of Working of Aerosol System

The aerosol formulation consists of two components, the product concentrate and the propellant. The product concentrate is the active ingredient of the aerosol combined with the required adjuncts, such as antioxidants, surface active agents and solvents, to prepare a stable and efficacious product. The concentrate can be a solution, suspension, emulsion, semisolid, or powders. When the propellant is a liquefied gas or a mixture of liquefied gases, it frequently serves the dual role of propellant and solvent or vehicle for the product concentrate. In certain aerosol systems, compressed gases — carbon dioxide, nitrogen and nitrous oxide are employed as the propellant.

When a liquefied gas propellant or propellant mixture is sealed within an aerosol container with the product concentrate, equilibrium is quickly established between the portion of propellant that remains liquefied and that which vaporizes and occupies the upper portion of the aerosol container. The vapour phase exerts pressure in all directions — against the walls of the container, the valve assembly and the surface of the liquid phase, which is composed of the liquefied gas and the product concentrate. This pressure, upon actuation of the aerosol valve forces the liquid phase up the dip tube and expel out of orifice of valve into atmosphere. As propellant meets the air, it expands and evaporates because of drop in pressure, leaving the product concentrate as airborne liquid droplets or dry particles, depending upon the formulation. As liquid phase is removed from container, the equilibrium between propellant remaining liquefied and that in vapour state is re-established. Thus, even during expulsion of the product from the aerosol package, the pressure within remains virtually constant, and the product may be continuously released at an even rate with same propulsion. However, when liquid reservoir is depleted, the pressure may not be maintained, and gas may be expelled from the container with diminishing pressure until it is exhausted. Working of aerosol container is as shown in Fig. 9.2.

Formulation and Manufacture of Aerosols

The procedure for the manufacturing of pharmaceutical aerosol includes:

1. Preparation of product concentrate
2. Filling of aerosol container

Preparation of Product Concentrate

Depending on the type of system used for the formulation of aerosols, the product is dispensed either as a fine mist, wet spray, quick-breaking foam, stable foam, semi-solid and solid type.

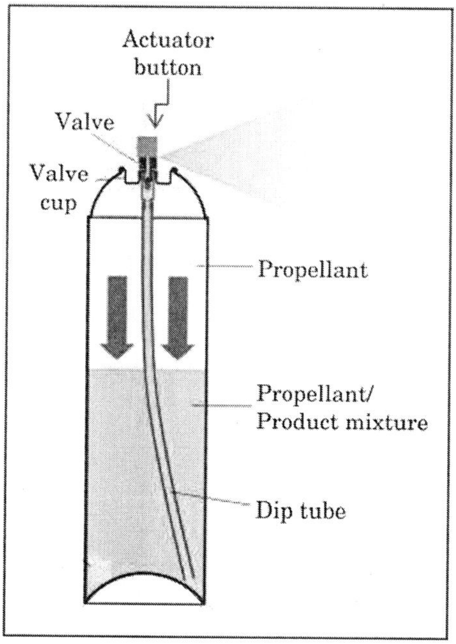

Fig. 9.2: Working of aerosol system

The type of aerosol system selected for formulation depends on the physical, chemical and pharmacological characteristics of active ingredients as well as the site of application of aerosol *i.e.*, topical, oral etc.

Various types of aerosol systems are:

1. Two-phase system or solution system
2. Three-phase system or water-based system
3. Suspension or dispersion system
4. Foam system
   (a) Aqueous stable foams
   (b) Non-aqueous stable foams
   (c) Quick breaking foams
   (d) Thermal foams
5. Intranasal system.

1. *Two-phase system or solution system*

In a two-phase system or solution system, the active ingredients are dissolved in the liquid propellant or mixture of propellants. When the active ingredients are dissolved in propellants in such cases the addition of solvents is not required. Two-phase system is used to formulate a large number of aerosols.

Propellant 12 helps in producing very fine particles, hence it is used generally in the formulation of a solution. Even other propellants are incorporated along with propellant 12 which have vapour pressure lower than that of propellant 12. This results in decreasing the pressure of the system hence, large particles are produced. The addition of less volatile solvents such as acetone, ethyl alcohol, ethyl acetate, glycerine and propylene glycol helps in reducing the vapour pressure.

The propellants used in the system ranges from 5% - 95% (5% in the production of foams and 95% are used for inhalation products). The vaporization rate of propellants depends on the boiling point of the solvents *i.e.*, boiling point of solvent used may lead to a decrease in rate of vaporization and increasing the chilling effect of propellants. The general formulation of two-phase system or solution system is shown in Table 9.5.

Table 9.5: General formulation of two-phase system or solution system.

Ingredient	*Quantity (% w/w)*
Active ingredients	10 – 15%
Propellants 12/11(50:50) (or)	85 – 90%
Propellants 12/11(30:70)	85 – 90%

This type of formulation is used for oral inhalation aerosol systems. Different ratios of propellants 12/114 also used *i.e.,* 45:55 or 55:45 for this purpose. The pressure of the system increases if the amount of propellant 12 is increased. Metal containers are used to pack propellant 12/11 in the ratio of 30:70 and propellant 12/114 in the ratio of 20:80 or 10:90. Examples of two-phase system are shown in Table 9.6 and Table 9.7.

Table 9.6: Example of two-phase system or solution system (a).

Ingredients	*Quantity (% w/w)*
Isoproterenol HCL	0.25%
Ascorbic acid	0.10%
Ethanol	35.75%
Propellant (dichlorodifluoromethane)	63.90%

This formulation is packed in15-30 ml stainless steel, aluminium or glass containers.

Table 9.7: Example of two-phase system or solution system (b).

Ingredient	*Quantity (% w/w)*
Octyl nitrite	0.1%
Ethanol (or ethyl alcohol)	20%
Propellant 114(or dichlorotetrafluoroethane)	49.2%
Propellant 12 (or dichlorodifluoromethane)	30.7%

Propellant 114 is used along with propellan 12 to reduce the vapour pressure of propellant 12.

2. Three-phase system or water-based system

The three-phase system consists of propellant phase, a water phase and vapour phase as the propellants are immiscible with water.

Water is used to replace non-aqueous solvents which are used in the formulation. Ethanol is used as a co-solvent to solubilise the propellant in water. Ethanol also helps in producing small particles as it has surface tension lowering properties.

The products produced by three-phase system are dispensed either in the form of spray or foam. A spray is produced if the system consists of emulsion in which the active ingredients and the solvent are dispersed and propellant exists as an external phase. At the time of dispensing, the propellant vaporizes and hence minute particles of active ingredients are produced.

This system also utilizes surfactants to a large extent. Surfactants help in proper homogenous dispersion. Only those surfactants are used which are less soluble in water and highly soluble in non-polar solvents. They are mostly used in the range of 0.2-0.5%.

For example esters of glycol, glycerol with long chain fatty acids and esters of sorbitol with oleic, stearic, palmitic and lauric acids.

The proportion of propellant can be in the range of 25-60% or it can be 5%. The proportion of propellant depends on the type of product. If the product contains a large amount of water and less amount of propellant, then fine particle size can be obtained by using mechanical breakup actuator along with vapour tap valve.

3. Suspension or dispersion system

To overcome the difficulty faced by the use of co-solvent, various new systems have been developed. The suspension system is one among them which consists of active ingredients dispersed in propellant or mixture of propellants. Surfactants or suspending agents are also utilized to slow the settling of dispersed active ingredients. This system is used for oral inhalation purposes. Examples of suspension or dispersion system are shown in Table 9.8 and Table 9.9.

Table 9.8: Suspension or dispersion system (a)

Ingredient	*Quantity (% w/w)*
Epinephrine bitartrate	0.50%
Sorbitan trioleate	0.50%
Propellant 114 (or dichlorotetrafluoroethane)	49.50%
Propellant 12(or dichlorodifluoromethane)	49.50%

Epinephrine bitartrate has particle sizes in the range of 1-5 μ which are less soluble in propellants. But they are capable of producing a therapeutic effect in the lungs due to their solubility with fluids present in the lungs.

Table 9.9: Suspension or dispersion system (b)

Ingredient	*Quantity*
Isoproterenol sulfate	33.3 mg
Oleyl alcohol	33.3 mg
Myristyl alcohol	33.4 mg
Propellant 114(or dichlorotetrafluoroethane)	7.0 g
Propellant 12(or dichlorodifluoromethane)	7.0 g

Isoproterenol sulfate remains in the propellant vehicle for a long time in order to dispense a proper dose.

The suspension system stability can be enhanced in the following ways:

1. Moisture content in the system is controlled.
2. Active ingredient derivatives are used which have low solubility in the propellant vehicle.
3. Particle size should be less than 5 μ.
4. The density of propellants and suspending agents are adjusted in order to make them equal in the system.
5. By using suitable dispersing agents.

After the formation of a suspension, some particles tend to agglomerate in the system due to factors such as solubility, moisture or particle size growth. When large agglomerates are formed, it leads to caking of suspension. At higher temperatures, there is an increase in the rate of agglomeration which can lead to flocculation (where the particles are loosely bound) or aggregation (where the particles are bound together tightly or fused). These particles stick to the wall of the container. This ultimately leads to valve clogging which leads to improper dosage and the particles damage the metal container.

Agglomeration is avoided by controlling the moisture content of suspending agent and propellant as they affect the stability of the aerosol system. The moisture content should be below 300 ppm. Before the actual manufacturing, the suspending agent and the propellants are dried. This is done by making the propellants pass through various desiccants (which absorb moisture).

In order to reduce agglomeration, surfactants and lubricants are also added.

Lubricants: Isopropyl myristate and mineral oil.

Surfactants: Sorbitan trioleate (HLB value is less than 10), sorbitan monooleate and sorbitan sesquioleate. Usually, they are used in the concentration of 0.01-1% for effective activity.

Even valve clogging can be avoided by the use of vapour tap valves.

4. *Foam system*

This system consists of active ingredients, aqueous or non-aqueous vehicle, surfactant and propellant. These systems are dispensed in the form of quick–breaking foams or stable foams which depends on the type of formulation and ingredients used.

In this system, the liquefied propellants are emulsified and exist as internal phase. This type of system is preferred for those ingredients which cause irritation as well as when the aerosol is to be applied to a limited area.

Various types of foam systems:

(a) Aqueous stable foams
(b) Non-aqueous stable foams
(c) Quick-breaking foams
(d) Thermal foams

Aqueous stable foams: In this type of system, the propellant proportion is usually 3-5% w/w. propellants as A-46, A-70 are used in the formulation. Stiff and dry foam is obtained if the quantity of propellant is increased, and wet foams are obtained by using low concentrations of propellants.

Preparation of emulsion base and example of aqueous stable foams are shown in Table 9.10 and Table 9.11 respectively.

The emulsion base is formulated in the aerosol by the following formula.

Steroids, antibiotics and other materials are formulated and dispensed by using this type of system. This system utilizes both hydrocarbons and fluorocarbons as propellants. But fluorocarbons cannot be formulated in this system unless permission is obtained from FDA.

The techniques used for formulating aerosol emulsions are similar to that of non-aerosol emulsions where surfactants of some solubility in propellants are also utilized.

Table 9.10: Preparation of emulsion base

Emulsion base	*Quantity (% w/w)*
Myristic acid	1.33%
Stearic acid	5.33%
Cetyl alcohol	0.50%
Lanolin	0.20%
Isopropyl myristate	1.33%
Triethanolamine	3.34%
Glycerin	4.70%
Polyvinylpyrrolidone (PVP)	0.34%
Water (purified)	82.93%

Table 9.11: Example of aqueous stable foams

Ingredients	*Quantity (% w/w)*
Active ingredient	2%
Emulsion base	94 – 95%
Hydrocarbon propellant A-46	3 – 4%

Non-aqueous stable foams: Various glycols such as polyethylene glycol are utilized for formulating such system. Example of non-aqueous stable foams is shown in Table 9.12.

Table 9.12: Formulation table of non-aqueous stable foams.

Ingredients	*Quantity (% w/w)*
Glycol	91 – 92.5%
Emulsifying agent	4%
Hydrocarbon propellant	3.5 – 5%

Emulsifying agent used in this system are glycol esters *i.e.*, propylene glycol monostearate. Even medicinal agents are added in the base.

Quick-breaking foams: Propellant exists as an external phase in this system. The product is dispensed in the foam which then turns into liquid form. This type of system is used for topical administration where the active ingredients are applied to a small or large area without using any mechanical force for dispensing. Example of quick-breaking foams is shown in Table 9.13.

Table 9.13: Formulation table of quick-breaking foams.

Ingredients	***Quantity (% w/w)***
Ethyl alcohol	46 – 66%
Surfactant	0.5% – 5%
Water	28 – 42%
Hydrocarbon propellant	3 – 15%

Cationic, anionic or non-ionic type of surfactants can be used in the formulation which should be soluble in both water and alcohol. Stability of foam is improved by varying the proportions of ingredients used in the formulation.

Thermal foams: This system helps in producing warm foams which are used for shaving purpose and also to dispense hair colours and dyes. But its use is inhibited due to lack of effectiveness, problem in usage and high cost. It also leads to corrosion problem. But these warm foams are found to be useful in formulating medicated foams where heat is applied.

5. *Intranasal system*

Different intranasal preparations are intranasal gels, nasal drops, non-pressurized nasal sprays, inhalants, ointments and creams. These preparations help in administering and depositing the drug into the nasal passageways. The production of pressurized metered nasal aerosol gained popularity due to the following reasons.

a) Particle size is small

b) More patient compliance

c) It maintains the sterility of the dose

d) It helps in delivering a measured amount of dose

e) The rate of penetration of the drug is more into the nasal passageway whereas penetration in the lungs is less.

f) Dosage is low compared to systemic preparation.

g) Irritation to the mucous membrane is less.

h) The product can be formulated in several ways.

Examples:

(a) Dexamethasone sodium phosphate is formulated in the form of pressurized aerosol suspension which is used in the treatment of allergic or inflammatory conditions of the nose.

(b) Beclomethasone dipropionate is formulated in the form of pressurized aerosol suspension and used in the treatment of seasonal and perennial rhinitis (nose inflammation).

The general formula for the intranasal system is shown in Table 9.14.

Table 9.14: General formula for intranasal system.

Ingredients	*Quantity (% w/w)*
Active ingredients	Up to 1%
Dispensing agents, additives and solvents	Up to 1%
Propellant 12/11 (60 : 40)	Up to 98%

The active ingredients used in the formulation should be micronized. The adapters of the intranasal aerosol product are short and narrow which helps in reducing vaporization of propellants before coming in contact with the mucosa. This, in turn, helps in achieving a low percentage of smaller particles. It is desirable as it minimizes the number of particles entering respiratory airways. However this system suffers from some drawbacks like additives cause irritation, leakage occurs from the nasal passageways and viscosity of the vehicle may impose problems.

Filling of Aerosol Container

Filling of aerosol formulation into the aerosol container is one of the important steps in the manufacturing the pharmaceutical aerosol. Filling of aerosol formulation into the aerosol container is carried out by different methods such as pressure filling, cold filling and compressed gas filling. These can be achieved by using specialised apparatus:

1. Pressure filling apparatus.
2. Cold filling apparatus.
3. Compressed gas filling apparatus.

Pressure filling apparatus

It consists of a pressure burette which regulates the small amount of liquefied gas into the aerosol container under pressure. An inlet valve is present at the bottom or top of the pressure burette, which incorporates the propellant into the container and flows with its own vapour pressure in the container. Then the trapped air escapes out from the top valve. The propellants which have low pressure stops flowing as the pressures of burette and container become equal. If further additional propellant is to be added, then the upper valve is attached to the nitrogen cylinder through a hose (rubber pipe) which helps in the flow of the propellant into the container. Otherwise, compressed air is provided to the upper valve of the container for further addition of propellant.

Procedure: Pressure filling method involves filling of the concentrate into the container at room temperature. Then the valve is placed on the container and crimped. Through the opening of the valve, the propellants are added or it can be added: "under the cap".

The use of rotary filling machines and new filling heads where the propellants are filled through the valve stem, the production level is increased. The trapped air in the container and air present in headspace is removed before filling the propellant. This is done so as to protect the products from getting adversely affected.

Advantages

1. Solution, emulsions and suspensions can be filled by this method as chilling of these products are not carried out.
2. Moisture contamination is less.
3. The production level can be increased.
4. Loss of propellant is less.
5. A wide variety of materials can be filled by this method, except some type of metering valves which are handled by cold filling method.

Cold filling apparatus

The apparatus used for cold filling purpose is simple compared to pressure filling apparatus. It consists of an insulated box in which the copper tubings are placed. The tubings are coiled to increase the area for cooling. The cooling unit must be filled with dry ice/acetone prior to use to give sufficient cooling effect. This system can be used with metered valves as well as with non metered valves.

Hydrocarbon propellants cannot be filled into aerosol containers using this apparatus because a large amount of propellant escapes out and vaporizes. This may lead to formation of an explosive mixture at the floor level. Fluorocarbons do not form any explosive mixture although their vapours are heavier than air.

Procedure: Non –aqueous products and product which can withstand low temperature are used in this method. The product concentrate is chilled to a temperature of -40°F and filled into already chilled container. Then the chilled propellant is added completely in one stage or two stages. The filling of propellant depends upon the amount of propellant used.

Another method is to chill both the product concentrate and propellant in a separate pressure vessel and then filling it into the container. The valve is placed and crimped on the container. Then test for leakage and strength of container is carried out by passing the container into a heated water bath, where the contents of the container get heated to 130°F after this, they are air-dried, and the caps are placed on the container and labelled.

The cold-filling method is no longer used, as it has been replaced by pressure filling method.

Compressed gas filling apparatus

The filling of compressed gas does not require any large types of equipment. They can be easily handled in the laboratory. To reduce the pressure of the compressed gas (high pressure), a pressure reducing valve is required.

The apparatus consists of a delivery gauge. A flexible hose pipe which can withstand high gauge pressure *i.e.*, 150 pounds per square inch is attached to the delivery gauge along with the filling head. A flow indicator is also present in specialized equipment.

Procedure: The product concentrate is filled into the container and valve is placed and crimped on the container. The air is removed from the container with help of a vacuum pump. Filling head is put in the opening of the valve and the gas is allowed to pass. The gas stops flowing if the pressure of the delivery and the pressure within the container become equal. Carbon dioxide and nitrous oxide are used if the gas is required in more quantity or for the solubility processes. High solubility can be obtained by shaking the container manually or with the help of mechanical shakers.

Evaluation of Aerosols

As described above pharmaceutical aerosols are pressurized dosage forms that upon actuation emit a fine dispersion of liquid and/or solid materials containing one or more active ingredients in a gaseous or liquid medium. In the evaluation of aerosol formulation both quality related to the aerosol packaging and safety, physicochemical properties, performance and biological activity of aerosol content to be taken into the consideration. Hence, evaluation of aerosol can be studied under two headings *viz*: 1) Quality control tests for pharmaceutical aerosols (quality related to the aerosol packaging) 2) Testing of pharmaceutical aerosols (safety, physicochemical properties, performance and biological activity of aerosol content).

Quality Control Tests for Pharmaceutical Aerosols

Following quality control tests are conducted for the evaluation of quality related to the aerosol packaging:

1. Containers
2. Propellants
3. Valves, actuators and dip tubes
4. Weight checking of the containers.
5. Test for leakage
6. Spray test

Containers

(a) Both coated and uncoated containers are properly checked so that there is no defect in the lining.

(b) By determining the degree of conductivity of an electric current, the metals can be identified.

(c) The glass containers are properly checked for flaws.
(d) Dimensions of the neck and other components of the valve should be according to the specifications mentioned.
(e) Weight of the empty bottle is also properly checked.

Propellants

(a) A sheet of detailed specifications is provided to the users before using the propellants.
(b) A sample of propellant is tested in the laboratory where vapour pressure, density is determined and compared to specification mentioned.
(c) With the help of gas chromatography techniques, propellants or propellant blend can be identified by determining their composition simultaneously.
(d) The purity and acceptability of the propellants are tested by determining moisture, halogens and non-volatile residues level.

Actuators, valves and dip tube

Various physical and chemical examinations are carried out on actuators, valves and dip tube. The valves are tested so that they are fit to be used. Three test solutions (Table 9.15, Table 9.16 and Table 9.17) are prepared so that the variations occurring in the valve delivery due to different formulation can be removed. These solutions consist of different range and concentration of propellant which are used in the preparation of aerosols. These solutions are prepared in bulk quantity and stored in tight containers. From these bulk solutions, the test solution is taken into test units in such a way that the proportion of ingredients remains the same.

Procedure

(a) 25 valves are selected which are placed on suitable containers.
(b) These containers contain the required test solution (*i.e.*, test solution 1, 2 or 3) which may be filled through pressure method.
(c) To this container, a button type actuator is attached. The actuator consists of orifices which are 0.020 inch or larger. This actuator remains in place throughout the test.

Table 9.15: Test solution-1

Ingredients	***Weight in % (w/w)***
Isopropyl myristate	0.10%
Dichlorodifluoromethane (Propellant 12)	49.95%
Dichlorotetrafluoroethane (Propellant 114)	49.95%
Specify gravity of the test solution-1 at 25°C is 1.384	

Table 9.16: Test solution-2

Ingredients	***Weight in % (w/w)***
Isopropyl myristate	0.10%
Alcohol (USP)	49.90%
Dichlorodifluoromethane (Propellant 12)	25.0%
Dichlorotetrafluoroethane (Propellant 114)	25.0%
Specify gravity of the test solution 2 at 25°C is 1.092	

Table 9.17: Test solution-3

Ingredients	***Weight in % (w/w)***
Isopropyl myristate	0.10%
Trichloromonofluoromethane (or propellant 11)	24.90%
Dichlorodifluoromethane (Propellant 12)	50.25%
Dichlorotetrafluoroethane (Propellant 114)	24.25%
Specify gravity of the test solution 3 at 25°C is 1.388	

(d) The product in the container is allowed to attain a temperature of 24-26°C by placing the container in such an atmosphere (*i.e.*, temperature of 24–26°C) and weight is checked.

(e) A single delivery is completely dispensed by pushing the valve for at least 2 seconds. The same procedure is repeated ten times.

(f) After dispensing a single delivery, the container is weighed.

(g) The difference between the two weights calculated gives the delivery in milligrams.

(h) In order to get the delivery in micro-litres, the delivery weight in milligrams is divided by specific gravity of the test solution.

(i) The test procedure is carried out on two individual deliveries from each valve of the 25 test solution prepared.

(j) Acceptance value for valve is given in Table 9.18.

Table 9.18: Acceptance value for valves

Delivery in μl	*Limits*
54 μl or less	± 15%
54 μl -200 μl	± 10%

The acceptance limit value is considered for 50 individual deliveries.

(i) Of the 50 individual deliveries, if four or more are outside the limits for the specified valve delivery, the valves are rejected.

(ii) If three individual deliveries are outside the limits, another 25 valves are sampled, and the test is repeated. The lot is rejected if more than one delivery is outside the specifications.

(iii) If two deliveries from one valve are beyond the limits, another 25 valves should be taken. The lot is accepted if not more than one delivery is outside the specifications.

Weight checking of the container

Periodic checking of the weight is done while filling procedure is carried out. The product concentrate is filled into the container, removed from the filling line and then weighed. The same procedure is carried out after filling the propellant into the container. Finally, after the filling operation is completed, the finished container is again weighed to ensure the filling accuracy.

Test for leakage

Methods are followed to check the crimping of the valve in order to check leakage if present in the container.

The dimension of the crimp is measured in a metal container to check whether they meet the specifications mentioned. The valve closures are tested for its proper efficiency. This is done by passing the filled containers through the water bath and periodically checking the water bath temperature and recording the results.

Department of Transport Test (DOT) is performed for aerosols and small receptacles containing compressed gas to check leak proofness. This is performed by immersing aerosol container in a hot water bath and inspecting it for leakage.

Spray test

Spray testing is carried out because.

(a) It helps in clearing the dip tube of the container which contains pure propellants. These propellants are filled into containers by pressure through the stem, body and a dip tube.
(b) It helps in clearing the dip tube of the container which contains pure concentrate. These products are filled by pressure into the container by under the cap method.
(c) It helps in proper checking for any defects present in the valve and pattern of the spray.

Testing of Pharmaceutical Aerosols

Several tests are performed to check the proper functioning of aerosols and safety measures during its use and storage. They are given in Table 9.19.

Flammability and combustion test

Flashpoint test: The apparatus used for determining flash point is standard tag open cup. In this test, the product to be filled in an aerosol

Table 9.19: Tests to check the proper functioning of aerosols and safety measures

I. Flammability and combustion test
- Flashpoint test
- Flame projection test

II. Physico-chemical properties test
- Vapour pressure
- Density
- Moisture content
- Propellant identification

III. Performance test
- Valve discharge test
- Pattern of spray
- Metered valves
- Reproducibility of dosage
- Net contents
- Stability of foam
- Determination of particle size

IV. Biological test
- Therapeutic activity test
- Toxicity test

container is chilled to a temperature of about -25°F. The chilled product is then transferred to the apparatus (*i.e.*, standard tag open cup) after transferring, the chilled product temperature is slowly increased and flash point is determined at the temperature when the vapour starts burning (ignites).

This method is still used although the results obtained are of limited value. This is because flash point obtained by this method is from flammable components only. Example: Hydrocarbon propellants present in topical aerosols.

Flame projection test: This test is carried out to know the effect of formulation of aerosol on an open flame. This is done by spraying the product on the flame for at least 4 seconds. The length of the extended flame is measured with the help of a ruler.

Test for physico-chemical properties

Vapour pressure: By using the pressure gauge, water bath or test gauges, vapour pressure of the aerosol can be measured. The air present in the headspace of the container shows variation in the pressure from container to container. Accurate vapour pressure can be determined with the help of a can puncturing device.

Density: Hydrometer or a pycnometer helps in measuring the accurate density of the aerosols. Modifications are done on these methods in order to incorporate liquefied gas, as these methods were used to determine density of non-aerosol products. A glass pressure tube is used. The metal flanges and hoke valve are attached to the pressure tube which helps in the introduction of liquid under pressure. The hydrometer is kept on the pressure tube and sufficient sample is added through the valve which rises the hydrometer half the length of the tube. In this way, the density can be read directly on the hydrometer. High-pressure cylinders of capacity 500 ml help in determining the specific gravity of the aerosols.

Moisture content: By the use of Karl Fischer and gas chromatography techniques, moisture content of the aerosols can be determined.

Propellants identification: By using the methods such as gas chromatography and infrared spectrophotometer, the propellants are identified and even the composition of each propellant in a blend can be determined.

Performance test

Valve discharge test: A standard aerosol container of known weight is taken and the product is dispensed for certain period of time. After dispensing, the container is weighed. The discharge rate can also be expressed in grams per second.

Spray pattern: The method used for determining spray pattern utilizes a paper which is treated with the mixture of dye and talc. The dye can be oil soluble or water-soluble depending on the type of aerosol formulation to be tested. The product is sprayed on the paper and particle which strikes causes the dye to go into the solution. The dye gets absorbed on the paper and determines the spray pattern.

Metered valves: The metered valves are tested for determining the reproducibility of dosage when the valve is pressed each time and dose received by the patients.

Reproducibility of dosage: This can be determined with the use of assay technique where one or two doses are dissolved in a solvent. The solutions are then assayed which determines the amount of ingredients present.

Another method can also be used for determining the reproducibility of dosage. The filled containers are accurately weighed. Then several doses are dispensed and the containers are again weighed. The average dose is obtained which is the ratio of difference in weight and number of doses dispensed. This procedure is again repeated and the results obtained are compared. Dose determination is difficult as the whole dose not reach the respiratory tract. Hence, an artificial respiratory system is developed for determination of dose received by the patients.

Net contents: One of the methods involves weighing the tared (empty) container which are placed on filling line and comparing its weight with the filled containers. The difference in the weight gives the net content or the product placed in the aerosol container.

Other methods are also used like weighing the filled container and then dispensing contents from the container which are also weighed. Another method is opening the container and removing the product. These tests are not considered as they are unable to present accurate results.

Stability of foam: Depending on the type of aerosol formulation, the stability of foam varies *i.e.*, from a few seconds to one hour or more. The stability of the foam can be determined by:

(i) Visual evaluation

(ii) Determining the time taken for a certain mass to penetrate into the foam

(iii) Determining the time taken for a rod to penetrate into the foam

(iv) Rotational viscometer.

Determination of particle size: Cascade impactor and light scatter decay methods are used for determining the particle size.

(i) Cascade impactor: The principle involved in this method is that the particles are projected through nozzles. These particles slide at very high velocity. The larger particles are collected from the stage where velocity is low and smaller particles are collected from stage where velocity is high. This apparatus is useful for analyzing particle which has a diameter in the range of 0.1-30 μ and retains in the respiratory tract. Modifications are done in the apparatus to improve its efficiency for determining particle size.

(ii) *Light scatter decay*: This method is used for determining the particle size in epinephrine aerosols. When the aerosol settles due to sudden changes, there is a change is the intensity of the light of the Tyndal beam. This change is measured in order to determine the particle size. The median diameter of the mass of particle size of epinephrine ranges from 2.7-3.5 μ.

1. About 70-78% particles have a diameter less than 5 μ.
2. 88-93% particles have a diameter less than 7 μ.
3. 98-100% particles have a diameter less than 10 μ.

Biological test

This test is performed to evaluate the efficiency of the aerosol products. Biological test performed on aerosol are similar to tests performed on non-aerosol products. Biological test is carried out to know the therapeutic activity and toxicity of the aerosol.

(a) Therapeutic activity test: The therapeutic activity is determined by a various test which is as follows :

(i) By determining the dosage of the product inhalation aerosols.

(ii) The particle size distribution is also determined.

(iii) The topical aerosols are applied on test areas and determination of absorption of active ingredients is carried out.

(b) Toxicity test: This test is carried out to know the effects of topical and inhalation aerosols. The application of topical aerosols on the affected area may cause irritation or may give a chilling effect which depends on the type and proportion of propellant used in the formulation. The test includes recording the change in temperature of the skin after the aerosol is sprayed on the skin for a certain period. The temperature is recorded by using recorded thermometers which are attached by thermistor probes.

The inhalation toxicity of topical aerosols is determined by exposing animals (test) to the vapours of the aerosol formulation.

Stability Testing of Aerosols

Stability is considered important in the formulation of aerosols. Factors such as effect of the product on the container and valve, effect of the container and valve on the product are considered. As the valve consists of different components and made up of different materials such as rubber (natural or synthetic) plastic and stainless steel, hence any slightest change in these components (*i.e.,* arrangement in the valve assembly) can lead to the production of a defective package. Stability testing is considered important as material and the drug may react with each other. These reactions are difficult to determine (since many components come in immediate contact with the drug). Hence, all these materials are studied separately as well as collectively. Even the coatings applied and valve of the container may react with the product, therefore different subcomponents of the valves and coating applied are also studied.

Stability testing is carried out on the following:

1. Product concentrate and propellants
2. Container of the aerosol
3. Valve of the aerosol

Product concentrate and propellants: Various physicochemical properties such as colour, density, odour, pH, refractive index, total weight, viscosity, spray rate, assay of active ingredients and infrared or gas chromatography curves are determined. These values or observations are used for comparison purposes when the product is evaluated each time. Usually, the product concentrate and propellant samples are placed in the sides so that they come in contact with the valve and container. In case if three-piece metal cans are used, then care must be taken as the samples having liquid as well as gas in it may come in contact with the side seams (joining).

Container of the aerosol: The contents of the container are chilled to 0°F or less. This is done for removing the contents and the container can be easily opened. Then the examination of corrosion present on the container is carried out. The changes present on aluminium, tin plate or steel (tin-free) can be easily observed with the naked eye or with the help of a microscope. Even detection of small pin holes is easy. The lacquer may get soft, dissolved, peeled or blistered by the effect of concentrate; hence examination is carried out for the presence of any internal lacquering on the container. Side-seam (joining) and the headspace of the container are carefully examined as these areas get easily affected. For glass containers examination is not carried out, but for a plastic container, testing is carried out as it may undergo leaching or sorption.

Valve of the aerosol: Valves are checked for its proper functioning. They should properly dispense the product and should be easily closed. The function of valve can be easily determined during dispensing. The value cup along with subcomponents of the valve are properly examined to check any softening, cracking, elongation or distortion present in the valve. These effects lead to defective valves which cannot function properly. The dip tube should be properly examined for any elongation or cracking and if these effects are present then it should be corrected.

Applications of Aerosols

Pharmaceutical applications of aerosols are as follows:

1. Aerosols can be used for both local and systemic effects.
   a. Aerosols exhibit local action in nose, throat, lungs, eye, ear, vagina, rectum etc.

b. Aerosols exhibit systemic effect when it passes from the lungs and gets absorbed into the bloodstream.

2. The drug administered through aerosols gives a quick response and rapid action.
3. Close control of the dose of drug can be possible by MDI's.
4. Administration of both liquid and solid form of the drug can be achieved.
5. Stability and sterility of the product are maintained during storage even after opening the valve since it is a closed system.
6. The drug is well protected from light and air in an aerosol formulation.
7. Aerosols are used to formulate several agents include local analgesics, antiseptics, fungicides, antibiotics and anti-inflammatory agents.
8. Aerosols are available in non-pharmaceutical preparations like deodorants, perfumes, cosmetics, hair sprays, toothpaste and shaving creams.
9. They are also available as household products such as spray starch, waxes, polishes, cleaners and lubricants.

Glossary

Aerosols	Pressurized dosage forms
Propellants	It is responsible for the development of pressure within the container, supplying the necessary force to expel the product when the valve is opened
Compressed-gases	Propellants like nitrogen, oxygen and carbon dioxide are used as compressed gases
Aerosol-container	Containers must withstand the pressure as high as 140 to 180 psig (pounds per sq. inch gauge) and temperature of about 54.44°C.
Valves	The function of the valve assembly is to permit expulsion of the contents of the can in the desired form, at the desired rate.
Metered dose inhalers (MDI)	Metering values are used when the formulation is potent medicament and measured amount of product need to be expelled from the container
Ferrule	It helps in attaching the valve properly to the container
Spring	It holds the gasket and brings back the valve in its closed position after the actuator is pushed or depressed
Actuators	Actuators are specially designed buttons placed on the valve stem. This helps in easy opening and closing of the valve

Product-concentrate	Product concentrate consists of active ingredients or a mixture of active ingredients along with surfactants, antioxidant, solvents etc.
Gasket	It helps in sealing the stem orifice when the valve is closed

QUESTION BANK

Q. I: Multiple Choice Questions

1 Identify the correct Non-flammable propellant

a) Trichloromonofluoromethane c) Dimethyl ether

b) Dichlorodifluromethane d) Difluoromethane

2 The dip tube in the aerosol container is made from one of the following

a) Polypropylene c) Aluminium

b) Glass d) Stainless steel

3 Which one of the following device is used to increase the efficacy of drug delivery *via* aerosols?

a) Tube spacers c) Actuator

b) Metered valve d) Pressure valve

4 Among the propellants used in aerosols, one of the following is used for topical pharmaceutical aerosols

a) Trichloromonofluoromethane c) Dichlorotetrafluoroethane

b) Dichlorodifluoromethane d) Propnane

5 The identification of propellants in pharmaceutical aerosols is carried out by

P) Gas chromatography R) Pycnometer

Q) Tag-open cup apparatus S) IR Spectrophotometer

a) P, Q c) Q, R

b) P, S d) R, S

6 Measurement of particle size in pharmaceutical aerosols is by

P) Cascade impactor R) Karl Fischer method

Q) Light scatter decay S) IR spectrophotometry

a) P, Q b) Q, R

c) R, S d) P, S

7 ______ is not component of the aerosol system

a) Propellant c) Actuator

b) Dip tube d) Paddle

8 The metered dose aerosol does not contain

a) Dip tube c) Activator stem

b) Metering chamber
d) None of the above

9 Filling of aerosols with liquefied propellants is done by

a) Cold fill process
b) Pressure fill process
c) Both (a) and (b)
d) None of the above

10 Aerosols may be tested for ______

a) Spray pattern
b) Weight variation
c) Reproducibility of the dosage form
d) All of the above

11 Which of the following material is used in the manufacture of aerosol container?

a) Glass
b) Plastic
c) Metal
d) All of the above

12 ______ aerosol contain the highest amount of water

a) One phase system
b) Two-phase system
c) Three phase system
d) None of the above

13 _______is attached to the aerosol container, hold the valve in place

a) Spring
b) Dip tube
c) Mounting cup
d) Actuator

Q. II: Very Short Answer Questions **2 Marks**

1. Write different components of an aerosol valve.
2. Metal as material for the aerosol container
3. Define aerosols. Name the type of aerosol systems.
4. Give the pharmaceutical applications of aerosols.
5. Add a note on particle size analysis of aerosols.
6. Functioning of cup valve in aerosols.
7. Briefly explain metered valve aerosols

Q. III: Short Answer Questions **5 Marks**

1. What are propellants? Classify with suitable examples.
2. Explain the various methods of filling of pharmaceutical aerosols
3. Explain the formulation of aerosol products giving the characteristics of each type of formulation.
4. How stability studies are conducted on aerosols products.
5. Write a note on working principle of aerosol system.
6. Discuss on containers for aerosols.
7. What are the advantages and applications of aerosols?

Q. IV: Long Answer Questions **10 Marks**

1. Give a detailed account of testing of pharmaceutical aerosols
2. Explain the general formulation, manufacturing and quality control tests for aerosol products
3. Explain in detail evaluation of aerosol products.

Chapter 10

Packaging Material Science

INTRODUCTION

Packaging is the means of economically providing containment, protection, presentation, identification, information, convenience and aids patient compliance, or a product during storage, distribution, display and use. In some cases, the pack is essential for the administration of medicine.

Pharmaceutical packaging enables the packaged medicine's requirements of efficacy, safety, uniformity, reproducibility, integrity, purity and stability to be maintained throughout the product's shelf - life. Furthermore, some pharmaceutical packaging is essential for the product's use and the drug's administration, *i.e.,* the pack is the delivery device. Examples of this are pressurized metered dose inhalers, nasal sprays, transdermal patches and pre-filled syringes.

The role of packaging seems to be constantly expanding, for example, anti-counterfeiting, branding and providing distinguishing features to the drug product to avoid errors as well as in the monitoring patient adherence.

Function of Package

1. ***Protection:*** A good package protects the container from static and dynamic force during transportation and storage. Vibration is mainly responsible for cracking of emulsion which can be inhibited by using good package. It also protects the contents from biological hazards, moisture, temperature, environmental gases, humidity etc. light-sensitive material can be protected from light by using amber coloured bottles.

2. ***Identification:*** Packaging provides information regarding product such as date of manufacturing, expiry date, use, batch no., warnings if any etc. It also provides an easy to identify the product for *e.g.,* coloured fluted bottles is used for packaging external preparation.

3. ***Storage and transport:*** Packaging plays an important role in the storage and transportation of product. Package shape should be such that it can be handled easily. It must be so designed that they can be stored in an efficient manner *i.e.*, safely one above the other.

4. ***Other functions*****:** Other functions of package include protection from theft, compression, impact, patient compliance, effective tool for marketing etc.

The Pharmaceutical Pack

A pharmaceutical pack protects and delivers safe, efficacious drug product. At the same time, it provides identification and information, enabling patient compliance and convenience. To assure these the pharmaceutical product can be packed by the primary package, proper closures, secondary package and tertiary package.

1. *Primary package*

The primary pack is in direct contact with the product during storage and delivery. The main aim of the primary package is to protect the formulation from environmental, chemical, mechanical and/or other hazards.

The wide range of pharmaceutical products, such as solid powders, granules, tablets, capsules, semisolids (*e.g.,* creams, ointments, gels), liquids (such as solutions, suspensions, emulsions). Some of which are sterile, obviously require a great diversity, both in primary pack design and in packaging materials. The latter include paper, glass, plastics, rubber, metal or combination materials such as laminates. Examples of primary packs include blister packs, strip packs, sachets, bottles, ampoules, vials, bags, tubes and syringes.

The primary pack may contain many doses (*i.e.,* be a multiple-unit pack, *e.g.,* a bottle containing many tablets) or a single dose (*i.e.,* be a single-unit pack, *e.g.,* blister pack, sachet).

The primary pack must be compatible with the product and take nothing out of the product and add nothing in. Drug absorption or adsorption into the pack would reduce product potency, while chemicals leaching out of the pack and into the product could induce drug degradation. In addition, the primary pack must protect the product against atmospheric factors, such as extremes of temperature, light, moisture, oxygen, carbon dioxide, particulates (*e.g.,* dust, dirt), as well as biological hazards, such as microorganisms, insects and rodents and enable product stability.

The primary pack is considered as ideal if it offers:

i) Child-resistance to restrict children's access to the product
ii) Tamper-resistant and tamper-evident to improve the product's security from pilferage and deliberate contamination and safeguard the product's legitimate user
iii) Compatibility with the product and take nothing out of the product and add nothing in
iv) Sufficient mechanical strength so as to withstand handling, filling, closing and transportation
v) It should be of such shape that can be elegant and also the contents can be easily drawn from it.
vi) In case of terminal sterilization-the container must bear heat when it is subjected for sterilization
vii) The desired degree of protection from environmental hazards
viii) The closure should be of non-toxic nature and chemically stable with container contents.

Types of containers used as primary packages

Airtight container: A container that is impermeable to solids, liquids and gases under ordinary conditions of handling, storage and transport. If the container is intended to be opened on more than once, it must be so designed that it remains airtight after re-closure.

Hermetically sealed container: A container that is impervious to air or any other gas under normal conditions of handling, shipment, storage and distribution, *e.g.,* sealed glass ampoule, gas cylinder etc.

Light-resistant container: A container that protects the contents from the effects of light by virtue of the specific properties of the material of which it is made. Alternatively, a clear and colourless or a translucent container may be made light-resistant by means of an opaque (light-resistant) covering and/or stored in a dark place; in such cases, the label on the container should bear a statement that the opaque covering or storage in dark place is needed until the contents have been used up.

Multidose container: A container that holds a quantity of the preparation suitable for two or more doses.

Tamper-evident container: A container fitted with a device or mechanism that reveals irreversibly whether the container has been opened.

Tightly-closed container: Tightly-closed container protects the contents from contamination by extraneous liquids, solids or vapours, from loss or deterioration of the article from effervescence, deliquescence or evaporation under normal conditions of handling, shipment, storage and distribution. A tightly-closed container must be capable of being tightly re-closed after use. Where a tightly-closed container is specified, a hermetically sealed container may be used for a single dose of an article. A gas cylinder may be considered to be a metallic, tightly-closed container designed to hold gas under pressure.

Well-closed container: A well-closed container protects the contents from extraneous solids and liquids and from loss of the article under normal conditions of handling, shipment, storage and distribution.

One container may serve as one or more container property, for example, the ambered coloured bottle used for packing the liquid dosage form may act as an airtight, light-resistant, multidose, tamper-evident, tightly-closed and well-closed container. Different types of containers are shown in Fig. 10.1.

Primary package for solid dosage forms

Strip package: In this, the contents are sealed in a packet. The package is made up of two layers of film. A strip containing many pockets and each pocket contains a single dose of medicament.

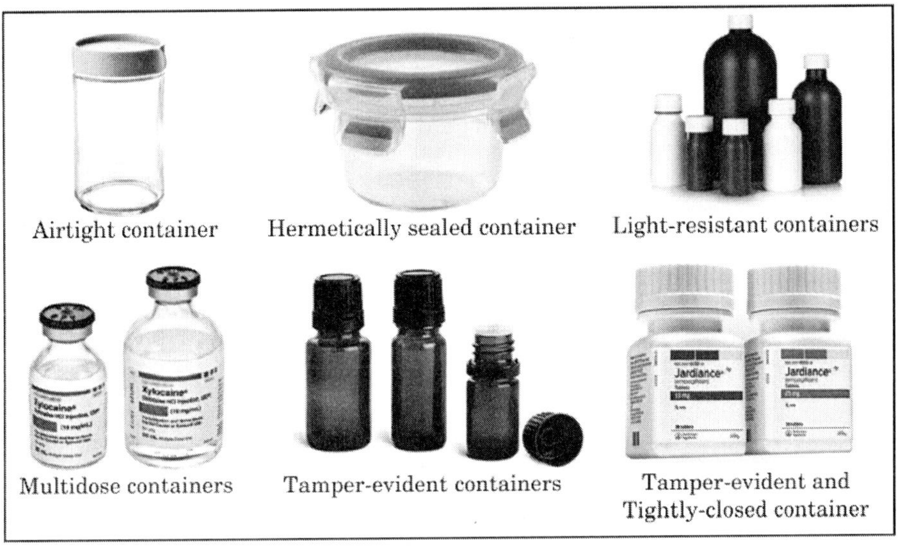

Fig. 10.1: Different types of containers

Blister package: It is made up of the base layer (PVC layer) with cavities which contain the pharmaceutical product. This type of package provides greater protection than a strip package. The lid is made up of aluminium or paper foil. The package is sealed by combining lid and base with the application of heat and pressure. Strip and blister packages are shown in Fig. 10.2.

Primary package for semi-solid dosage forms

Semi-solid dosage forms include creams, pastes, ointments etc. the containers used for semi-solid dosage forms include collapsible tubes.

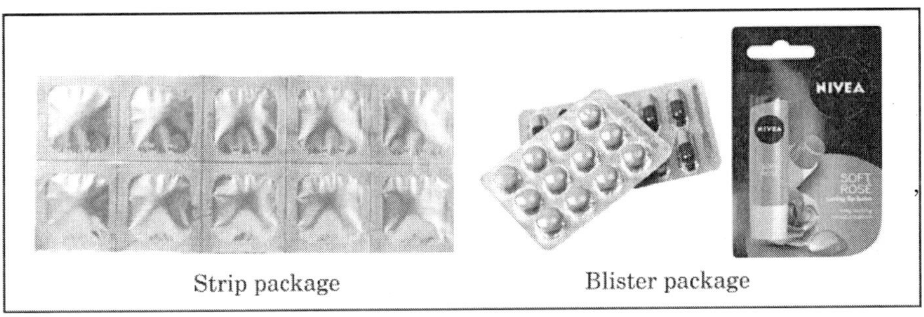

Fig. 10.2: Strip and Blister package

Plastic containers are also very popular nowadays. Another type of products is also available in the market for *e.g.,* Pressurized products for these types of products the package made up of stainless steel, aluminium etc. is used. The package used must be strong enough to withstand pressure built up in the container.

2. *Closures*

Closure is a device – *e.g.,* stopper, lid, top or cap – which is used to close a container and is an integral part of the pack. The word 'pack' therefore covers both the container and the closure. Without the latter, the functions of a pack, such as containment, presentation, protection and convenience, cannot be fulfilled and like the container, the closure must be inert, compatible with the contents, and protect the latter against environmental hazards, such as oxygen, light, moisture, etc.

An effective closure system prevents the loss of material from the container, prevents the environmental contamination of the product and prevents the microbes to enter inside the container.

Certain closures must maintain sterility, *e.g.,* in multi-use parenteral vials. A good seal between the container and the closure prevents anything from leaking out or gaining access into the pack and is obtained by a snug fit between the inner face of the closure and the external face of the container finish. Resilient liners inside the closure are sometimes used to achieve a snug fit, although many plastic closures are internally moulded to achieve a good seal and are liner- free.

The closure has to be user- friendly, allow easy opening to legitimate consumers and be easy to reclose (for multi-unit packs), as well as child-resistant, tamper resistant and tamper-evident. Closures may also include dispensing devices, *e.g.,* a pump on bottles containing creams. The outer surface of the closure may also be ribbed to allow good grip when opening by twisting. Pharmaceutical closures are mostly made of plastic (thermosets and thermoplastics), although metal is also used, *e.g.,* on parenteral vials.

Closures are available in different designs

Threaded screw type: These are made up of aluminium, tin or plastic. As the name indicates they contain threads which get engaged with the threads present on the neck of container. These types of closures provide the effective seal which protects the product from physical and chemical reaction. Plastic caps are more popular than metal because plastic is resistant to corrosion.

Lug cap: The difference in lug cap and thread cap is that in thread cap, continuous threads are present but in lug cap threads are present in intermittent fashion. Another difference is that lug cap requires only a quarter turn. Lug caps are mainly used in storage of food products.

Crown caps: These caps are made up of metal and commonly used for beverages bottles. These also provide an effective seal and cannot be open with hands. These cannot be seal again.

Roll on closures: Roll on closure contains the aluminium roll-on cap which can be easily sealed, opened and closed. These are available in resealable, non- sealable and pilfer proof type forms. These are available for use on glass or plastic bottles and jars for food, beverages, chemicals and Pharmaceuticals.

Pilfer-proof: In this additional length extends below to threaded portion which forms a bridge. When the closure is removed then the bridge break and the additional portion remains in place on the neck of container which shows its opening.

Tamper–evident closures: Tamper evident closures are designed to prevent accident and intentional tampering to create safe packaging. The main concept of the tamper-evident packaging is increasingly being recognized in pharmacopoeias. Various types of tamper-evident packaging are used in pharmaceutical industries are bottles with inner mouth seals, tape seals, breakable cap ring system etc.

Child resistant closures: Child-resistant packaging is special packaging used to reduce the risk of children ingesting dangerous items. This is often accomplished by the use of a special safety cap. It is required by regulation for prescription drugs, over-the-counter medications. In some jurisdictions, unit packaging such as blister packs is also regulated for child safety.

The same closure serves different purpose threaded screw type of closure may act as pilfer-proof, tamper–evident and childresistant closure.

Different types of closures are shown in Fig. 10.3.

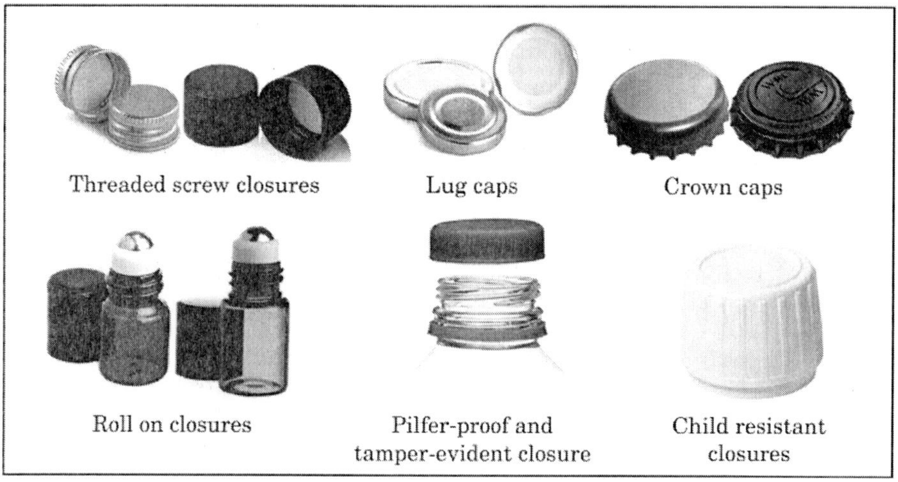

Fig. 10.3: Different types of closures used in pharmaceutical packaging

3. *Secondary package*

The secondary pack (*e.g.,* a carton box or a glass bottle) contains the primary pack, as well as ancillary components, such as dispensing spoons and information leaflets.

A secondary packaging component generally serves one or more of the following additional functions:

- Provides protection from excessive transmission of moisture or solvents into or out of the packaging system.
- Provides protection from excessive transmission of reactive gases (atmospheric oxygen, inert headspace filler gas, or other organic vapours) into or out of the packaging system.
- Provides light protection for the packaging system.
- Provides protection for a packaging system that is flexible or needs extra protection from rough handling.
- Provides an additional measure of microbiological protection (*i.e.*, by maintaining sterility or by protecting the packaging system from microbial intrusion).

4. *Tertiary package*

It is used for warehouse storage and transport shipping. The most common form is a palletized unit load that packs tightly into the container. For example shippers, pellets etc.

Packaging Materials

Once the function(s) of the desired packaging has been defined, selection of the packaging material is the first step in the packaging process. The commonly used materials for packaging pharmaceutical products include glass, plastic, metals, rubber, paper etc.

Glass

Glass containers are very commonly used for storing pharmaceutical products. These containers are intended to come into direct contact with pharmaceutical products.

Advantages

i) Impermeable to water vapours, air etc.
ii) Available in various sizes and shapes.
iii) Have efficient mechanical strength and rigidity.
iv) Transparent so the contents can be easily seen from outside for *e.g.,* in case of parental products.
v) Can be converted into light-resistant glass by mixing with metal oxides.
vi) Have an elegant appearance than the plastic containers.
vii) Able to withstand temperature and pressure during sterilization.
viii) Can be easily labelled.
ix) Can be easily sealed which can provide hermetic sealing.

Disadvantages

i) Have heavyweight which increases their transportation cost.
ii) Breakable.
iii) Can easily leach alkali to aqueous solutions if not properly treated with chemicals.

Composition and manufacturing process of glass containers

Glass is produced by heating together various inorganic substances to form a molten mass and then rapidly cooling the latter which solidifies in a non-crystalline state. Sand (or more properly silicon dioxide; silica) which is the main constituent of sand), limestone (calcium carbonate) and soda ash (sodium carbonate) are heated to very high temperatures (*e.g.,* 1500°C) in a furnace. The ingredients melt and gradually react and form a homogeneous molten mass.

In addition to silica, soda ash and limestone, other compounds are added in trace amounts to achieve certain properties in the glass formed. For example:

- Alumina (Al_2O_3) increases the hardness, durability and clarity of the glass
- Selenium or cobalt oxides improve clarity
- Lead oxide gives clarity and sparkle (but makes glass soft)
- Boron compounds give low thermal expansion and high heat-shock resistance
- Arsenic trioxide and sodium sulphate are added to reduce blisters in the glass.

Opacity and different colours are achieved by the inclusion of a range of compounds, as shown in Table 10.2.

Table 10.2: Additives that are generally used to achieve different colours of glass.

Colour	*Possible additives*
Amber	Iron oxides, manganese oxides, carbon oxides, sulphur compounds
Browns	Iron oxides, carbon oxides, sulphur compounds
Greens	Iron oxides
Yellow	Greens uranium oxides
Yellow	Lead with antimony
Deep blue	Cobalt oxide
Light blue	Copper compounds
Reds	Gold chloride, selenium compounds, copper compounds
Amethyst	Manganese oxides
Black	Mixture of manganese, cobalt and iron
White	Tin compounds, antimony oxides

The latter is then converted into glass containers by one of two basic methods: blow moulding or tubular glass fabrication. Blow moulding, the older method is when a 'gob' (a small piece of highly viscous molten glass) of glass is moulded into a container. The second method is used to manufacture ampoules and vials. Once a homogeneous molten glass mass is formed at high temperature, the molten mass is converted into glass tubing as it moves out of the furnace. The tubing is cut to prescribed lengths and the individual glass tubes are then converted into ampoules or vials.

Types of glasses

Four types of glass –as types I, II, III and NP glass – are used to package pharmaceuticals.

Type I: Borosilicate glass: This is the best pharmaceutical grade and is produced by adding boron oxide to glass, hence this glass is also called borosilicate glass. It is the most inert glass, shows the least amount of leaching of glass components and is used in ampoules and vials or liquid parenteral products. Due to its lowest coefficient of thermal expansion, this glass is highly resistant to temperature changes, *e.g.,* during severe sterilization procedures. Type I glass is used to package slightly acidic solutions (standard glass can increase the alkalinity of its contents). This glass is also the most expensive to produce.

Type II: De-alkalized soda lime glass: This is the next (lower) grade and is made from the same materials as standard glass (soda lime glass) but its surface is treated with sulphur dioxide. The latter reacts with the oxides found on the glass surface, for example, sodium oxide is converted to sodium sulphate, which can then be removed by washing the glass. Such surface treatment, thus, reduces the amount of ions that can leach out of the glass. Hence, type II glass is also referred to as treated soda lime glass or dealkalized soda lime glass. Type II glass is suitable for solutions that can be buffered to remain below pH 7. At higher pH, the oxides in the glass (which are free to move) are more easily leached out.

Type III: Regular soda lime glass: This type of glass contains metal oxides, sodium oxides, aluminium, earth oxides mainly calcium oxides. This is the next (lower) grade and is standard soda lime glass and is analogous with glass used in food packaging. It is used to package large volumes (normally >100 ml). The large volume to surface area of product in contact with the glass surface limits the amount of glass components that can leach into the product. The main disadvantage is that it can leach alkali in the preparation. So it is used to store liquid formulations which are not alkali sensitive. It is also used to store all types of solid dosage forms.

NP (non-parentral) glass: This is the lowest grade and is called non-parenteral glass, and, as the name suggests, is not used or packaging parenteral products, as small volumes of the latter would be easily contaminated by sodium and other materials leaching out of the glass. This type of glass is not used for autoclaved products because autoclaving will accelerate the glass erosion reaction. NP glass is, however, suitable for packaging large volumes (normally >100 ml) of topical products like creams and of oral products, such as mouthwashes.

Plastics

Plastics are very commonly used for packaging pharmaceutical products. These constitute about 20% of the weight of all pharmaceutical packaging. Plastics can be easily moulded to required shape. Hence, plastics are widely used as containers (*e.g.*, bottles, trays), closures (*e.g.*, screw-tops), cling films, carrier bags, sacks, overwraps, etc. Plastics are also widely used to package medicines in a variety of containers, such as:

- Bottles for solid and liquid products
- Tubes for creams, ointments and gels
- Pouches to contain individual suppositories
- Blister packs
- Bags to contain intravenous solutions and parenteral nutritional products
- Bottle closures.

Advantages

i) Plastics are unbreakable.

ii) Plastics have less weight than glass and so their transport cost is also very less.

iii) Plastics are available in various size and shapes.

iv) Can be easily moulded into the desired shape.

v) Provide good protection power against chemical hazards.

vi) Plastics do not have alkali leaching property as in glass containers.

vii) Have suck back feature.

Disadvantages

i) The main disadvantage is permeation. The atmospheric gases, vapours or liquid from surrounding environment can easily migrate into a plastic container.

ii) Permeation causes problem of oxidation and/or hydrolysis and can degrade the product which is sensitive to hydrolysis and/or oxidation.

iii) They also have leaching problem, for *e.g.,* dyes which are used as colouring agent may migrate into product from the container.

iv) Another problem is sorption; sorption is the process of removal of one or more constituents from the product by packaging material. This can affect the therapeutic efficacy of the product.

v) The preservative can also be absorbed by the container material. This may change the flexibility of the container.

Materials used for making plastic containers

Polyethylene: Polyethylene is a very commonly used polymer. It is available in high density, medium density and low-density grades. Mainly high-density polyethylene is used for pharmaceuticals. Polyethylene containers are transparent and flexible. It provides protection against moisture but poor protection against oxygen and other environmental gases. The containers prepared from polyethylene cannot be sterilized by heat but can be easily sterilized by autoclave. Polyethylenes have a melting point range of 120-150°C. It has an excellent chemical resistance, it means it provides protection against strong acid and alkali. It is used to prepare plastic bag, plastic films, bottles etc.

Polypropylene: It is very popularly used in Pharmaceutical container. It has many qualities of polyethylene. It has a melting point of 170°C which is higher than polyethylene and makes it suitable for sterilization at a high temperature. It has very good resistance power to almost all types of chemicals. It is superior to low-density polyethylene. The main drawback of polypropylene is its less clarity which can be improved by making thin walls containers. Another drawback is its brittleness at low temperature and this can also be improved by mixing it with some proportion of polyethylene.

Polyvinylchloride (PVC): It has high clarity and good oxygen barrier. It is the third most widely produced polymer after polyethylene and polypropylene. It can be made softer and flexible by incorporation of plasticizers. The heat stability of PVC is very poor and its melting point is 160°C. It has good insulation properties but inferior to polyethylene and polypropylene. PVC can be used for making containers used for blood and blood components, catheters, bypass sets, hemodialysis sets etc. The main advantages of PVC include its transparency, light weight, softness, suitability for sterilization and biocompatibility.

Polyamide (Nylon): It is macromolecules having repeated units linked by amide bonds. Nylon is mainly artificially made. It can be produced by the interaction of a diamine and a dicarboxylic acid. It has the main advantage of good chemical resistance, high strength, good toughness, high heat resistance, good water resistance etc. it can be autoclaved easily. The main disadvantage is high moisture absorbtivity, attacked by an oxidizing agent, strong acids and alkalis etc.

Polystyrene: It is made from petroleum. It is non-biodegradable, light and rigid. Its main advantages are inexpensive, resistant to acids, strong alkalis and strong oxidizing agents, high heat resistance, expandable etc. The main disadvantage is that it can leach styrene and benzene when come in contact with warm food, oils, alcohols etc. which causes contamination of the product.

Polycarbonate: Polycarbonate is resistant to dilute acids, oxidizing or reducing agents, salts, oils (fixed and volatile), greases, and aliphatic hydrocarbons. It is attacked by strong acids, reducing agents, amines, ketones, aromatic hydrocarbons, and some alcohols. It has the highest impact strength and inexpensive. It is clear and very good heat resistance power. It is mainly used for manufacturing of surgical equipment.

Metals

Metals are very commonly used as packaging material in the form of cans (*e.g.,* pressurized metered dose inhaler (pMDI) containers), tubes (or creams, ointments, gels), pouches (or powders, granules, liquids, suppositories), blister packs and closures.

Advantages

i) Metals are mechanically strong and can withstand the high internal pressure containers for example in pMDI.
ii) Metals are impermeable to gases and light and are malleable
iii) Metals can be tailored in hardness and flexibility with respect to the desired container.
iv) Malleability allows the metal collar to be crimped in place and flexible pouches and metal tubes to be crimped closed.
v) The metal's malleability also means that when metal tubes are squeezed to expel the product, *e.g.,* a cream, the tube does not spring back into its original shape and air is not sucked back into the container.
vi) Metals are shatterproof, lightweight (due to the act that it is strong even when thin layers are used).
vii) Labels are not required to be pasted because labels can be printed directly on the surface.

Disadvantages

i) They may leach metal particles into product.
ii) They may react with certain drugs or chemicals and produce a toxic product, hence surface is coating is required.
iii) They are costlier than plastic.

Material used for making metal package

Aluminium: Aluminium is very commonly used because of its lightweight and elegant appearance. They are less expensive than tin. The transparent coating of oxide formed on surface of aluminium on reaction with oxygen protect the metal from further oxidation but some complexing agent and product of high or low pH can cause corrosion on reaction with an oxide coating. Aluminium is used for preparation of ointment tube, tablets and capsule strips, screw caps etc.

Tin: It is expensive than amongst other metals used for pharmaceutical containers preparation. It is resistant to chemical attack. It offers a good appearance and it is chemically inert. It is used for preparation for food containers.

Lead: It is inexpensive than amongst all other metals. It is soft in nature. So usually 3% antimony is added in lead to increase its hardness. The main disadvantage of lead is that there is possibility of lead poisoning if taken internally. So, before its use, it should be coated with an inner lining of inert metal or polymer. It is used for non-food products such as paints, inks, lubricants etc.

Types of metal containers

Collapsible tubes: These are made up of aluminium, tin or lead. They are used to pack semisolid preparation. Aluminium tubes are used for dispensing of toothpaste and creams. Lead is not used for pharmaceutical purpose because of risk of lead poisoning. In case of aluminium collapsible tubes, there are chances of minimum contamination of the remaining portion of tube content because of the absence of suck back mechanism.

Metal containers for solid dosage forms: Aluminium is mainly used for this purpose. So the containers for tablets and capsules are light in weight and also strong enough.

Metal foil: These foils are used for wrapping of individual suppositories or pessaries. The metal foil is also used for strip and blister packing of tablets and capsules.

Rubber and elastomers

These are extensively used as stoppers (closures on parenteral containers). When used as a closure they allow a hypodermic needle to enter the container, and reseal when the needle is removed. They are soft enough to mould and conform to the opening of the container and allow a tight seal. The materials used must therefore be resilient, resistant to coring (must not fragment when penetrated by a needle) and compatible with the pack contents. The terms rubbers and elastomers are sometimes used interchangeably differentiate between the two words as follows:

- Elastomers are polymers that can be stretched and which return to their original length once the force is removed

- Rubbers are formulations of these elastomers and in addition to the elastomer polymer, contain a number (2 to 10) of substances such as fillers, vulcanising agents, cure accelerators, activators, plasticizers, lubricants, antioxidants and pigments.

Many types of rubbers are used for pharmaceutical packaging purpose for *e.g.,* butyl rubber, nitrile rubber, silicon rubber etc. Butyl rubber is very commonly used because of its low absorption property and also they are cheaper than other synthetic rubber but it decomposes above 130°C. Nitrile rubber has oil resistant and heat resistant property but it can absorb the preservative from the preparation. Silicon rubbers have very low absorption and permeability of water and are stable for a long time. But they are very expensive.

A rubber is prepared by mixing a base polymer with additives. The selection of base polymer and additives depends upon the type of rubber properties to be desired. The resultant rubber is non vulcanized compound.

Additives used in preparation of rubber

Fillers: Two types of fillers are used. Reinforce for *e.g.,* carbon black and other is non reinforce for *e.g.,* calcium carbonate. Carbon black is mostly used due to this most of the rubbers are black.

Plasticizers: They are used to improve the flow of rubber during their processing for *e.g.* oils and paraffins.

Vulcanizing agent: Vulcanization is a process of conversion of rubber molecule into a network by formation of cross links. Vulcanizing agents are used for introducing cross-linking. For example sulphur.

Accelerators: They are used to increase the rate of cross-linking reaction and optimize the vulcanizate properties by reducing sulphur content. For example thiazoles.

Activators: They activate the vulcanizing process. For example zinc oxide, stearic acid.

Pigments: These are used as a colouring agent to colour rubber compounds. For examples cadmium, iron etc.

Paper and paperboards

Paper is one of the oldest pharmaceutical packaging materials. It has diverse applications including labels and leaflets, collapsible and rigid cartons, bags and sacks and sachets. Unlike the other packaging materials, glass, metal and plastic, paper is not usually used in the manufacture of the primary pack, *i.e.,* the container holding and in direct contact with the pharmaceutical product. An exception is a sachet, which is the primary pack, where the paper is separated from the product by a layer of another material. A number of coatings may be applied to the paper to improve its surface properties, such as to reduce its porosity and liquid penetration rate (using gelatin, starch, modified resins or waxes), or increase its opacity, gloss, brightness and printability (using clay, calcium carbonate or titanium dioxide).

Paperboards are also used as a secondary package which is thicker than paper and heavy in weight. Examples of paperboards are a whiteboard, solid board, chipboard, fiberboard. These boards are mainly laminated using polyethylene or waxes. Chipboard is obtained from recycled paper. Bleached sulphate boards are the example of solid boards which are laminated with polyethylene.

Advantages

Paper has many advantages as a packaging material:

- Relatively low cost and readily available
- Generally of non-toxic origin
- Easily recycled
- Readily torn or cut open, an advantage when the paper is used in sachets
- Its 'dead old' (ability to hold a crease) allows the making of cartons and bags as well as its use or patient information leaflets
- Rigidity and strength allow its use in cartons. At the same time, it can act as a slight cushion to protect the primary pack
- Easily printed and coated
- As can be seen from its method of production, nature and properties of the finished paper can be controlled, such that paper may be 'tailor-made' or specific applications. For example, its opacity and colour can be varied by the use of additives; its

porosity can be adjusted to allow diffusion of steam or sterilization while maintaining a barrier to microorganisms.

Disadvantages

- No barrier properties against moisture, gases and odours
- Moisture-sensitive
- No heat- or cold-seal properties and hence, cannot be sealed without adhesives or special coatings
- Poor transparency and gloss compared to certain plastic films.

To overcome such disadvantages, paper can be combined with other materials. For example, paper can be further coated by polymers or laminated to plastic or to aluminium foil to improve its barrier properties to gases and moisture, and to create heat sealing ability when used in the primary pack.

Laminates

A laminate is made by bonding together two or more plies (layers) of different materials, such as paper, plastic and metal. The aim is to combine the desirable properties of the different plies into a single packaging structure. A minimum amount of material is used and the laminate is cost-effective.

Laminates are used to produce pharmaceutical packs such as sachets, blister packs, tubes, pouches, etc. An example is a structure consisting of paper/ metal oil/polythene plies, used or sachet packaging. The paper provides strength, printability and the ability to easily tear the package, the oil provides an excellent barrier to light, moisture and gases and the polythene enable heat sealability.

Factors Influencing Choice of Containers

Selection of the primary packaging material is the first step in the packaging process and takes into account:

- Dosage form
- Route of administration
- Drug/product stability
- Need of terminal sterilization

- Visual inspection of the packaged medicine
- Patient compliance and convenience
- Aesthetics
- Cost,
- Environmental- friendliness, etc.

Dosage form: It is primarily related to the physical state, *e.g.,* solid, liquid or gas and whether it is sterile, non-sterile, unit dose or multi-dose.

Liquids, which are in constant intimate contact with the primary pack, as opposed to solids such as tablets and capsules, require greater quality from a pack in order to 'take nothing out of the product or add nothing in'.

Injectable liquids require even greater quality from the pack compared to oral liquids, to maintain sterility and freedom from other possible contaminants, such as extraneous particulates.

Semi-solids need to be able to be dispensed from the container, under slight pressure, *e.g.,* squeezing of a tube. Drugs which are sensitive to atmospheric conditions such as sunlight need a packaging material which stops light transmission into the pack.

Route of administration: The route of administration may make certain packaging features desirable or necessary. The mode of dispensing and of packaging of formulation is related to the route or mode of administration.

To help the administration, the pack may be required to act as a dispersing aid or a device, *e.g.,* an aerosol, or have accessories which can either be made part of the pack or used as a separate unit, *e.g.,* a dropper assembly. Finally, the pack may either become part of a device, *e.g.,* a cartridge tube which may be used with a reusable or disposable syringe, or have a separate device which administers the product once removed from the pack, *e.g.,* a hand- or power-operated nebuliser.

Drug/product stability: Prior to formulation of the drug entity, the drug substance should be challenged by a range of factors such as light, temperature range, oxygen, carbon dioxide, water/moisture, so that modes of degradation or physicochemical change can be established.

These obtained data helps to select proper container for packaging the final formulation. For example type I glass is used to package slightly acidic solutions, Light-resistant containers are used to pack light sensitive formulations, airtight containers are used for moisture sensitive formulation etc.

Need of terminal sterilization: Medicines which are terminally sterilized in their final packs need to be made from materials that can withstand the sterilization procedure. For example, large volume parenteral like sodium chloride injections are packed in glass or plastic container which is stable during the moist heat sterilization process.

Visual inspection of the packaged medicine: To make packaged medicine visible from outside the transparent containers are used, for example, parental products are packed in transparent containers so that it helps to visual observation of particulate matter in the formulation (clarity test).

Patient convenience and compliance: The container used has to be user-friendly, allow the easy opening to legitimate consumers and be easy to reclose (for multi-unit packs). Use of metred dose inhaler is the best example of packaging the formulation which compliance patient convenience and compliance.

A unit dose eye drop which both eliminates the need for a preservative and reduces risks associated with cross-infection, by administering only a single dose. A unit dose pack also offers a number of other convenience factors, *i.e.,* no risks associated with opening and reclosing, size of pack, etc.

Patient convenience and compliance can be aided by the use of blister packaging, which allows transport of the required doses (rather than the whole bottle) and which can also be printed with information to aid memory, for example, or contraceptive pills.

However, convenience can also be extended to warehousing and production as well as the end user, *i.e.,* in terms of incoming materials, reel-fed packs need less storage space than glass, metal and plastic containers.

The other factors taken into the consideration during the selection of proper container for pharmaceutical formulations include aesthetics, cost and environmental- friendliness etc.

Legal and Official Requirements for Containers

Like the medicine, the pharmaceutical packaging is subject to regulation and approval by government drug regulatory agencies.

- The packaging is considered part of the product and manufacturers must submit large amounts of data to show that the packaging is safe, efficacious and performs as claimed.
- The regulatory bodies produce guidance documents to assist manufacturers, such as on labelling, patient information leaflets, closures and the testing of containers.
- When FDA evaluates a drug, the agency must be firmly convinced that the package for a specific drug will preserve the drug's efficacy as well as its purity, identity, strength and quality for its entire shelf life.
- As per Federal food, drug and cosmetic act it is the responsibility of the manufacturer to prove the safety of packaging material and to get approval before using it for any food or drug product.
- The FDA does not approve containers as such, but only the materials used in the container. A list of substances considered "Generally Recognized as Safe" (GRAS) has been published by the FDA in the opinion of qualified experts they are safe under specified conditions, assuming they are of good commercial quality.
- A material that is not included under GRAS are prior sanction and is intended to be used with food, must be tested by the manufacturer and the data must be submitted to the FDA.
- The FDA regulations related to drugs states that containers, closures and other components, parts of drug packages to be suitable for their intended use, must not be reactive, additive or absorptive to an extent that the identity, strength, quality or purity of the drug will be affected.
- Any drug container must be approved for such use, along with the drug before going on the market the drug manufacturer must include data on the container and package components in contact with pharmaceutical product in its New Drug Application (NDA).
- If the FDA can determine that the drug is safe and effective and that the package is suitable, it approves the drug and

package. Once approved, however, the drug package may not be altered in any manner without prior FDA approval.

- In the case of plastics most resin manufactures maintain Master File on their resins with the FDA. Upon request from the resin manufacturer, the FDA uses this file as a reference to support a New Drug Application that which a drug manufactures files.

Some Important Labelling Requirements

Product labels must contain the following information:

- Name, trade name or description
- Name and complete address of manufacturer/packer, importer, country of origin of the imported food
- Net weight, number or volume of contents in metric units
- Distinctive batch, lot or code number
- Month and year of manufacture and packaging
- Month and year by which the product is best consumed
- Information about pharmaceutical and industrial products must be in english
- If food products have been genetically modified (GM) this must be indicated in the label.

Stability Aspects of Packaging Materials

As regulators increasingly look for proof of pharmaceutical product stability throughout the supply chain, it is critical for manufacturers ensure that pharmaceuticals maintain stable temperatures and endure handling from warehouse-to transit–to the shelf. The ultimate proof of suitability of the container closure system and the packaging processes established by full shelf-life stability studies. Stability study is termed as a complex process because of the involvement of a variety of factors influencing the stability of a pharmaceutical product. These factors include stability of the active ingredient(s); interaction between active ingredients and excipients, manufacturing process followed, type of dosage form, container/closure system used for packaging. Light, heat and moisture conditions encountered during shipment, storage and handling.

Following a pharmaceutical package, stability testing are performed for the proper selection of packaging material and storage condition for the product.

Shock and vibe testing: Dropping, rotational edge dropping and rotational flat drop tests to simulate real-world exposure of the package to shock forces by forklifts, package handling or other factors in the pharmaceutical package's distribution cycle.

Vibration testing: Packages and products experience a wide range of dynamic forces and stresses during distribution that could harm a product. It performs vibration tests on samples to simulate the stresses and forces a package/product would experience during the distribution process.

Package strength testing: Package strength testing is conducted to measure and ensure that the components of the package will not separate when specific forces are applied. The testing of flexible components such as pouches, seal peel or burst testing are methods used to prove the strength of the package.

Package integrity testing: It uses established tests to test the integrity of a pharmaceutical package. Such tests include dye leak, visual inspection, vacuum leak and bubble leak testing to inspect the package's integrity capabilities. The integrity of seals in case of vials and bottles is determined by Leaker's test, water hammer test and spark tester probe.

Distribution simulation testing: Packages experience many different forces during the shipping and distribution process. It is the product manufacturer's responsibility to evaluate and document the ability of the package to withstand the distribution and storage environments.

Compression strength testing: Packages behave differently when exposed to compressive forces. It uses testing capabilities to apply compressive forces to packages and products and provide a comprehensive report with data on the strength of a package.

Quality Control Tests for Packaging

A container for a pharmaceutical product is intended to contain a drug substance or drug product with which it is or may be in direct contact.

Containers must be chosen with care and after taking into consideration the nature of the pharmaceutical product and the likely effects of transportation and storage, even for short periods of time.

A container should be designed so that the contents may be removed in a manner suitable for the intended use of the article in it. It should also provide an adequate degree of protection, minimize the loss of constituents and should not interact physically or chemically with the contents in a way that will alter their quality to an extent beyond the limits given in the individual monograph, or present a risk of toxicity.

Quality control test for packaging can be classified by taking the following points into consideration:

1. Type of packaging material used for the manufacturing of containers
2. Type of formulation to be packed
3. Design container or type of container
4. Physical tests, chemical tests, mechanical tests, optical tests and microbiological tests

Any of the above mentioned quality control tests conducted for packaging is performed to assure:

- Protection of content
- Compatibility with content
- Safety
- Performance

Protection of content

Pharmaceutical packages encounter various hazards such as a) Mechanical hazards – shock, compression, puncture, vibration etc. b) Environmental hazards-temperature, pressure, moisture, gases, light, etc., c) Biological hazards- contamination with microorganisms.

There are various tests to ensure that the resultant packaging or container used for pharmaceutical products is complying with its specification.

- A container intended to provide protection from light or offered as a light-resistant container must meet the requirements of the USP Light Transmission test. The procedure requires the use of a spectrophotometer, with the required sensitivity and accuracy, adapted for measuring the amount of light transmitted by the plastic materials used for the container.

- The ability of a container closure system to protect against moisture can be ascertained by performing the USP Water Vapour Permeation test. The USP sets limits to the amount of moisture that can penetrate based upon size and composition of the plastic components (HDPE, LDPE, or PET).
- The integrity of the container can be evaluated in several ways. A couple of the most common tests are dye penetration and microbial ingress.
- Container closure systems stored in a dye solution and exposed to pressure and vacuum cycles are examined for dye leakage into the container.
- The microbial ingress is similar in fashion but determines the microbial contamination of the contents when soaked in a media contaminated with bacteria.
- Other quantitative tests that can be run are vacuum/pressure decay, helium mass spectrometry and gas detection.

Compatibility

- Components compatible with a dosage form will not interact sufficiently to change the quality of the product or its components.
- A leachability study designed to evaluate the amount and/or nature of any chemical migrating from the packaging material to the pharmaceutical product should be determined. The study should evaluate substances that migrate into the pharmaceutical product vehicle for the length of the shelf-life claim. The drug product should be evaluated at regular intervals, such as at one, three, or six months or at one or two years until the length of the shelf life claim has been met.
- Analytical techniques such as liquid chromatography/mass spectrometry to evaluate nonvolatile organics, gas chromato-graphy/mass spectrometry (GC/MS) to evaluate semi-volatile organics, and Inductively Coupled Plasma (ICP) spectroscopy to detect and quantitative inorganic elements should be a part of this study.
- Coupling MS to LC and GC methods provides a definitive and effective tool for identifying unknown impurities and degradation products.

- Other changes such as pH shifts, precipitates, and discolouration, which may cause degradation of a pharmaceutical product, must be evaluated.
- Changes in the physical characteristics of the container, such as brittleness must be evaluated using thermal analysis and hardness testing.
- An infrared (IR) scan of each plastic component should also be included. An IR scan can fingerprint the materials and also provide proof of identity, which will later become part of quality control.

Safety

- All packaging components should be constructed of materials that will not leach harmful or undesirable amounts of substances to which a patient will be exposed during drug treatment.
- Determining the safety of a packaging component is not a simple process and a standardized approach has not been established.
- However, an extraction study should be one of the first considerations. Isolation is accomplished through sample preparation, followed by incubation in solvents at well-defined and well-controlled times and temperatures.
- Sample preparation is an area in which an experienced chemist's knowledge of chemical procedures is indispensable.
- Prior to performing any of the chemical tests, it is important to have precise information on the synthesis of the polymer itself. This includes descriptions of the monomers used in the polymerization, the solvents used in the synthesis, and the special additives that have been added during material production.
- For containers used to package drugs ranked with a high degree of concern, such as inhalation aerosols and injectables, this type of information is imperative.
- Knowledge of degradation products that may be released into the drug product is also important. Some potential extractable chemicals from packaging materials are water soluble, while others are soluble only in non-polar environments.
- For the packaging which is in contact with the drug products, extraction in both polar and non-polar environments is relevant.

- The USP includes physicochemical tests for plastics based on water extracts; while water, alcohol, and hexane extracts are required for polyethylene containers under controlled temperature and time parameters (70°C for 24 hours for water and alcohol and 50°C for 24 hours for hexane). These tests are particularly useful in defining materials as rich or poor in extractable chemicals.
- The tests categorize material extracts in general terms, such as nonvolatile residue (total extractable), residue on ignition, buffering capacity, heavy-metals content, and turbidity.

Biological reactivity is the second part of safety testing and is designed to test extractable chemicals for toxicological properties.

- FDA's guidance document suggests that the USP biological reactivity tests can determine the safe level of exposure *via* the label-specified route of administration.

Performance

- The fourth attribute of suitability of the container closure system, performance and drug delivery, refers to its ability to function in the manner for which it was designed. There are two major considerations when evaluating performance.
- The first consideration is functionality that may be to improve patient compliance, minimize waste, or improve ease of use.
- The second consideration is drug delivery, which is the ability of the packaging system to deliver the right amount or rate.
- Packaging systems that address this consideration are pre-filled syringes, transdermal patches, dropper or spray bottles and metered-dose inhalers.

Drug-Container Considerations for Quality Control Tests

1. ***Permeation:*** The transmission of gases, vapours or liquid through packaging materials can have an adverse effect on self-life of the drug. Permeation of water vapour and oxygen through the container wall into the drug can be a problem if the dosage form is sensitive to hydrolysis and oxidation. Temperature and humidity are important factors influencing the permeability of oxygen and water through containers.

2. *Leaching:* Leaching or migration of small quantities of ingredients from the container to the product may lead to drug contamination and may affect its efficacy, safety and/or stability.

3. *Sorption:* It may be defined as bonding of a solute to a container material. This process involves the removal of constituents from the drug product by the packaging material. Sorption may lead to a serious problem for drug preparation in which important ingredients are in solution. Since drug substances of high potency are administered in small doses, losses due to sorption may significantly affect the therapeutic efficacy of the preparation.

4. *Chemical reactivity:* Certain ingredients that are used in container formulations may react chemically with one or more components of a drug product. At times ingredients in the formulation may react with the container. Even micro quantities of chemically incompatible substance can alter the appearance of the container or the drug product.

Quality Control Tests for Glass Containers

Glass is a common material used in either non- sterile or sterile liquid dosage forms. It leaches alkali from its surface. Leaching of alkali can be reduced but cannot be made zero. Hence, evaluation of chemical resistance of glass containers is performed before using it for a particular product. The evaluation of chemical resistance of glass containers is donc under controlled conditions of accelerated temperature and time.

(A) Powdered glass test: From the glass containers, alkaline constituents (oxides of sodium, potassium, calcium, aluminium, etc.) are leached into purified water under conditions of elevated temperatures. When the glass is powdered the leaching of alkali can be enhanced.

Principle involved in the powdered glass test to estimate the amount of alkali leached from the glass powder. The amount of acid that is necessary to neutralize the released alkali (a specified limit) is specified in the pharmacopoeia. The basic analysis is acid-base titration using methyl red indicator.

Method: In this test, the containers are washed, dried and crushed, sieved and again crushed through a nest of sieves. Which is then washed with acetone and dried, 10 g of this crushed glass is mixed with high purity water in a conical flask and exposed to a standard regimen of autoclaving at 121°C for 30 minutes. The water is then separated in another container; to it are added washing of the specimens made using purified water. The pooled sample is titrated using 0.02N sulphuric acid using methyl red solutions as an indicator. The type of glass and test limit are given in Table 10.3.

(B) Water attack test: This test is used only with containers that have been exposed to sulphur dioxide fumes under controlled humidity conditions. Such a treatment neutralizes the surface alkali. Now the glass becomes chemically more resistant. The principle involved in the water attack test is to determine whether the alkali leached from the surface of a container is within the specified limits or not. Since the inner surface is under test entire container (ampoule) has to be used. The amount of acid that is necessary to neutralize the released alkali from the surface is estimated, the leaching of alkali is accelerated using elevated temperature for a specified time. Methyl red indicator is used to determine the endpoint. The basic is acid-base titration. Table 10.3 shows limits of alkalinity for glass containers.

Table 10.3: Types of glass and their test limits

Tests	*Containers*	*Limits of 0.02 N H_2SO_4*
1. Powdered glass test	Type I	1.0 ml
	Type III	8.5 ml
	Type NP	15.0 ml
2. Water attack test	Type II (100 ml or less)	0.7 ml
	Type II (over 100 ml)	0.2 ml

Method: The containers are filled up to 90% of their overflow capacity. The containers are exposed for autoclaving at 121°C for 60 minutes. The contents of the container are pooled and titrated with 0.02N sulphuric acid using methyl red solutions as an indicator.

Quality Control Tests for Plastic Containers

(A) Leakage test: Fill ten containers with water. Fit with intended closures and keep them inverted at room temperature for 24 hours. There are no signs of leakage from any container then it passes leakage test.

Table 10.4: Quality control test for paper and board

Tests	***Description***
Moisture content	All the substances will be measured at a temperature specified for the test
Folding endurance	Hold the test piece back and forth until rupture occurs
Air permeability	Important for using lightweight uncoated paper on a machine having vacuum pick up system
Tensile strength	The maximum tensile force per unit width that a paper or board will withstand before breaking
Tear strength	The mean force required to continue the tearing of an initial cut in a single sheet of paper.
Stiffness	The degree of resistance offered by the paper/board when it is bent
Burst resistance	The maximum uniformly distributed paper, applied at a right angle to the surface of a test piece paper and board will stand under conditions of test Hydraulic pressure is applied to the diaphragm, bulging it until test paper bursts.

(B) Collapsibility test: This test applicable to containers which are to be squeezed in order to remove the contents. A container by collapsing inwards during use yields at least 90% of its nominal contents at the required rate of flow at ambient temperature.

(C) Clarity of aqueous extract: Select unlabelled, unmarked and non-laminated portions from suitable containers, taken at random sufficient to yield a total area of sample required taking into account the surface area of both sides cut these portions into strips none of which has a total area of more than 20 cm^2. Wash the strips free from extraneous matter by shaking them with at least two separate portions of distilled water for about 30 seconds in each case, then draining off the water thoroughly.

(D) Transparency test: Fill five empty containers to their nominal capacity with diluted suspension as described in IP 1966. The cloudiness of the diluted suspension in each container is detectable when viewed through the containers as compared with a container of the same type filled with water.

(E) Water vapour permeability test: Fill five containers with a nominal volume of water and heat seal the bottles with an aluminium foil-poly ethylene laminate or other suitable seal. Weigh accurately each container and allow to stand for 14 days at a relative humidity of 60 ±

5% and a temperature between 20 and 25°C reweigh the containers. The loss in weight in each container is not more than 0.2%.

(D) Biological tests: The USP has provided its procedures for evaluating the toxicity of plastic materials essentially the tests consist of three phases:

- *Implantation test*: Implanting small pieces of plastic material intramuscularly in rabbits.
- *Systemic injection test*: Injecting eluates using sodium chloride injection, with and without alcohol intravenously in mice and injecting eluates using polyethylene glycol 400 and sesame oil intraperitoneally in mice.
- *Intracutaneous test*: Injecting all four eluates subcutaneously in rabbits. The reaction from test samples must not be significantly greater than non-reactive control samples.

Quality Control Tests for Metal Containers

Metals have a number of advantages over other packaging materials. Like glass, metal is nearly totally impermeable to gas and water. In addition, metal containers are extremely strong and are shatterproof. For applications requiring malleability such as collapsible tubes, metal offers relatively easy manufacturing and very easy use. Metals can also be fashioned into more complex delivery systems such as metered-dose inhalers, dry powder inhalers, aerosol administration devices and even ready-to-use needles.

Metals are prone to the development of "pinhole" defects during manufacturing that can drastically compromise their barrier properties — especially in particularly thin sections. Not only can these defects be deleterious to the container, but they can also compromise the quality of the pharmaceutical.

Quality control Tests for Paper, Paperboard and Cardboard

Because paper, paperboard and cardboard offer virtually no moisture or gas barrier, they are typically part of the secondary pharmaceutical container. The tests pieces of paper and board are conditioned for the tests to be carried out in standard conditions. They are temperature: 23ºC ±1ºC, relative humidity: 50% ± 2%. Some of the tests performed are given in Table 10.4.

Quality Control Test for Closures

The closure is normally the most vulnerable and critical component of a container as far as stability and compatibility with the product is concerned. Following tests are performed for closers:

(A) Penetrability: This is measured to check the force required to make a hypodermic needle penetrate easily through the closure. It is measured by using the piercing machine. The piercing force must not exceed a stated value. If it exceeds that stated value, the hypodermic needle can be damaged as a result of undesirable hardness of the closures.

(B) Fragmentation test: This test is performed on 20 closures. Each closure is penetrated with a hypodermic needle in a piercing machine five times within a limited area and needle is washed to transfer any fragment present. The contents are filtered through the coloured paper that contrasts with the rubber and the fragments counted. On an average, there should not be more than three fragments per unit.

(C) Self-sealability test: Applicable to multidose containers fill 10 vials with water close them with prepared closures and secure with a cap. For each closure use, a new hypodermic needle and pierce 10 times each time at different site immerse the vials upright in methylene blue (0.1%) solution and reduce external pressure for 10 minutes. Restore the atmospheric pressure and leave the vials immersed for 30 minutes. Rinse the outside of the vials. None of the vials contains any trace of coloured solution.

(D) Extractive test: In this test, the closure is boiled with water for four hours under reflux and the water evaporated to dryness. The residue must not exceed the specified amount.

(E) Compatibility test: This test is performed to check the compatibility of the rubber closures with various types of the substances since it is necessary to ensure that there is no interaction between the contents of the bottle and the closure.

The quality control tests for packaging specific for parenteral preparation and aerosols are described in the respective chapters.

Glossary

Primary package	Primary package are those packages which are in direct contact with the Pharmaceutical formulation
Secondary package	The package external to the Primary package is known as secondary package
Tertiary package	Tertiary Package is used for warehouse storage and transport shipping
Airtight container	A container that is impermeable to solids, liquids and gases under ordinary conditions of handling, storage and transport
Hermetically sealed container	A container that is impervious to air or any other gas under normal conditions of handling, shipment, storage and distribution
Light-resistant container	A container that protects the contents from the effects of light by virtue of the specific properties of the material of which it is made
Multidose container	A container that holds a quantity of the preparation suitable for two or more doses
Tamper-evident container	A container fitted with a device or mechanism that reveals irreversibly whether the container has been opened.
Tightly-closed container	A tightly-closed container protects the contents from contamination by extraneous liquids, solids or vapours, from loss or deterioration of the article from effervescence, deliquescence or evaporation under normal conditions of handling, shipment, storage and distribution
Well-closed container	A well-closed container protects the contents from extraneous solids and liquids and from loss of the article under normal conditions of handling, shipment, storage and distribution
Threaded screw type	As the name indicates they contain threads which get engaged with the threads present on the neck of container
Lug cap	The difference in lug cap and thread cap is that in thread cap, continuous threads are present but in lug, cap threads are present in intermittent fashion
Crown caps	These caps are made up of metal and commonly used for beverages bottles. These also provides an effective seal and cannot be open with hands. These cannot be seal again
Roll on closures	Roll on closure contains the aluminium roll-on cap which can be easily sealed, opened and closed.
Pilfer proof	In this additional length extends below to threaded portion which forms a bridge. When the closure is removed then the bridge break and the additional portion remains in place on neck of container which shows its opening
Tamper–evident closures	Tamper evident closures are designed to prevent accident and intentional tampering to create safe packaging

Child resistant closures	Child-resistant packaging is special packaging used to reduce the risk of children ingesting dangerous items. This is often accomplished by the use of a special safety cap

QUESTION BANK

Q. I: Multiple Choice Questions

1 Disposable syringes are made up of
 a) Polypropylene c) Glass
 b) Transparent polystyrene d) Poly tetrachloro ethylene

2 Water attack test is used to identify the alkalinity in
 a) Type I glass c) Type III glass
 b) Type II glass d) All the 3 types

3 Water resistance of glass containers are tested by measuring:
 a) Amount of alkali released into water c) Estimation of silicate levels
 b) Amount of acid released into water d) Turbidity

4 Powdered glass test is carried out for all kinds of glass EXCEPT
 a) Borosilicate glass c) Soda lime glass
 b) Treated soda lime glass d) General purpose

5 In which type of packaging system the product is in direct contact with packaging material?
 a) Primary Package c) Tertiary Package
 b) Secondary Package d) All of the above

6 _____ fitted with a device or mechanism that reveals irreversibly whether the container has been opened
 a) Tightly-closed container c) Well-closed container
 b) Tamper-evident container d) None of these

Q. II: Very Short Answer Questions 2 Marks

1. Define pharmaceutical packaging.
2. Define primary and secondary packaging.
3. What are the most important primary packaging materials?
4. What are the functions of secondary packaging?
5. What are tamper evident closures?

Q. III: Short Answer Questions **5 Marks**

1. What are the criteria for the selection of materials for pharmaceutical packaging?
2. Short note on the evaluation of a pharmaceutical container closure system.
3. Write a note on child resistant and tamper-proof packages.
4. Write any two quality control tests for glass containers.
5. Explain folding endurance test for packaging materials.
6. Write a note on labeling requirements.
7. Write quality control tests on rubber closure.
8. Add a note on quality control tests for paper and paper boards.

Q. IV: Long Answer Questions **10 Marks**

1. Explain in detail hydrolytic resistance test for glass.
2. Explain in detail powdered glass test.
3. Give details of glass as the packaging material.
4. Discuss the legal and official requirements for containers
5. Discuss the stability aspects of packaging materials

Answers Keys

CHAPTER 1: PREFORMULATION STUDIES

1	b	2	c	3	d	4	a	5	b
6	a	7	c	8	d	9	c	10	a
11	b	12	a	13	b	14	d	15	a
16	d								

CHAPTER 2: TABLETS

1	a	2	a	3	a	4	a	5	c
6	b	7	d	8	b	9	a	10	d
11	a	12	c	13	d	14	b	15	d
16	b	17	b	18	b	19	a	20	c
21	a	22	b	23	b	24	a	25	d
26	a	27	a	28	c	29	c	30	d
31	d	32	b	33	a	34	b	35	b
36	c	37	b	38	b	39	a	40	d
41	c	42	a	43	c	44	d	45	a
46	c	47	d	48	c				

CHAPTER 3: LIQUID ORALS

1	b	2	c	3	a	4	c	5	d
6	b	7	a	8	d	9	c	10	a
11	b	12	c	13	c	14	d	15	c
16	a	17	a						

CHAPTER 4: CAPSULES

1	c	2	b	3	d	4	d	5	d
6	d	7	c	8	a	9	b	10	c
11	c	12	d	13	b	14	b	15	a
16	b	17	d	18	a	19	d	20	a
21	a	22	a	23	b	24	d	25	c
26	c	27	b	28	a	29	a	30	a
31	a	32	d	33	a	34	d	35	b
36	c	37	a	38	c	39	b	40	a
41	b	42	a	43	a	44	b	45	d

CHAPTER 5: PELLETS

1	c	2	c	3	a	4	d	5	b

CHAPTER 6: PARENTERAL PRODUCTS

1	a	2	b	3	a	4	d	5	a
6	d	7	b	8	c	9	d	10	b
11	d	12	b	13	d	14	b	15	c
16	b	17	b	18	c	19	c	20	b
21	c	22	b	23	d	24	b	25	b
26	c	27	d	28	a	29	b	30	a

CHAPTER 7: OPTHALMIC PREPARATIONS

1	a	2	a	3	a	4	b	5	d
6	c	7	a	8	c	9	c	10	d
11	a								

CHAPTER 8: COSMETICS

1	a	2	b	3	c	4	d	5	a
6	a	7	a	8	c	9	a	10	a
11	a	12	d	13	d	14	a	15	c
16	b								

CHAPTER 9: PHARMACEUTICAL AEROSOLS

1	a	2	a	3	b	4	d	5	b
6	a	7	d	8	d	9	c	10	d
11	d	12	c	13	c				

CHAPTER 10: PACKAGING MATERIAL SCIENCE

1	a	2	b	3	a	4	b	5	a
6	b								

Appendix 1

Defination and Examples of Some Commonly Used Additives

ADSORBENTS

Adsorbent is the additive used in the tablet formulation which adsorbs the semisolid or liquid excipients and avoids cohesiveness of tablet powder to allow proper tablet compression.

Bentonite	Magnesium silicate
Kaolin	Silica (cab-o-sil, syloid, aerosil)
Magnesium carbonate	Starch
Magnesium oxide	Tricalcium phosphate

ANTIADHESIVES

These agents prevent the sticking of tablet material (powder or granules) to the punch and to some extent to the tablet die wall. Hence, it avoids the tablet processing problems of sticking and picking which occurs due to the presence of excess moisture.

Colloidal silica	Metallic stearates
Corn starch	Sodium lauryl sulfate
Magnesium stearate	Talk

ANTIFOAMING AGENTS

An agent which counters the formation of foams can be termed as antifoaming agents. Generally, surfactant with HLB value between 1.5 to 3 is good foam killers.

Arlacel C
Atlas G 1706
Ethylene glycol fatty acid ester
Glyceryl mono stearate
Propylene glycol mono stearate
Span 65
Span 85

ANTIOXIDANTS

These are the substances which are added to the formulation to prevent degradation of the therapeutic agent due to oxidation

Acetone
Ascorbic acid
Ascorbyl palmitate
Benzoin
Beta- Naphthol
Butylated hydroxyl anisole
Butylated hydroxyl toluene
Citric acid
Cysteine hydrochloride
Ethyl gallate
Gallic acid
Glycerin
Maleic acid
Monoisopropyl citrate
Propyl gallate
Sodium bisulfite
Sodium metabisulfite
Sodium sulfite
Sodium thiosulfate
Thiosorbitol
Thioglycerol
Thiourea
Hydroquinone
Isosorbic acid
Lecithin
Thioglycolic acid
Alpha tocopherol
Trihydroxy butyrophenone

BINDERS

Binders are also called as pharmaceutical glue, as they cause adhesion of powder particles to form granules. They are incorporated to produce cohesive bonding between granules during the process of compaction to form a tablet.

Acacia
Alginates
Carboxymethylcellulose
Hydroxypropylcellulose
Methylcellulose
Polyvinylpyrrolidone
Sorbitol
Ethylcellulose
Gelatin
Glucose
Sucrose
Starch
Tragacanth
Vinyl acetate copolymers

COATING MATERIALS

These are the materials used for coating of tablets to protect against decomposition by atmospheric oxygen or humidity, to provide desired release pattern, to mask taste or odour or for aesthetic purposes.

Aminoalkyl acrylate copolymer	Organic acids like benzoic, salicylic, naphthoic, fumaric, uric, glutamic, aspartic, etc.
Cellulose acetate phthalate	Polyethyleneglycols
Cellulose acetate	Polyvinylacetates
Epoxy resins	PVP
Ethyl cellulose	PVP modified shellac
Ethyl cellulose wax mixtures	Shellac
Gelatin	Sodium CMC
Half esters of maleic anhydride copolymers	Sodium ethylcellulose sulfate
Hydroxypropyl methyl cellulose	Styrene-maleic acid copolymers
Hydroxy ethylmethyl cellulose	Sugars
Hydroxypropylcellulose	Terpolymers
Lipid cellulose mixtures	Zein

COLOURANTS

Colourants are the agents which imparts colour to the dosage forms like tablets, capsules, syrups etc.

I. Natural

Alizarin	Hesperidin
Anattenes	Indigo
Caramel	Quercetin
Beta-carotene	Riboflavin
Carbon black	*Rubia tinctorum*
Carmic acid	Rutin
Chlorophyll	Saffron
Cochineal	Titanium dioxide
Curcumin	Turmeric
Ferric oxides (red and yellow)	Tyrian purple

II. Synthetic

Alizarin cyanine	Indigo carmine 73015
Amaranth I N 16185	Napthol blue black 20470
Brilliant blue FCS 42090	Orange G 16 30
Carmoisine 14720	Ponceaux 4 R 16255
Eosine G 45380	Quinizarine 61565
Erythrosin 45430	Quinoline yellow SS 47000
Fast red E 16045	Resorcin brown 20170
Fast green FCF 42053	Sudan III 26100
Green S 44090	Sunset yellow FCF 15185
Green F 61570	Tartrazine 19140

COMPLEXING AGENT

These are the substances that form stable water-soluble complexes (Chelates) with metals; used in some liquid pharmaceuticals as stabilizers to complex heavy metals that might promote instability. In such use they are also called as sequestering agents.

Boric acid for glycerine, epinephrine	Na-CMC for quinine, diphenhydramine, pyribenzamine etc.
Caffeine for organic acids, benzocaine, riboflavin etc.	PEG for phenols, barbiturates, organic acids, iodine
Dextrins for vitamin A palmitate	Protamine sulfate for heparin
Dimercaprol (BAL) for heavy metals	PVP for procaine HCl, salicylates,hexylresorcinol, antibiotics,cortisones, xanthines
DTPA (Diethylene-triamine penta acetic acid) for heavy metals	Saccharin for xanthenes, amides,phenolic compounds
EDTA and its salts for heavy metals	Surfactants for chlorobutanol, banzocaine, acetyl salicylic acid.
EDTA for papaverine, morphine, ascorbic acid, antibiotics, epinephrine, prednisolone etc.	Tolonium chloride for heparin
Methyl cellulose for benzoic acid and hydroxybenzoates	

DILUENTS

Diluents are inert substances which add the necessary bulk to a formulation to prepare tablets of the desired size. Certain drugs like aspirin, antibiotics etc, exert their therapeutic action in sufficiently high doses, hence do not require diluents or binders. Highly potent drugs such as digoxin, clonidine hydrochloride etc., exerts their therapeutic effect in very low doses, hence their bulk is increased by adding diluents.

Amylose	Magnesium carbonate
Bentonite	Magnesium oxide
Calcium carbonate	Mannitol
Calcium sulphate	MCC
Dicalcium phosphate-dihydrate	PVP
Food grade and amorphous cellulose	Sorbitol
Glycine	Starches
Hydroxylated starches like emdex celutab	Sucrose
Inositol	Sucrose based preparations like dipac, Nu-tab, sugar tab etc
Lactose	Tribasic calcium sulfate

DISINTEGRANTS

Disintegrating agents are added to promote tablet breakup after administration. This is seen when the tablet comes in contact with an aqueous environment or GI fluid. Disintegrating agents act in opposition to binding agents. Stronger the binder used stronger the disintegrating agent is required to disintegrate the tablet so as to release the medicament.

Agar	Hemicellulases (when gums are binders)
Alginic acid	Invertases (when sucrose is binder)
Alginates	Karaya gum
Amylases (When starches are binders)	Locust bean gum
Bentonite Carageenases (When alginates, methylcelluloses are binders)	Microcrystalline cellulose

Cellulases (When celluloses are binders)
Carboxy methyl cellulose
Effervescent combinations (organic acids like citric, tartaric in combination with sodium carbonate)
Guar gum
Explotab
Primagel
Pectin
Proteases (when gelatin or zein is binder)
Tragacanth
Veegum

EMULSIFYING AGENTS

Emulsifying agents are used to promote and maintain dispersion of finely divided particles of liquid in a vehicle in which it is immiscible. End product may be liquid emulsion or semisolid emulsion

I. Surfactants for monomolecular film

Alkyl polyoxyethylene sulfates
Benzalkonium chloride
Cetrimide
Dioctylsodium sulfosuccinate
Lauryldimethylbenzylammonium chloride
Lecithin
N-cetyl N-ethyl morpholinium ethosulfate
PEG 400 monostearate
Polyoxyethylene laurylether
Polyethylene glycol monostearate
Propylene glycol monolaurate
Polyoxyethylene monolaurate
Polyoxyethyelene alkylphenol
Polyoxyethylene sorbitan monolaurate (Tween 20)
Polyoxyethylene sorbitan monopalmitate (Tween 40)
Polyoxyethylene sorbitan monooleate (Tween 80)
Polyoxyethylene laurylether (Brij 35)
Potassium oleate
Sodium oleate
Sodium lauryl sulfate
Sorbitan monolaurate (Span 20)
Glyceryl monstearate (GMS)
Sorbitan sesquioleate (Alacel C)
Potassium laurate
Potassium stearate
Sorbitan monopalmitate (Span 40)
Sorbitan monostearate (Arlacel 60)
Sodium laurate
Triethanolamine oleate
Triethanolamine stearate

II. Surfactants forming multimolecular films

Aacacia	Hectorite
Agar	Magnesium hydroxide
Alginates	Pectin
Attapulgite	Silica gel
Bentonite	Tragacanth
Gelatin	Veegum

FLAVOURING AGENTS

These are used to impart pleasant flavour and often odour to a preparation.

Almond	Oil of bergamot
Amyl acetate	Oil of caraway
Anethol	Oil of cardamom
Apple	Oil of cinnamon
Apricot	Oil of clove
Banana	Oil of coriander
Benzaldehyde	Oil of fennel
Black current	Oil of lavender
Blueberry	Oil of lemon
Burgundy	Oil of narcissus
Butterscotch	Oil of nutmeg
Cherry	Oil of orange
Chocolate	Oil of peppermint
Custard	Oil of rose
Ethyl acetate	Oil of rosemary
Ethyl vanillin	Oil of spearmint
Eucalyptol	Oil of thyme
Eugenol	Orris root
Ginger	Palmarosa
Grape	Peach
Hyacinth	Phenyl ethyl alcohol
Jasmine	Pineapple
Lemongrass	Plum
Liquorice	Raspberry

Mango
Maple
Melon
Methyl salicylate
Narcissus
Neroli
Oil of anise
Saffron
Sandalwood
Strawberry
Thymol
Vanillin
Violet

FLOCCULATING AGENTS

Flocculating agents are added to enhance particle re-dispersibility in the dispersion medium. In contrast to deflocculated particles, flocculated suspensions can always be re-suspended with gentle agitation.

Electrolytes like KH_2PO_4, $AlCl_3$, NaCl etc.
Ionic and non-ionic surfactants
Hydrocolloids

GLIDANTS

These are the agents which are added to tablet formulation to improve the flow property of granules/powders.

Aerosil
Colloidal silica
Corn starch
Talc

LUBRICANTS

These are added to a tablet formulation to decreases the friction between the granules and the die wall of tablet press. Lubricants are required during tablet compression and ejection.

Boric acid
Corn starch
DL-leucine
Magnesium lauryl sulfate
Metallic stearates
PEG 4000
PEG 6000
Polyvinylpyrrolidone
Sodium acetate
Sodium benzoate
Sodium chloride
Sodium lauryl sulfate
Sodium oleate
Stearic acid
Talcum
Waxes with high melting points

PRESERVATIVES

These are the agents used in liquid or semisolid preparations to prevent growth of microorganisms

2,2'-thiobis (4,6-dichlorophenol)	Methyl chlorothymol
4:3:4-trichlorosalicylanilide	Monomethylol dimethyl hydantoin
8-hydroxyquinoline	Monothioglycerol
Benzalkonium chloride	Nitromerosol
Benzoic acid and benzoate	Ortho and para chlorbenzoic acid
Benzylalcohole	p- chlor phenylpropanediol
Beta- phenylethylalcohol	Parachlor metacresol
Beta-p-chlorophenoxyethyl alcohol	Parachlor metaxylenol
Beta-phenoxy propyl alcohol	Parahydroxybenzoate
Betaphenoxyethylalcohol	P-chlorphenylglyceryl ether
Boric acid and its salt	Phenol
Cetrimide	Phenol hexachlorophene
Cetylpyridinium chloride	Phenyl mercuric nitrate and other salt of phenyl mercuric acid
Chlorbutanol	Potassium hydroquinoline sulfate
Cresol	Propionic acid
Dihydroacetic acid	Salicylic acid and salicylate
Dichlorometaxylenol	Sorbic acid and its salts
Dichlorophen	Sulphurous acid
Dimethyldidodeceylammonium chloride	Tetrachlorsalicylanilide
Ethyl vanillin	Thimerosal
Formaldehyde	Trichlorocarbanilide
Formic acid	Trichlorsalicylanilide
Hibitane	Vanillin

SOLUBILISING AGENTS

These are the agents which improve the solubility of poorly water soluble drugs

Atlas G 1690
Atlas G 1794
Brij 35
Ipegal CA 630
Myrj 45
Myrj 49
Myrj 51
Myrj 52
PEG 400 monostearate
Sodium oleate
Triethanolamine oleate
Tween 20
Tween 40
Tween 60
Tween 80

SOLVENTS

Solvents used to dissolve another substances in preparation of a solution; may be aqueous or non aqueous

Acetone
Alcohol
Amylene hydrate
Carbon tetrachloride
Chloroform
Ether
Ethyl acetate
Ethanolamines (mono and tri)
Isopropyl alcohol
Methyl isobutyl ketone
PEG 400
Petroleum ether
Propylene glycol
Water

SUSPENDING AGENTS

These are agents which increases the viscosity and reduces the sedimentation rate of particles in a vehicle in which they are not soluble.

Acacia
Agar
Alginates
Attapulgite
Bentonite
Carboxymethyl cellulose
Carbopol
Carbomer
Cellulose powder
Chondorus
Gelatin
Guar gum
Hectorite
Hydroxyl ethyl cellulose
Hydroxy propyl cellulose
Methyl celluloses
Microcrystalline cellulose
Polyvinyl alcohol
Povidone
Psyllium seed gum
Pectin
Tragacanth
Veegum

SWEETENING AGENTS

These agents are used to impart sweetness to a preparation

Aspartyl phenylalanine	Lactose
Cyclamates	Maltose
Dextrose	Mannitol
Fructose	Saccharin
Glycerin	Sorbitol
Glycyrrhizin	Sucrose
Honey	Xylitol

VEHICLES

Vehicles are carrying agents used in formulating a variety of liquids for oral and parenteral administration

1:3 butylene glycol	Mineral oils like liquid paraffin
Dimethyl acetamide	N-(Beta-hydroxyethyl)
Dioxalanes	Polyethylene glycols
DMSO	Propylene glycol
Ethanol	Silicones like dimethyl polysiloxanes
Glycofural	Vegetable oils, such as corn oil, cotton seed oil, castor oil, olive oil,coconut oil etc.
Glycerol	Water
Lactamide	Methyl phenyl polysiloxanes

WETTING AGENTS

Wetting agent are the one which removes adsorbed air from the surface of particle and easy penetration of the vehicle into the pores. They also act by reducing the interfacial tension existing between solid and liquid components.

Alginates	Tragacanth
Bentonite	Sorbitan esters
Cellulose derivatives	Span 20 and Span 40
Polysorbates	Sodium lauryl sulphate (SLS)

APPENDIX 2

LIST OF SORTED OUT PREVIOUS GATE/GPAT QUESTIONS FROM 2006 TO 2019

GATE 2006

Q.9. Certain suspensions with a high percentage of dispersed solids exhibit an increase in resistance to flow with increasing rates of shear: Such system actually increase in volume when sheared and are termed as

(A) Thixotropic (B) Dilatant

(C) Plastic (D) Newtonian

Q.10. In the process of sugar coating of tablets the colorants are added in one of the following steps

(A) Syrup coating (B) Polishing

(C) Subcoating (D) Seal coating

Q.26. During compression of moisture-critical granules a hygroscopic substance used to maintain a proper moisture level is

(A) Sorbitol (B) Talc

(C) Acacia (D) Tragacanth

Q.28. Which one of the following is used as a local anaesthetic in the formulation of parenteral product?

(A) Acetic acid (B) Benzyl alcohol

(C) Ethyl alcohol (D) Sorbitol

Q.29. In the formulation of suspensions for soft gelatin encapsulation base adsorption of the solid to be suspended is expressed as

(A) The number of grams of liquid base required to produce a capsulatable mixture when mixed with 1 g of solid

(B) The number of ml of liquid base required to produce a capsulatable mixture when mixed with 1 g of solid

(C) The number of grams of solid base required to produce a capsulatable mixture when mixed with 1 g of solid

(D) The number of mgs of liquid base required to produce a capsulatable mixture when mixed with 10 g of solid

Q.44. Abrasive and humectant compounds in the formulation of toothpaste are

(P) Dicalcium phosphate (Q) Sodium lauryl sulphate

(R) Sorbitol syrup (S) Tragacanth

(A) P, Q (B) Q, R

(C) P, S (D) P, R

Matching Exercises: Match Group I with Group II and identify the correct combination

Q. 61.

Group-I (Film defects)	Group-II (Explanation)
(P) Orange peel effect	(1) Inadequate spreading of the coating solution before drying causes a bumping effect on the coating
(Q) Blistering	(2) It is the result of drying coated tablets in ovens, due to too rapid evaporation of the solvent from the core and the effect of high temperature on the strength, elasticity and adhesion of the film
(R) Cracking	(3) Occurs when the processing temperature used is too high for a particular formulation
(S) Bloom	(4) Occurs if internal stresses in the film exceed the tensile strength of the film

(A) P-1, Q-2, R-4, S-3 (B) P-2,Q-3, R-1,S-4

(C) P-3, Q-4, R-2, S-1 (D) P-4,Q-1, R-3,S-2

Q.62.

Group-I (Term)	Group-II (Example)
(P) Hydrophilic suppository base	(1) Nitrocellulose
(Q) Polymorphism	(2) Titanium dioxide
(R) Film former used in the formation of nail Lacquer	(3) Cocoa butter
(S) Opaquant extender	(4) Polyethylene glycol

(A) P-1, Q-2, R-3, S-4 (B) P-2, Q-1, R-3, S-4

(C) P-3, Q-4, R-2, S-1 (D) P-4, Q-3, R-1, S-2

GATE-2007

Q.3. The duration of action of a sublingual nitroglycerin tablet is

(A) 8-10 h (B) 4-8 h

(C) 10-30 min (D) 3-5 min

Q.20. What is the concentration of NaCI required to make 1% solution of cocaine HCl Isotonic with blood plasma? Freezing point of 1% w/v solution of NaCI is -0.576° C and freezing paint of 1% w/v cocaine HCI is -0. 09°C.

(A) 0.746% w/v (B) 0.9% w/v

(C) 0.5 w/v (D) 0.373% w/v

Q.31. In the preparation of ointments, macrogols are used as

(A) Water soluble base (B) Hydrocarbon base

(C) Absorption base (D) Oleogenous base

Q.32. An antioxidant commonly used in the formulation of a non-aqueous parenteral preparation is

(A) Thioglycollic acid (B) Ascorbic acid

(C) Sodium metabisulpite (D) Butylated hydroxy toluene

Q.34. With regard to the Standards for Sterile Water for Injection, IP. the 'residue on evaporation' limit is

(A) Higher than Water for Injection, IP (B) Lower than Water for injection, IP

(C) Same as that of the Water for injection (D) No such standard is prescribed in the monograph

Q.45. Zeta potential

(P) is the difference in potential between the surface of the tightly bound layer and the electroneutral region

(Q) is the potential at the solid surface of the suspended particle

(R) can be positive, zero or negative

(S) is the electrothermodynamic potential

(A) P, R (B) P, S

(C) Q, R (D) P, Q

Q.46. Two of the official standard for uncoated tablets as per IP are

(P) Shape

(Q) Friability

(R) Disintegration time

(S) Uniformity of weight

(A) P, Q (B) P, S

(C) Q, R (D) R, S

Matching Exercises: Match Group I with Group II and identify the correct combination

Q. 61. Group-I — Group-II

(P) Crystal growth — (1) Griffin

(Q) pH scale — (2) Sorensen

(R) HLB scale — (3) DLVO theory

(S) Interparticular force — (4) Ostwald ripening

(A) P-4, Q-2, R-1, S-3 — (B) P-3, Q-1, R-2, S-4

(C) P-2, Q-4, R-3, S-1 — (D) P-1, Q-3, R-4, S-2

GATE 2008

Q.20. Drave's test is associated with the measuring the efficiency of

(A) Detergents — (B) Wetting agents

(C) Suspending agents — (D) Absorbent

Q.30. A super disintegrant in tablet formulation is

(A) Sodium starch glycolate — (B) Starch

(C) PVP — (D) Mg-.Aluminium silicate

Matching Exercises: Match Group I with Group II and identify the correct combination

Q.60. Group-I — Group-II

Industrial dryers — Pharmaceutical materials dried

(P) Drum dryer — (1) Antibiotic solution

(Q) Fluidised bed dryer — (2) Tablet granules

(R) Spray dryer — (3) Gelatin

(S) Freeze dryer — (4) Suspension of kaolin

(A) P-1, Q-3, R-4, S-2 — (B) P-4, Q-2, R-3, S-1

(C) P-4, Q-2, R-1, S-3 — (D) P-3, Q-2, R-4, S-1

Q.62. Group-I — Group-II

Types of coating — Coating material

(P) seal coating — (1) HPMC

(Q) Sub coating — (2) Carnauba wax

(R) Polishing — (3) Gelatin

(S) Film coating — (4) PEG 4000

(A) P-4, Q-3, R-2, S-l — (B) P-4, Q-2, R-3, S-1

(C) P-2, Q-4, R-1, S-3 — (D) P-1, Q-3, R-2, S-4

GATE 2009

Q.11. The official dissolution test apparatus contains cylindrical vessel and the lower edge of the blade is positioned from inside bottom of the vessel at

(A) 18 to 22 mm (B) 23 to 27 mm

(C) 20 to 24 mm (D) 25 to 29 mm

Q.22. In multistation punching machine, the upper as well as lower punches are connected by

(A) Cams (B) Turrets

(C) Wire meshes (D) Revolving belts

Q.23. As per the Drugs and Cosmetics Act, the HEPA filters are required to filter the air in the pharmaceutical manufacturing unit. Grade A filter is used for

(A) Aseptic preparation and filling (B) Background room used for preliminary activities

(C) Filtering liquid preparations (D) Handling of components after washing

Matching Exercises: Match Group I with Group II and identify the correct combination

Q.42.

Group I	Group II
Equipment	To determine
P. Cascade impactor	1. Flash point
Q. Tag Open Cup apparatus	2. Sedimentation rate
R. Pycnometer	3. Particle size
S. Rheometer	4. Density of liquid

(A) P-3, Q-1, R-4, S-2 (B) P-1, Q-3, R-2, S-4

(C) P-4, Q-2, R-3, S-1 (D) P-2, Q-3, R-1, S-4

Q.44.

Group I	Group II
Transdermal drug delivery system	Method of penetration
P. Membrane modulated system	1. Drug is homogenously dispersed in polymer and then moulded into a patch
Q. Diffusion controlled system	2. Drug reservoir is encapsulated in rate controlling polymer patch

R. Matrix dispersion system	3. Drug is dispersed in hydrophilic polymer and then cross linked with lipophilic polymer by high shear mechanical force
S. Microreservoir system	4. Drug is directly dispersed in polymer patch

(A) P-2, Q-4, R-1, S-3
(B) P-1, Q-2, R-3, S-4
(C) P-1, Q-4, R-2, S-3
(D) P-4, Q-1, R-3, S-2

Q.43.

Group I Classification	Group II Penetration enhancer
P. Ionic surfactant	1. Terpenes
Q. Nonionic surfactant	2. Polyoxyethylene-20-cetyl ether
R. Non surfactant	3. Polyethylene-9-lauryl ether
S. Chelating agent	4. Citric acid

(A) P-3, Q-2, R-1, S-4
(B) P-2, Q-3, R-1, S-4
(C) P-3, Q-4, R-1, S-2
(D) P-4, Q-2, R-3, S-1

GPAT 2010

Q.34. Humectants added in cosmetic preparations generally act by
(A) Hydrogen bond formation
(B) Covalent bond formation
(C) Complex formation
(D) The action of London forces

Q.36. Bloom strength is used to check the quality of
(A) Lactose
(B) Ampoules
(C) Hardness of tablets
(D) Gelatin

Q.41. The healing agent used in hand creams is
(A) Soft paraffin
(B) Urea
(C) Bees wax
(D) Stearyl alcohol

Q.44. Which one of the following is the commonly used bulking agent in the formulation of freeze dried low dose drug products?
(A) Sodium chloride
(B) Mannitol
(C) Starch
(D) HPMC

Q.46. Which filler can NOT be used for the preparation of tablets for amine containing basic drugs to avoid discoloration of the tablets?
(A) Dicalcium phosphate
(B) Microcrystalline cellulose
(C) Starch
(D) Lactose

Q.47. The ability of human eye using illuminated area to detect a particle is limited to

(A) 0.4 micron (B) 25 micron

(C) 50 micron (D) 10 micron

Q.49. The role of borax in cold creams is

(A) Anti-microbial agent (B) To provide fine particles to polish skin

(C) *In-situ* emulsifier (D) Antioxidant

Q.85. Coulter counter is used in determination of

(A) Particle surface area (B) Particle size

(C) Particle volume (D) All of A, B, *C*

Q.87. The temperature condition for storage of drug products under cold temperature is given as:

(A) Temperature between 8ºC and 25°C (B) Temperature below 2°C

(C) Temperature at 0°C (D) Temperature between 2°C and 8°C

Q.95. Class 100 area is referred to

(A) Manufacturing area (B) Aseptic area

(C) Clean room (D) Ware house

Q.100 In which of the following techniques the sample is kept below triple point?

(A) Lyophilization (B) Spray drying

(C) Spray congealing (D) Centrifugation

GPAT 2011

Q.25. Which one of the following drying methods is commonly used in pharma industry for drying of soft shell capsules?

(A) Truck drying (B) Fluid bed drying

(C) Vacuum drying (D) Microwave drying

Q.28. Which water is used for hand washing in a change room of pharmaceutical manufacturing plant?

(A) Potable water (B) Purified water

(C) Disinfectant water (D) Soap water

Q.32. The minimal effective flow rate of air in Luminar Flow hood should be not less than how many cubic feet per minute?

(A) 10 (B) 50

(C) 100 (D) 1000

Q.36. Which of the followings act as a non-ionic emulsifying agent?

(A) Triethanolamine oleate (B) Polyoxyethylene sorbitan monooleate

(C) N-Cetyl-N-ethylmorpholinium ethosulfate (D) Dioctyl sulfosuccinate

Q.38. By addition of which of the followings the shells of soft gelatin capsules may be made elastic?

(A) Polyethylene glycol (B) Sorbitol

(C) Propylene glycol (D) Dibutyl phthalate

Q.39. Department of Transport Test (DOT) is performed for which of the followings?

(A) Strip packing (B) Aerosols

(C) Injection packing (D) Glass containers

Q.42. The first stage of wetting on addition of a granulating agent to the powders is characterized by which one of the followings?

(A) Capillary state (B) Pendular state

(C) Funicular state (D) Droplet state

Q.43. The degree of flocculation of a suspension is 1.5 and the sedimentation volume is 0.75. What will be the ultimate volume of deflocculated suspension?

(A) 2.0 (B) 1.5

(C) 0.75 (D) 0.5

Q.48. According to USP, the speed regulating device of the dissolution apparatus should be capable of maintaining the speed within limits of what % of the selected speed?

(A) 1% (B) 2%

(C) 4% (D) 5%

Q.50. What is Primogel?

(A) Substituted HPMC for direct compression (B) Modified microcrystalline cellulose for direct compression

(C) Hydro gelling polymer for gel formation (D) Modified starch for disintegration

Q.51. Choose the correct statement

Statement [P]: Soft gelatin capsules contain 12-15 % moisture.
Statement [Q]: Hard gelatin capsule shells contain 6-10 % moisture.

(A) Both of the above statements P & Q are true (B) Both of the above statements P & Q are false

(C) Statement P is true and Q is false

(D) Statement P is false and Q is true

Q.52. A drug whose solubility is 1 g/L in water, when given orally at a dose of 500 mg is absorbed upto 95% of the administered dose. The drug belongs to which class according to the BCS classification?

(A) Class I

(B) Class II

(C) Class III

(D) Class IV

Q.125 A tooth paste contains stannous fluoride and calcium pyrophosphate along with other formulation constituents. Choose the correct statement out of the followings?

(A) Stannous fluoride is an anticaries agent while calcium pyrophosphate is a dentifrice

(B) Stannous fluoride is a dentifrice while calcium pyrophosphate is a desensitizing agent

(C) Stannous fluoride is a desensitizing agent while calcium pyrophosphate is an anticaries agent

(D) Both are dentifrices while calcium pyrophosphate is additionally a desensitizing agent

GPAT-2012

Q.103 Based on Henderson-Hasselbalch equation, at what pH value a weak acid would be 99.9% ionized?

(A) At pH equivalent to pka + 3

(B) At pH equivalent to pka - 3

(C) At pH equivalent to pka - 1

(D) At pH equivalent to pka + 1

Q.104 Some statements about crystals are given below: Choose the corrected combination of statements about crystals.

[P]: The crystal lattice is constructed from repeating units called unit cells.

[Q]: The external appearance of a crystal is described by crystal habits, such as needles, prisms, rosettes etc.

[R]: Polymorphism is the ability of a compound to crystallize as more than one distinct crystalline species with different internal lattice.

[S]: Hydrates are always more soluble than anhydrous form of the same drug

(A) Statement P, Q and S are correct but R is wrong

(B) Statement P, Q and R are correct but S is wrong

(C) Statement Q, R and S are correct but P is wrong

(D) Statement R, S and P are correct but Q is wrong

Q.105 Speed disc automizer rotates at a speed of:

(A) 3000-5000 revolutions per min

(B) 3000-50000 revolutions per min

(C) 300-50000 revolutions per min

(D) 300-5000 revolutions per min

Q.108 The Gold coating on a USP Dissolution apparatus - I basket should be:

(A) Not more than 2.5 μ in thickness

(B) Not more than 0.001 mm in thickness

(C) Not more than 0.025 μ in thickness

(D) Not more than 0.1 mm in thickness

Q.109 Containers used for aerosols should withstand a pressure of:

(A) 130-150 Psig at 130°F

(B) 140-180 Psig at 130°F

(C) 140-170 Psig at 120°F

(D) 120-140 Psig at 120°F

Q.111 Determine the correctness or otherwise of the following Assertion [a] and the Reason [r]:

Assertion [a]: For an API of approximately same particle size, the angle of repose will increase with departure from spherical shape.

Reason *[r]:* Angle of repose is a function of surface roughness and particle size. With constant particle size, increase in roughness increases angle of repose.

(A) Although [a] is true but [r] is false

(B) Both [a] and [r] are false

(C) Both fa] and [r] are true and [r] is the correct reason for [a]

(D) Both [a] and [r] are true but [r] is NOT the correct reason for [a]

Q.112 Study the following two statements: Choose the correct answer.

[X]: When used as granulating agent PEG 6000 improves dissolution rate of the dosage form as it forms a complex with a better solubility.

[Y]: Sodium CMC when used as a binder affects dissolution rate of the dosage form as it is converted to less soluble acid form at low pH of the gastric fluid.

(A) Both X and Y are correct

(B) X is incorrect and Y is correct

(C) X is correct and Y is incorrect

(D) Both X and Y are incorrect.

Q.128 Which of the following colours is NOT permitted to be used in drugs by Drugs and Cosmetic Act 1940?

(A) Chlorophyll

(B) Riboflavin

(C) Tartrazine

(D) Amaranth

Q.129 At equal concentrations which one of the following mucilages will possess maximum viscosity?

(A) Maize starch (B) Rice starch

(C) Wheat starch (D) Potato starch

Q.133 The integrity of seals in case of vials and bottles is determined by some tests. Some of them are given below:

[P]: Leaker's test

[Q]: Water hammer test

[R]: Spark tester probe

(A) P & Q (B) Q & R

(C) P & R (D) P, Q & R

Q.145 How much quantity (in grams) of sodium chloride is needed to make 30 ml of 2% of isotonic drug (sodium chloride equivalent 0.20) solution?

(A) 0.60 (B) 0.27

(C) 0.15 (D) 0.12

Q.146 Read the following statements about lyophilization: Choose the correct combination of statements.

[P]: Lyophilization cannot be done in final containers like multiple dose containers.

[Q]: Lyophilized product needs special methods for reconstitution.

[R]: Lyophilization causes protein denaturation in tissues.

[S]: Lyophilization is suitable for drying the thermolabile products.

(A) P is true and Q, R & S are false (B) Q is true and P, R & S are false

(C) R is true and P, Q & S are false (D) S is true and P, Q & R are false

GPAT-2013

Q.26. Which of the following would cause increase in the binding strength at the dry granulation process in significant degree

(A) Carboxymethylamylpectinglycolate (B) Macrogol-4000

(C) Magnesium stearate (D) Lactose

Q.27. The correct statements concerning coacervation microencapsulation

1. Coacervation always leads to monophase microcapsule
2. When the gelatin is used for microcapsules's wall material, the coacervation is bound to happen on consequence of alcohol or salt (sodium sulphate) effect

3. Only gelatin can be used for microcapsules's wall
4. Simple or compound coacervation can be distinguished according to the number of macromolecular colloids taking part in the process
5. The pH conditions of the system and the solubility of auxiliary materials do not have any effect on the separation of the microcapsule

(A) only1 and 4 are correct (B) only 2 and 3 are correct

(C) only 1 and 5 are correct (D) only 2 and 4 are correct

Q.33. All are true EXCEPT

(A) Soft soap give emulsions with a basic pH in the basic range

(B) Hard soaps form water-in-oil emulsions

(C) Water soluble polymers favour the formation of water-in-oil (w/o) emulsions

(D) On HLB system, lower numbers are assigned to lipophilic compounds while higher number are assigned to hydrophilic compounds

Q.45. Which is the most prominent amino acid in the gelatin?

(A) F (B) W

(C) G (D) Y

Q.46. Which aerosol particles will be deposited in alveoli?

(A) > 20 μ (B) < 0.6 μ

(C) 2 and 6 μ (D) 1-2 μ

GPAT-2014

Q.20. Which sugar is suitable for diabetic patient?

(A) Fructose (B) Lactose

(C) Mannitol (D) Sucralose

Q.34. Evaluation of colour in the tablet is done by

(A) Reflectance spectrophotometer (B) Tristimulus colorimeter

(C) Microreflectance photometer (D) All of the above

Q.35. The disintegration time of the effervescent tablet is:

(A) 2 min (B) 2.5 min

(C) 3.5 min (D) 5 min

Q.36. Identify the false statement/s about magmas:

P. The addition of suspending agents to magmas is always necessary

Q. Magmas differ from gelsin that their suspended particles are bigger

R. Magmas are two phase systems

S. Magmas basically are gels

(A) P and Q (B) Q and R

(C) only P (D) only S

Q.39. Globule size of parenteral emulsion should be

(A) 0.1-0.5 μ (B) 0.5-5 μ

(C) 5-10 μ (D) Any of the above

Q.47. Regarding the role of surfactants in pharmaceutical suspension for oral administration, which of the following statements are false

(A) Surfactants decrease the water contact angle of dispersed drug particles

(B) Surfactants promote flocculation

(C) Surfactants with high HLB stabilise oral suspensions

(D) Surfactants increases the viscosity of the continuous phase of pharmaceutical suspensions

Q.53. Which of the following plastic is transparent and flexible?

(A) Silicon rubber (B) PVP

(C) HDPED (D) PE

Q.78. The oil used in parenteral product cannot contain

(A) WFI (B) Paraffin oil

(C) Peanut oil (D) Glycerin

Q.102 Which of the following is not added to chewable tablet?

(A) Glidant (B) Disintegrant

(C) Lubricant (D) Antiadhesive

Q.111 The drug formulated as suspension follows _____ order of reaction

(A) Zero (B) Pseudo zero

(C) First (D) Pseudo first

GPAT-2015

Q.1 Polymorphs in pharmaceutical solids are detected by which technique?

(A) MS (B) LC-MS

(C) Solid state NMR (D) Coulter-conter

Q.20 When HLB value of surfactant is 10 to 11, it acts best as:

(A) Solubilizer (B) O/W emulsifier

(C) W/O emulsifier (D) Detergent

Q.53 An acceptable emulsion should be stable with no visible signs of separation at 45°C or 50°C for at least how many days?

(A) 10-15 days (B) 15-30 days

(C) 60-90 days (D) 90- 120 days

Q.82 Which of the following is not used as enteric coating materials ?

(A) Cellulose acetate phthalate (B) Pectin

(C) Acrylate polymers (D) Polyvinyl acetate phthalate

Q.93 Slugs are prepared in which kind of granulation technique?

(A) Wet granulation (B) Dry granulation

(C) Steam granulation (D) Melt granulation

Q.104 Which of the following is correct about parenteral nutrition?

(A) Parenteral nutrition solutions are hypertonic solutions and IV fluids are isotonic

(B) Parenteral nutrition solutions and IV preparations are isotonic solutions

(C) Parenteral nutrition solutions are hypertonic solutions and IV fluids are isotonic

(D) Parenteral nutrition solutions can be supplemented with medications

Q.110 Which of the following is not a plasticizer ?

(A) Steary alcohol (B) Triacetin

(C) Pullulan (D) Castor oil

GPAT-2016

Q.49. Which of the following is an irreversible phenomenon related to stability of emulsion

(A) Cracking (B) Creaming

(C) Coalescence (D) Flocculation

Q.75. A drug of low water solubility when given orally is absorbed up to 90% of the administered dose. The drug belongs to which class according to BCS classification ?

(A) Class IV (B) Class III

(C) Class II (D) Class I

Q.76. Which problem can arise if the material to be compressed into tablet tends to adhere to die walls?

(A) Picking (B) Sticking

(C) Capping (D) Marbling

Q.78. Eudragits are:

(A) Phthalate polymers
(B) Cellulose polymers
(C) Acrylate polymers
(D) Amide polymers

Q.94. Which of the following is a solid dosage form excipient which can play the role of a diluents, a disintegrant, a glidant, a lubricant and a pore/ channel former?

(A) Lactose
(B) Microcrystalline cellulose
(C) Ethyl cellulose
(D) Eudragit RL100

Q.97. The propellant commonly used in topical is:

(A) Trichloromonofluoromethane
(B) Trifluoromonofluoroethane
(C) Dichlodifluoromethane
(D) Isopropyl alcohol

Q.104 What is the significance of term overfill?

(A) It is similar to overage
(B) It is excess volume to be filled in containers as vials, ampoules to avoid loss by degradation
(C) It is excess filling of container as vials, ampoules to avoid loss during use
(D) It is violation of packaging regulation as per GMP

Q.113 The term used to describe unequal distribution of colour on a tablet is

(A) Chipping
(B) Mottling
(C) Lamination
(D) Double impression

Q.114 Match the events in tablet manufacturing process with the effects found in tablets

1) Rapid drying of coated tablets after coating	(P) Increased disintegration time
2) Use of highly viscous solutions	(Q) Weight variation
3) Improper feed rate from hopper	(R) Orange peel
4) Excessive compression force	(S) Blistering

(A) 1-R, 2-S, 3-Q, 4-P
(B) 1-R, 2-S, 3-P, 4-Q
(C) 1-S, 2-R, 3-Q, 4-P
(D) 1-R, 2-P, 3-S, 4-Q

GPAT 2017

Q.22. Antioxidant used as blocking agent in sterile product is

(A) Ascorbic acid esters
(B) Sodium bisulphate
(C) Ascorbic acid
(D) EDTA

Q.38. Which among the following is a class-I method, used for rendering a solution of drug isotonic with body fluids

(A) Cryoscopic method (B) White-Vincent method

(C) Sprowls method (D) Hammerlund method

Q.45. Type IV dissolution apparatus as per USP is

(A) Flow through cell (B) Paddle type apparatus

(C) Reciprocating cylinder (D) Paddle over disk apparatus

Q.53. Hot stage microscopy is an important tool in pre-formulation studies for the study of

(A) Pseudopolymorphism (B) Particle size measurement

(C) Microbial contamination (D) Compaction behaviour

Q.57. Which of the following technique is not useful to detect the polymorphs

(A) DSC (B) HPLC

(C) PXRD (D) Melting point determination

Q.103 Free flowing powders show a flatter cone and have ______

(A) Smaller angle of repose (B) Larger angle of repose

(C) Intermediate angle of repose (D) None of the above

Q.111 As per I.P. if the solubility range of a solute is 30 to 100 parts, it will be

(A) Soluble (B) Freely soluble

(C) Sparingly soluble (D) Slightly soluble

Q.120 Foaming during liquid filling can be reduced by following ways, except

(A) Increase in speed of the filling line (B) Minimised product turbulence

(C) Closed system filling (D) Defoaming device

GPAT 2018

Q.18. The agent used to prevent the dental carries is:-

(A) Sodium fluoride (B) Strontium chloride

(C) Zinc chloride (D) Dicalcium phosphate

Q.56. Substance used to reduce friction during tablet compression and facilitate ejection of tablets fromthe die cavity is called as:

(A) Lubricant (B) Glidant

(C) Anti-adherent (D) Humectant

Q.58. The proportion of NaCl liquid to give 1.5% solution of drug isotonic with blood plasma is:- (Thefreezing point of 1% w/v solution of drug is -0.122 and NaCl is -0.576°C)

(A) 0.79% (B) 0.585%

(C) 0.9% (D) 0.5%

Q.61. As the dielectric constant values increases, the polarity of the solvents ________

(A) Decreases (B) Increases

(C) Remains constant (D) Decreases and then remains constant

Q.62. The angle of repose is calculated by __________.

(A) tan α= Radius/Height (B) tan α= 1+Radius/Height

(C) tan α= 1-Radius/Height (D) tan α= Height/Radius

Q.65. Vials and bottles are regularly not subjected to following test:-

(A) Sterility test (B) Clarity test

(C) Leaker (chamber) test (D) Pyrogen test

Q.66. A material which is insoluble and inert and used in matrix tablet formulation is:-

(A) Polyethylene (B) Stearyl alcohol

(C) Polyethylene glycol (D) Triglycerides

Q.69. Which test is done for USP Type-I glass containers for injections?

(A) Water attack test (B) Powdered glass test

(C) Powdered glass followed by water attack test (D) Water attack followed powdered glass test

Q.70. Isoelectric point of Type A gelatin is ________.

(A) pH 7.0 (B) pH 4.7

(C) pH 9.0 (D) pH 7.4

Q.71. What is the effective ratio of methyl paraben and propyl paraben for anti-microbial activity?

(A) 1:1 (B) 5:1

(C) 2.5:1 (D) 10:1

Q.74. The friability issue of the tablet can be solved by different ways EXCEPT:-

(A) Increasing the upper punch pressure of tablet machine

(B) Addition of more tablet binder to granules

(C) Increasing the moisture content of granules

(D) Adjusting the lower punch pressure of tablet machine

Q.76. In a free-flowing powder, the bulk density and tapped density would be close in value, therefore, the Carr index would be:-

(A) Small (B) Medium

(C) Large (D) None

GPAT 2019

Q.1. Containers may be rendered free from pyrogens by adequate cleaning and by:

(A) Autoclaving at 121°C for 15 min (B) Heating at 210°C for 3-4 hours

(C) Autoclaving at 121°C for 1 hour (D) Heating at 100°C for 3-4 hours

Q.2. Which of the following oxide is not used for achieving amber colour to glass?

(A) Manganese (B) Iron

(C) Cobalt (D) Carbon

Q.3. In tablet, hydroxy propyl methyl cellulose is used as

(A) Diluent (B) Film former

(C) Disintegrant (D) Binder

Q.4. Which one of the following is the property of micro-emulsion?

(A) Globule size more than 1 micron (B) They have poor stability

(C) They exhibit viscoelestic gel phase, when internal phase is added in excess

(D) They have milky yellow color

Q.5. In case of aerosol testing, valve delivering acceptance criteria for a volume of 54 μL or less is:

(A) 75% (B) ± 5%

(C) ±10% (D) ±15%

Q.6. "Shake well" label must be placed on the containers of:

(A) Ophthalmic suspension (B) Occusert

(C) Ophthalmic solution (D) Ophthalmic gels

Q.7. Microcrystalline cellulose is also called as

(A) Sugar tab (B) Nutab

(C) Emdex (D) Avicel

Q.8. For bitter drugs in paediatric formulation, excellent flavouring agent will be

(A) Raspberry syrup (B) Orange syrup

(C) Lemon syrup (D) Black current syrup

Q.9. Which polymorphic form of a drug candidate has highest melting point

(A) Unstable (B) Meta stable

(C) Hydrate (D) Stable

Q.10. Which of the following statement is NOT true regarding bulkiness?

(A) The reciprocal of bulk density is bulkiness

(B) Bulkiest substance will require container larger than required less bulky substance

(C) Smaller particles shift between the larger ones and increases bulkiness

(D) Bulkiness increases with decrease in particle size

Q.11. In pre-formulation study polymorphs can be detected by:

(A) Counter current chromatography (B) High performance liquid chromatography

(C) Refractometry (D) Differential scanning calorimetry

ANSWER KEY

GATE 2006

9	B	10	A	26	A	28	B	29	A	44	A
61	A	62	D								

GATE 2007

3	C	20	A	31	A	32	D	34	A	45	A
46	D	61	A								

GATE 2008

20	B	30	A	60	D	62	A

GATE 2009

11	B	22	A	23	A	42	A	43	A

GPAT 2010

34	A	36	D	41	B	44	B	46	D	47	B
49	C	85	D	87	D	95	B	100	A		

GPAT 2011

25	B	28	B	32	C	36	B	38	B	39	B
42	B	43	D	48	B	50	D	51	B	52	B
125	A										

GPAT 2012

103	A	104	B	105	B	108	A	109	B	111	C
112	B	128	B	129	D	133	D	145	C	146	D

GPAT 2013

26	B	27	D	33	C	45	C	46	D

GPAT 2014

20	D	34	D	35	D	36	C	39	A	47	D
53	D	78	B	102	B	111	A				

GPAT 2015

1	C	20	B	53	C	82	B	93	B	104	A
110	A										

GPAT 2016

49	A	75	C	76	B	78	C	94	B	97	B
104	C	113	B	114	C						

GPAT 2017

22	A	38	A	45	A	53	A	57	B	103	A
111	C	120	A								

GPAT 2018

18	A	56	A	58	B	61	B	62	D	65	C
66	C	69	B	70	C	71	D	74	D	76	A

GPAT 2019

1	B	2	C	3	B	4	C	5	D	6	A
7	D	8	A	9	D	10	C	11	D		

APPENDIX 3

MODEL QUESTION PAPER-I

Subject: Industrial Pharmacy

Class: B. Pharmacy Third Year (Sem-V)

Times: 3 Hours **Max. Marks: 75**

Q.I. Multiple Choice Questions **(20 x 1 = 2)**

1. If Carr's index of powder is 10% then the type of powder flow is
   a) Poor c) Very poor
   b) Excellent d) Good
2. In the process of sugar coating of tablets, the colourants are added in one of the following steps
   a) Syrup coating c) Sub coating
   b) Polishing d) Seal coating
3. During compression of moisture critical granules a hygroscopic substance used to maintain moisture level is
   a) Sorbitol c) Acacia
   b) Talc d) Tragacanth
4. In tablet coating process inadequate spreading of the coating solution before drying causes.
   a) Orange peel effect c) Blistering effect
   b) Sticking effect d) Picking effect
5. A dilution test can be used for identification of
   a) Suspension c) Emulsion
   b) Milk and magma d) All of the above
6. By addition of which of the following the shells of soft gelatin capsule may be made elastic?
   a) Polyethylene glycol c) Sorbitol
   b) Propylene glycol d) Dibutyl phthalate
7. Bloom strength is used to check the quality of
   a) Lactose c) Hardness of tablets
   b) Ampoules d) Gelatin
8. The standard moisture content specification for HGC is ______% w/w
   a) 13 – 16 c) 90
   b) 50 – 60 d) 5 – 10

9. The particle size of pellets should be in the range of
   - a) 100 to 300 μ
   - b) 300 to 600 μ
   - c) 600 to 1000 μ
   - d) 1000 to 1400 μ
10. What is the concentration of NaCl required to make 1% solution of cocaine HCL isotonic with blood plasma? Freezing point of 1% w/v solution of NaCl is –0.576° C and freezing point of 1% w/v cocaine HCL is –0.09° C
   - a) 0.746 % w/v
   - b) 0.9 % w/v
   - c) 0.5 % w/v
   - d) 0.373 % w/v
11. One thousand nanogram equals to
   - a) Centigram
   - b) Gram
   - c) Kilogram
   - d) Microgram
12. The colligative property of a solution is related to the:
   - a) Total number of solute particles
   - b) pH
   - c) Number of ions
   - d) Number of ingredients
13. Cryoscopic method is familiar in the calculation of isotonic solution. This method is based on
   - a) Freezing point depression of the drug
   - b) pH of the drug
   - c) Solubility of the drug
   - d) None of the above
14. A commonly used antioxidant for oil system is
   - a) Butylated hydroxyl toluene
   - b) Ascorbic acid
   - c) Sodium metabisulfite
   - d) Thyoglycol
15. A synthetic sweetening agent which is approximately 200 times sweeter than sucrose and has no aftertaste is
   - a) Saccharin
   - b) Aspartame
   - c) Cyclamate
   - d) Sorbitol
16. Identify the correct non-flammable propellant
   - a) Trichloro mono fluoromethane
   - b) Dichloro monoflurométhane
   - c) Dimethyl ether
   - d) Difluoromethane
17. The dip tube in the aerosol container is made from one of the following
   - a) Polypropylene
   - b) Glass
   - c) Aluminium
   - d) Stainless steel
18. Disposable syringes are made up of
   - a) Polypropylene
   - b) Transparent polystyrene
   - c) Glass
   - d) Poly tetrachloro ethylene

19. Water attack test is used to identify the alkalinity in
    a) Type I glass c) Type III glass
    b) Type II glass d) All the 3 types
20. The distribution of globule is not uniform in an emulsion. This stage is called as
    a) Creaming c) Caking
    b) Coalescence d) Breaking

OR

Q.I. Objective Type Questions **(10 x 2 = 20)**

1. Define pre-formulation. Enlist different pre-formulation parameters.
2. Differentiate disintegrants and super disintegrants with examples.
3. Give examples of two anti-oxidants and two preservatives used in liquid orals.
4. Write the pharmaceutical applications of soft gelatin capsules.
5. Enlist the application of pellets
6. What is the use of buffers in parenteral formulation?
7. Role of viscosity modifiers in ophthalmics
8. Define and classify cosmetic preparations
9. What are metered valve aerosols?
10. What are tamper evident closures?

Q. II. Answer any two of the following: **(2 x 10 = 20)**

1. Give a detailed account of different excipients used in the tablets and write their functions.
2. Discuss quality control test for parenterals
3. Write a brief note on soft gelatin capsules. Explain the construction and working of rotary die machine used in the manufacture of soft gelatin capsules.

Q. III. Answer any seven of the following: **(7 x 5 = 35)**

1. Give an account on applications of preformulation in development of solid dosage forms.
2. Add a note on tablet tooling
3. Explain formulation of elixir
4. Describe briefly the manufacturing of soft gelatin capsules
5. Add a note on preparation of sterile dry powder injections
6. Discuss the formulation of an eye ointment.
7. Discuss the formulation of cold cream and vanishing cream
8. Give testing of pharmaceutical Aerosols.
9. Write a note on powdered glass test.

MODEL QUESTION PAPER-II

Subject: Industrial Pharmacy

Class: B. Pharmacy Third Year (Sem-V)

Times: 3 Hours **Max. Marks: 75**

Q I: Multiple Choice Questions **(20 x 1=20)**

1. pH of the buffer system can be calculated by using
   - a) pH-partition theory
   - b) Noyes-Whitney law
   - c) Henderson-Hasselbalch equation
   - d) None of the above
2. The purpose of seal coating in sugar coating process for tablets is
   - a) To prevent moisture penetration into the tablet core
   - b) To round the edges and build up tablet weight
   - c) To impart the desired colour to the tablet
   - d) To give lustre to the tablet
3. The durability of a tablet to combined effect of shock and abrasion is evaluated by using
   - a) Hardness tester
   - b) Disintegration test apparatus
   - c) Friabilator
   - d) Screw gauge
4. In the preparation of multilayer tablets, one of the substances listed is used for hydrophilic matrix coating
   - a) C.M.C.
   - b) Shellac
   - c) Stearyl alcohol
   - d) Bees wax
5. ______ is needed for suspension, lotion, emulsion, creams and ointments to keep high container consistency and yet pour and spread easily when needed. It is also satisfactory for IM slow release yet easy to inject
   - a) Thixotropy
   - b) Rheopexy
   - c) Rheology
   - d) Newtonian flow
6. Which of the following is suitable as liquid fills for hard gelatin capsules?
   - a) Polyethylene glycols
   - b) Arachis oil
   - c) Fatty acid ester
   - d) All of the above
7. Type A gelatin exhibits an isoelectric point in the pH of ______
   - a) 4.4
   - b) 9
   - c) 5
   - d) 7

8. Drugs which are highly acidic in nature causes_____ of gelatin
   a) Hydrolysis of gelatin
   b) Tanning of gelatin
   c) Non-tanning effect on gelatin
   d) None of the above
9. Which of the following dosage form limits localised build-up of the drug in GIT?
   a) Pellets
   b) Tablets
   c) Capsules
   d) Granules
10. What is the proportion of NaCl required to render a 1.5 5 solution of drug isotonic with blood plasma? The freezing point of 1% w/v solution of drug is –0.122° C and that of NaCl is –0.576° C
    a) 0.65 %
    b) 0.585 %
    c) 0.9 %
    d) 0.5 %
11. An antioxidant commonly used in the formulation of a non aqueous parenteral preparation is
    a) Thioglycollic acid
    b) Ascorbic acid
    c) Sodium metabisulphate
    d) Butylated hydroxyl toulene
12. Which of the following is used as a local anaesthetic in the formulation of parenteral products?
    a) Acetic acid
    b) Benzyl alcohol
    c) Ethyl alcohol
    d) Sorbitol
13. Which of the following is used as a preservative in ophthalmic preparations
    a) Benzalkonium chloride
    b) Phenol
    c) Benzoic acid
    d) Chlorocresol
14. Surfactants are characterized by the presence of
    a) Water-soluble groups alone
    b) Fat solubilising groups alone
    c) Water and fat solubilizing groups in the same molecule
    d) Groups with a positive charge
15. Benzyl peroxide is
    a) An astringent
    b) An emollient
    c) A preservative
    d) A keratolytic
16. Which one of the following device is used to increase the efficacy of drug delivery via aerosols?
    a) Tube spacers
    b) Metered valve
    c) Actuator
    d) Pressure valve

17. Among the propellants used in aerosols, one of the following is used for topical pharmaceutical aerosols
    a) Trichloromonofluoromethane
    b) Dichlorodifluoromethane
    c) Dichlorotetrafluoroethane
    d) Propnane
18. Water resistance of glass containers are tested by measuring:
    a) Amount of alkali released into water
    b) Amount of acid released into water
    c) Estimation of silicate levels
    d) Turbidity
19. Powdered glass test is carried out for all kinds of glass EXCEPT
    a) Borosilicate glass
    b) Treated soda lime glass
    c) Soda lime glass
    d) General purpose
20. In the emulsion, which instability step can be prevented by an emulsifying agent?
    a) Breaking
    b) Coalescence
    c) Creaming
    d) Flocculation

OR

Q I. Objective Type Questions **(10 x 2 = 20)**

1. Write the goals and objectives of pre-formulation
2. What are disintegrants? Give two examples.
3. What is co-solvency? Give two examples of co-solvents.
4. Define base adsorption and minim per gram factor.
5. Enlist the different techniques of pelletization
6. Name the methods of adjustment of isotonicity.
7. Stabilizing agents used in eye drops
8. Add a note on sun protection factor
9. Different components of an aerosol valve. Give their functions
10. Define pharmaceutical packaging.

Q II. Answer any two of the following: **(2 x 10 = 20)**

1. Explain in detail about in-process and final product quality control tests for uncoated tablets.
2. Explain the excipients used in the manufacture of parenterals giving their functions and examples.
3. Explain in detail in-process and final quality control test for hard gelatin capsules.

Q III. Answers seven of the following: (7 x 5 = 35)

1. Write the significance of BCS classification of drugs
2. Add a note on film defects and their remedies
3. Discuss the stability of emulsion and suspension
4. Explain in detail extraction of gelatin
5. Write the significance of isotonicity in parenteral products
6. Discus in detail formulation requirements and method of preparation of eye lotions.
7. Write a note on lipsticks
8. Add a note on propellants used in aerosols
9. Give details of glass as the packaging material

MODEL QUESTION PAPER-III

Subject: Industrial Pharmacy

Class: B. Pharmacy Third Year (Sem-V)

Times: 3 Hours **Max. Marks: 75**

Q. I: Multiple Choice Questions **(20 x 1=20)**

1. The amorphous form of the drug is prepared by
   a) Rapid precipitation
   b) Lyophilisation
   c) Rapid cooling of liquid melts
   d) All of the above
2. Which filler cannot be used for the preparation of tablets for amine-containing basic drug to avoid discolouration of the tablets?
   a) Dicalcium phosphate
   b) Microcrystalline cellulose
   c) Starch
   d) Lactose
3. The first stage of wetting on addition of granulating agent to the powders is characterized by which one of the followings?
   a) Capillary state
   b) Pendular state
   c) Funicular state
   d) Droplet state
4. According to USP, the speed regulating devices of the dissolution apparatus should be capable of maintaining the speed within limits of what % of the selected speed?
   a) 1%
   b) 2%
   c) 4%
   d) 5%
5. The concentration of sucrose in simple syrup BP is
   a) 85 % w/w
   b) 60.70 % w/w
   c) 66.70 % w/w
   d) 40.74 % w/w
6. Ideally, solid fills for HGCs should exhibit which the following properties?
   a) Homogeneity of mix
   b) Low angle of repose
   c) Low shearing stresses during powder flow
   d) All of the above
7. Which of the following excipients are common components of the fill of SGCs?
   a) Lipophillic liquids
   b) Water miscible liquids
   c) Both a and b
   d) None of above
8. Drugs which are highly basic in nature causes
   a) Tanning effect on gelatin
   b) Hydrolysis of gelatin
   c) Both a and b
   d) None of the above

9. Pelletization of powder leads to all the followings EXCEPT
   a) Dose uniformity
   b) Improvement in flow property
   c) Reduction in dust formation
   d) Increased compressibility
10. How many grams of drug is required to prepare 500 ml of a 1: 2500 solution?
    a) 0.2
    b) 0.02
    c) 0.4
    d) 1.25
11. A co-solvent used in the preparation of parenteral product is
    a) Benzyl alcohol
    b) Methyl alcohol
    c) Dimethyl acetamide
    d) Phenol
12. Bulking agent used for parenteral preparation is
    a) Sodium metabisulphate
    b) Benzyl alcohol
    c) Carbolic acid
    d) Sorbitol
13. Eye lotions are supplied in ______ form
    a) Concentrated
    b) Diluted
    c) Powder
    d) All of the above
14. HLB system is used to classify
    a) Surfactants
    b) Preservative
    c) Antioxidants
    d) Sequestering agent
15. In cosmetic preparation, an antioxidant used in an aqueous system is
    a) Sodium formaldehyde sulphoxylate
    b) Phenol
    c) α-tocopherol
    d) Methylparaben
16. ______ is not a component of the aerosol system.
    a) Propellant
    b) Dip tube
    c) Actuator
    d) Paddle
17. Filling of aerosols with liquefied propellants is done by
    a) Cold fill process
    b) Pressure fill process
    c) Both (a) and (b)
    d) None of the above
18. In which type of packaging system the product is in direct contact with packaging material?
    a) Primary Package
    b) Secondary Package
    c) Tertiary Package
    d) All of the above
19. _____ fitted with a device or mechanism that reveals irreversibly whether the container has been opened
    a) Tightly-closed container
    b) Tamper-evident container
    c) Well-closed container
    d) None of these

20. For an ideal suspension, sedimentation volume should be :

a) Zero	c) Equal to one
b) Less than one	d) More than one

OR

Q. I. Objective Type Questions **(10 x 2 = 20)**

1. Give BCS classification of drugs
2. What are chewable tablets? Give their advantages
3. Define creaming and cracking of emulsions.
4. Mention the difference between type A and type B gelatin.
5. Give any four reasons for pelletization
6. How are isotonic solutions different from paratonic solutions?
7. Name any four preservatives used in ophthalmic preparations
8. List out the components of toothpaste with their use.
9. Metal as material for the aerosol container
10. Define primary and secondary packaging materials

Q. II. Answer any two of the following: **(2 x 10 = 20)**

1. Explain in detail wet and dry granulation techniques
2. Describe in detail the production facilities required to be maintained for parenterals.
3. Explain in detail in-process and final quality control test of a soft gelatin capsule.

Q III. Answer any seven of the following **(7 x 5 = 35)**

1. What is polymorphism? Add a note polymorphism of drugs
2. Describe the steps involved in sugar coating with suitable examples
3. Describe the different methods of filling of liquid oral dosage forms
4. Explain the working of rotary die machine with a neat labelled diagram
5. Compare pull sealing technique and tip sealing technique
6. Explain the formulation of eye drops
7. Discuss in detail the formulation of toothpaste
8. Explain the various methods of filling of pharmaceutical aerosols
9. Write quality control tests of rubber closure

Bibliography

1. Theory and practice of industrial pharmacy. Leon Lachman, Herbert A. Lieberman. Special Indian edition. C B S Publishers. New Delhi.
2. Aultons's Pharmaceutics. The design and manufacture of medicines. Michael E Aulton (Editor), third edition. Elsevier, Churchill Livingstone.
3. Bentley's Textbook of Pharmaceutics. E. A. Rawlins (Editor), 8th edition. Bailliere Tindall. London.
4. Cooper and Gunns's Dispensing for pharmaceutical students. S. J. Carter (Editor), 12th edition, C B S Publishers. New Delhi.
5. Modern cosmetics by E.G. Thomsen. Universal Publishing Corporation. Bombay.
6. Pharmaceutical dosage forms: Parenteral Medications Volume 1-3, second edition. Kenneth E. Avis, Herbart A. Liberman and Leon Lachman (Editors). Marcel Dekker. New York.
7. Ansel's Pharmaceutical Dosage forms and Drug Delivery systems. Loyd V. Allen, Jr. Nicholas G. Popvich, Howard C. Ansel (editors), Lippincott Williams & Walkins, 8th Edition. Baltimore, USA.
8. Applied Biopharmaceutics and Pharmacokinetics. Leon Shargel, Susanna Wu-Pong, Andrew B.C. Yu, fifth edition (Internation edition), Mc Graw Hill. Singapore.
9. Modern Pharmaceutics. Gilbert S. Banker and Christopher T. Rhodes (Editors), 4th Edition. Marcel Dekker, Inc. New York.
10. Pharmaceutical Packaging Technology, D. A. Dean, E. R. Evans and I. H. Hall (Editors), first edition. Taylor & Francis. London.
11. Pharmaceutical Technology and Biopharmaceutics. O.V.K Reddy, Pulse publications.
12. Pharmaceutical pre-formulation and formulation. Mark Gibson (Editor). CRC Press. USA.

13. Introduction to cosmetic formulation and technology, Gabriella Baki and Kenneth S. Alexander. John Wiley & Sons, Inc., Hoboken, New Jersey.
14. Physical pharmaceutics. C V S Subrahmanyam, 2nd Edition, Vallabh Prakashan New Delhi.
15. Encyclopedia of Pharmaceutical Science and Technology; Pelletization Techniques, Josephine Lay Peng Soh. 4th Edition.
16. Indian Pharmacopoeia 2007
17. GPAT: Companion. Nazma N. Inamdar, Milind P. Wagh. 14th Edition. Career Publications. Nashik.
18. Pharmaceutical Formulation. B.M. Mittal. Vallabh Prakashan. New Delhi

Subject Index

L

M

N

O

P

R

S